J. Michael Bruen, M.D.
Oct '96

ADVANCES IN Vascular Surgery

VOLUME 4

ADVANCES IN
Vascular Surgery

VOLUME 1

ADVANCES IN
Vascular Surgery

VOLUME 4

Editor-in-Chief
Anthony D. Whittemore, M.D.
Professor of Surgery, Harvard University Medical School; Chief, Division of Vascular Surgery, Brigham and Women's Hospital, Boston, Massachusetts

Associate Editors
Dennis F. Bandyk, M.D.
Professor of Surgery, University of South Florida College of Medicine; Director, Vascular Surgery Division, Tampa, Florida

Jack L. Cronenwett, M.D.
Professor of Surgery, Dartmouth Medical School; Chief, Section of Vascular Surgery, Dartmouth–Hitchcock Medical Center, Lebanon, New Hampshire

Norman R. Hertzer, M.D.
Chairman, Department of Vascular Surgery, Cleveland Clinic Foundation, Cleveland, Ohio

Rodney A. White, M.D.
Professor of Surgery, University of California at Los Angeles School of Medicine; Chief of Vascular Surgery, Associate Chairman, Department of Surgery, Harbor—University of California at Los Angeles Medical Center, Torrance, California

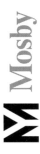 Mosby

St. Louis   Baltimore   Boston   Carlsbad   Chicago   Naples   New York   Philadelphia   Portland
London   Madrid   Mexico City   Singapore   Sydney   Tokyo   Toronto   Wiesbaden

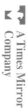
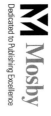

Mosby

Dedicated to Publishing Excellence

A Times Mirror
Company

Vice President and Publisher, Continuity Publishing: Kenneth H. Killion
Director, Editorial Development: Gretchen C. Murphy
Developmental Editor: Kris Horeis
Acquisitions Editor: Li Wen Huang
Manager, Continuity—EDP: Maria Nevinger
Project Supervisor: Rebecca Nordbrock
Assistant Project Supervisor: Sandra Rogers
Freelance Staff Supervisor: Barbara M. Kelly
Circulation Manager: Lynn D. Stevenson

Printed in the United States of America
Composition by The Clarinda Company
Printing/binding by The Maple-Vail Book Manufacturing Company

Mosby-Year Book, Inc.
11830 Westline Industrial Drive
St. Louis, Missouri 63146

Editorial Office:
Mosby-Year Book, Inc.
161 North Clark Street
Chicago, Illinois 60601

International Standard Serial Number: 1069-7292
International Standard Book Number: 0-8151-9408-0

Contributors

Samuel S. Ahn, M.D.
Associate Clinical Professor of Surgery, UCLA Center for the Health Sciences, Section of Vascular Surgery, Los Angeles, California

Robert C. Allen, M.D.
Assistant Professor of Surgery, Assistant Director of Surgical Education, Department of General Surgery, Section of Vascular Surgery, Baylor University Medical Center, Dallas, Texas

Michael Belkin, M.D.
Assistant Professor of Surgery, Harvard Medical School, Brigham and Women's Hospital, Boston, Massachusetts

Martin M. Brown, M.D., F.R.C.P.
Reader in Neurology, St. George's Hospital Medical School, London, England

Timothy A.M. Chuter, M.D.
Assistant Professor of Surgery, University of California, San Francisco

Anthony J. Comerota, M.D., F.A.C.S.
Professor of Surgery, Chief, Section Vascular Surgery, Director, Center for Vascular Diseases, Temple University Hospital, Philadelphia, Pennsylvania

Blessie Concepcion, B.S.
UCLA Center for the Health Sciences, Section of Vascular Surgery, Los Angeles, California

Michael S. Conte, M.D.
Assistant Professor of Surgery, Yale University School of Medicine, New Haven, Connecticut

Jack L. Cronenwett, M.D.
Professor of Surgery, Dartmouth Medical School; Chief, Section of Vascular Surgery, Dartmouth-Hitchcock Medical Center, Lebanon, New Hampshire

A.R. Downs, M.D., F.R.C.S.C., F.A.C.S.
Professor of Surgery, Department of Surgery, Health Sciences Centre, University of Manitoba, Winnipeg, Manitoba

Thomas J. Fogarty, M.D.
Professor of Surgery, Division of Vascular Surgery, Stanford University Medical Center, California

Gary W. Gibbons, M.D.
Clinical Chief, Division of Vascular Surgery, Chairman, Quality Assurance, Department of Surgery, New England Deaconess Hospital; Associate Clinical Professor of Surgery, Harvard Medical School, Boston, Massachusetts

Samuel Z. Goldhaber, M.D.
Cardiovascular Division, Brigham and Women's Hospital, Harvard Medical School, Boston, Massachusetts

R.P. Guzman, M.D., F.R.C.S.C., F.A.C.S., R.V.T.
Assistant Professor of Surgery, Department of Surgery, Health Sciences Centre, University of Manitoba, Winnipeg, Manitoba

Geoffrey M. Habershaw, D.P.M.
Chief, Division of Podiatry, New England Deaconess Hospital; Clinical Instructor in Surgery, Harvard Medical School, Boston, Massachusetts

Timothy R.S. Harward, M.D.
Associate Professor of Surgery, Section of Vascular Surgery, Department of Surgery, University of Florida College of Medicine, Gainesville

Richard L. Hughes, M.D.
Assistant Professor of Neurology, University of Colorado School of Medicine, Denver

James B. Knox, M.D.
Fellow in Vascular Surgery, Brigham and Women's Hospital, Boston, Massachusetts

David A. Kumpe, M.D.
Director of Interventional Radiology; Professor of Radiology and Surgery, University of Colorado School of Medicine, Denver

Michael L. Marin, M.D.
Assistant Professor of Surgery, Division of Vascular Surgery, Department of Surgery, Montefiore Medical Center, The University Hospital for the Albert Einstein College of Medicine, New York, New York

Joseph L. Mills, M.D.
Associate Professor of Surgery, Chief, Section of Vascular Surgery, University of Arizona Health Sciences Center, Tucson

Kenneth Ouriel, M.D.
Associate Professor of Surgery, The University of Rochester, Rochester, New York

Richard E. Parsons, M.D.
Fellow in Vascular Surgery, Division of Vascular Surgery, Department of Surgery, Montefiore Medical Center, The University Hospital for the Albert Einstein College of Medicine, New York, New York

Frank J. Veith, M.D.
Professor and Chief, Vascular Surgical Services, Division of Vascular Surgery, Department of Surgery, Montefiore Medical Center, The University Hospital for the Albert Einstein College of Medicine, New York, New York

Paul M. Walker, M.D., Ph.D., F.R.C.S.C.
James Wallace McCutcheon Chair, Surgeon-in-Chief, Vice President, Surgical Directorate, The Toronto Hospital, Canada

Anthony D. Whittemore, M.D.
Professor of Surgery, Harvard Medical School; Chief, Division of Vascular Surgery, Brigham and Women's Hospital, Boston, Massachusetts

Preface

More than 30 years after Dr. Tom Fogarty introduced his thrombo-lectomy balloon catheter, the field of minimally invasive vascular intervention is on the brink of an explosion in the application of translu-minal technology, an explosion only partially controlled. The editors ac-knowledge the engineering and entrepreneurial skills that have enabled Dr. Fogarty to provide continued impetus for the development of percu-taneous transluminal technology, and we are grateful for his historical contribution to this fourth volume of *Advances in Vascular Surgery*. Drs. Marin and Chuter represent two of the young investigators deeply in-volved in the early feasibility studies of the endoluminal approach to the management of aortic disease, following on its introduction by Dr. Parodi, who described his contribution in the first volume of this series. As these initial stent graft prototypes are more reliably seated in more anatomi-cally uniform aneurysms, there is continued thrust to intervene at a smaller diameter. Dr. Cronenwett lends a balanced view toward patient selection, placing in perspective the temptation to treat the small, more anatomically suitable cases.

Although balloon angioplasty of renal, peripheral, and coronary ar-teries are now commonplace, very little has been written regarding an-gioplasty of the mesenteric vasculature. Dr. Allen describes his consider-able experience with this technique, an experience balanced by Dr. Har-ward's contribution describing a more conventional surgical approach.

The surgical management of cerebral vascular disease, now better grounded than ever with respect to indications, is yet again in upheaval with the aggressive and uncontrolled anecdotal descriptions of carotid balloon angioplasty. Dr. Brown's European trial represents an early at-tempt at a controlled study; we are grateful for his chapter and look for-ward to results as they emerge. Dr. Kumpe has summarized the early ex-perience with thrombolytic therapy for acute stroke and draws interest-ing parallels to the role these agents play in acute myocardial infarction. With the small but reproducible incidence of stroke associated with ce-rebral angiography, the search for noninvasive means of extracranial ar-terial assessment continues, as evidenced by Dr. Knox's description of spi-ral CT.

Options for the management of infrainguinal disease include lytic therapy as summarized by Dr. Ouriel, who has been instrumental in two major studies. As summarized by Dr. Ahn, and despite hopes to the con-trary, results with directional atherectomy remain disappointing, paral-leling the course charted by thermal laser technology.

Conventional infrainguinal reconstruction using autogenous vein re-mains the primary choice for peripheral vascular reconstruction, yet in the absence of ipsilateral saphenous vein, the optimal ectopic source re-mains controversial. Drs. Downs and Guzman place their experience in

Winnipeg with the superficial femoral vein in perspective. Dr. Mills reports the current recommendations for graft surveillance, and Drs. Conte and Belkin describe the basis underlying our option to extend tibial reconstruction to patients with disabling claudication. Drs. Gibbons and Habershaw report their approach to the management of diabetic foot infections, a comprehensive approach developed from years of experience with patients from the Joslin Clinic in Boston.

As is true with arterial intervention, more aggressive yet minimally invasive techniques for the management of deep vein thrombosis and its complications are exemplified by Dr. Comerota's chapter on the management of phlegmasia and Dr. Goldhaber's discussion of current management of pulmonary embolus. Finally, Dr. Paul Walker has contributed an outstanding chapter in our Basic Science section describing the advances made in understanding reperfusion injury with an eye toward proactive intervention rather than passive management of complications.

Anthony D. Whittemore, M.D.
Editor-in-Chief

Contents

PART I

Endovascular Techniques

Endovascular Technology

Thomas J. Fogarty, M.D.

Professor of Surgery, Division of Vascular Surgery, Stanford University Medical Center, California

Although a relatively recent concept, endovascular technology has a rich and interesting history.[1] Diagnostic and therapeutic endovascular approaches can be divided into two 30-year periods. The first 30 years were marked by the introduction of endovascular *diagnostics* in 1929. Development of these modalities continues to this date. The basic contributions that laid the foundation for this technology, however, occurred between the years 1929 and 1959. During this relatively short period a significant number of cardiac and vascular diagnostic procedures were rapidly developed. Table 1 details a partial list of some of the more notable contributions made and the individuals involved in the development of these diagnostic endovascular technologies. In this earlier diagnostic era, the multispecialty contribution of the principal innovators is obvious. Specialists from the various disciplines included surgeons, radiologists, and cardiologists. The most recent contribution to endovascular diagnostic technology, intravascular ultrasound, was in fact pioneered by both a cardiologist, Paul Yock, and a vascular surgeon, Rodney White. Both of these specialists recognized the potential clinical usefulness of this intraluminal enabling technology.[2, 3] Intraluminal ultrasound not only provides a greater understanding of the pathophysiology of the atherosclerotic lesion but also allows interventionalists to diagnose and assess the results of therapy. Additionally, the use of ultrasound during the performance of endovascular procedures offers the most reliable means of documenting the completeness of the intervention in real time.

The second 30 years of endovascular technology emphasized *therapeutic* catheter-mediated approaches in the management of vascular pathology. This began in the early 1960s and continues into our current

TABLE 1.
Historical Developments in Endovascular *Diagnostics*

Developer	Year	Instrument	Use
Dos Santos	1929	Needle	Visualization
Forssman	1929	Coaxial catheter	Physiologic
Cournand	1941	Coaxial catheter	Cardiac diagnostic
Seldinger	1953	Guiding catheter	Percutaneous access
Sones	1959	Coaxial catheter	Coronary visualization

Advances in Vascular Surgery®, vol. 4
© 1996, Mosby–Year Book, Inc.

TABLE 2.
Historical Contributions to Endovascular
Therapeutics

Developer	Year	Instrument	Use
Fogarty	1963	Coaxial balloon	Removal
Dotter	1964	Coaxial catheter	Dilate
Gruntzig	1974	Coaxial balloon	Dilate
Palmaz	1985	Stent	Stent
Simpson	1988	Coaxial cutter	Removal
Parodi	1991	Stent graft	Graft

time. Table 2 highlights some of the developers and their contributions to the treatment phase of this endovascular revolution.

BALLOON CATHETER EMBOLECTOMY—FOGARTY

Endovascular technology directed to the management of acute arterial occlusion was the first therapeutic catheter technique to be accepted on a widespread clinical basis. A review of the literature from 1950 to 1960 clearly points out the extremely high mortality and morbidity associated with acute arterial occlusion before catheter development. The majority of patients sustained embolic occlusions secondary to rheumatic heart disease; this resulted in attendant mortality and amputation rates both exceeding 50%. All patients had severe underlying cardiac disease that went untreated because at that time no standard techniques or instrumentation was available to manage their multisystem pathology. The original report describing a less invasive approach for managing embolic occlusions was presented in 1963.[4] This first therapeutic endovascular instrument consisted of a pliable catheter body with a soft latex balloon located at the distal tip. The procedure for remote clot extraction was performed from a small groin incision through a common femoral arteriotomy. After distal insertion, the balloon catheter was passed beyond the acute occlusion, inflated, and then slowly withdrawn, extracting the embolic and thrombotic material. The balloon catheter technique for embolectomy marked the conversion of a previously complicated, prolonged major surgery into a minimally invasive and relatively easy-to-perform endovascular procedure accessed through small incisions under local anesthesia.

At the request of the editor, I will include a personal documentation of the events leading to the development of the Fogarty embolectomy catheter. Indeed, the background in which the catheter technique for embolectomy was developed was somewhat unusual and interesting inasmuch as it resulted primarily from the efforts of a fledgling medical student. I worked as a scrub technician in a local hospital while still a high school student. The opportunity to work with Dr. Jack Cranley on a part-time, but regular basis became available during my premedical and medical school education. This experience led to the all-too-frequent observation of unsuccessful attempts to revascularize limbs after acute arterial occlusion. Second operations were frequent and usually involved amputation. These failures occurred despite desperate efforts on the part of the surgical team and resulted from a lack of adequate instrumentation to treat the occlusion. The desire to change these outcomes prompted me to handcraft the first balloon catheter during my senior year in medical school. The basic unit consisted of a used 6-French ureteral catheter. The small finger of a size 5 latex glove was cut at the tip and used as the balloon. Using fly tying techniques, the finger tip was tied onto the distal tip of the 6-French ureteral catheter to form a balloon reservoir. The instrument was bench-tested in tapered test tubes in which blood had been allowed to clot. Shortly after these initial testing periods, I was accepted for an internship at the University of Oregon, where the handmade catheters were tested in two cadavers. During that same year I received notice that I would be drafted immediately after completion of my internship. Despite Dr. Bert Dunphy accepting me for a surgical residency at the University of Oregon, I was told that there would be no relief from my military obligation and I reluctantly returned to Cincinnati, Ohio, for induction after my internship. While waiting for induction, I again worked with Dr. John Cranley as a surgical assistant. The time for induction passed without any notice given of when I was to report for duty. Drs. Cranley and Dunphy discussed the situation, and it was decided that Dr. Dunphy would make an inquiry on my behalf. It was determined that my draft records had been lost in the transfer between the states of Oregon and Ohio. Dr. Dunphy convinced the military that my time would be better served by allowing me to complete the year with Dr. Cranley in the form of a fellowship and then return to the University of Oregon for further training in general surgery. It was during that year that Dr. Cranley and his colleagues performed the first balloon embolectomy. The first case was performed in 1961, and the initial experience along with seven additional cases was reported in *Surgery, Gynecology & Obstetrics* in 1963. It is of interest to note that the initial embolectomy report was rejected by three prominent peer-reviewed journals before being accepted by *Surgery, Gynecology & Obstetrics* for inclusion in the section "Surgeon at Work."

BALLOON ANGIOPLASTY—DOTTER, GRUNTZIG

Charles Dotter was a professor and the Chairman of Radiology at the University of Oregon. Upon my return to Oregon after my fellowship with Dr. Jack Cranley, Dotter talked to me about my earlier work and expressed an interest in treating chronic occlusion percutaneously. Dotter's initial concept for balloon angioplasty was applied in 1964[5] and involved co-axial catheters passed over one another with the intent of increasing the cross-sectional area of a chronically diseased vessel. Although this concept was crude, it did work on occasion and, in fact, was used much more commonly in Europe than the United States. Charles Dotter recognized the limitation of this rudimentary technology and requested that I make a balloon catheter that could be used to effect dilatation. At Dr. Dotter's request, in 1965 a balloon catheter was made that consisted of a latex balloon circumferentially covered by a second balloon that provided extra thickness and less compliance. After its initial use and success, Dr. Dotter requested of Dr. Dunphy that I spend 6 months' research time with the department of radiology to further refine the dilatation balloon catheter instrument and technique.

I was summoned to Dr. Dunphy's office and informed that if I were interested in a surgical residency, I would not be able to collaborate with Dr. Charles Dotter. Accordingly, balloon catheters were constructed for the most part in the evening and late night hours and delivered daily to the admitting desk where Dr. Dotter or one of his associates would pick them up for inclusion into their continuing clinical study. Although I was not able to formally engage in these actual clinical experiences, I would often see the results of their indiscretions and subsequently end up operating on these early angioplasty patients at all odd hours. The first dilatation balloon catheter that I made for Dr. Dotter in 1965 resulted in a successful clinical result, and angiographic study 14 years later documented continued vessel patency.[6]

In 1974, Dr. Andreas Gruntzig[7] extended the clinical applications of the balloon catheter concept; he emphasized that noncompliant balloons were required to dilate atherosclerotic lesions. This methodology was then subsequently applied to the coronary arterial system as well as the peripheral vasculature.

Catheter-mediated endarterectomy, or more appropriately, *atherectomy*, was introduced by Dr. John Simpson.[8] An interesting historical note relating to atherectomy centers around the fact that the initial development and clinical application resulted from a collaborative effort between Simpson and me. Although Dr. Simpson and I had originally been faculty colleagues at the Stanford University Medical Center, we left Stanford in the early 1970s to go into private practice. The timing and reasons for our departures were related in an unusual way. I left Stanford primarily because there were insufficient beds to accommodate a very busy clinical practice. With the vigorous urging and strong endorsement of Dr. Norman Shumway, I transferred my practice to Sequoia Hospital in Redwood City, California, in the hope that I could devote more time to clinical research. Dr. John Simpson followed several years later to the same institution. The reason for his departure related to his inability to carry out relatively independent clinical research as a Stanford faculty member. After a joint initial clinical evaluation of an atherectomy device in the peripheral arterial system, Dr. Simpson continued his work and applied the concept of atherectomy to coronary atherosclerotic pathology.[9] Although the original hope was that this instrumentation would have broad clinical applications, unfortunately, at this point in time atherectomy has less clinical usefulness than originally envisioned.

STENTS AND STENT GRAFTS—PALMAZ, PARODI

In 1985,[10] Palmaz introduced the concept of a balloon expandable vascular stent, and in 1986, his further studies documented the potential for an intraluminal vascular graft.[11] Stent technology has increasing applications not only in the peripheral vasculature but also in coronary and nonvascular pathologies. Although Volodos, a Russian surgeon, introduced the concept of a vascular stent graft in the Russian literature in 1986,[12] *clinical* utilization was reported in the North American literature by Dr. Juan Parodi in 1991. Parodi's extensive publications on the subject have made his name most widely associated with this device.[13] As the name implies, the stent graft is a combination of a vascular stent that provides support and an enveloping graft material that lines the spaces of the stent. The device is introduced via catheter, deployed, spanned across the pathology, and secured in place by a variety of different mechanisms. The approach is currently being investigated for the treatment of both aneurysmal and chronic occlusive disease. The stent graft is a promising new technology that will, we hope, once again convert a major operation into a less invasive procedure with reduced mortality and morbidity.

CONCLUSION

From a physician specialist standpoint, endovascular diagnostics and therapeutics have seen contributions from surgeons, cardiologists, radiologists, and bioengineers. From my perspective, endovascular therapeutics is a rapidly growing field that will have a significant place in the management of patients with peripheral vascular disease. The pathology that endovascular therapy seeks to correct represents today's most common medical afflictions. These atherosclerotic disease states have their highest incidence in well-developed countries and are a significant cause of the morbidity and mortality that affect our aging population. Less invasive approaches provide some of the answers that will address society's demands for quicker, safer, more simplified, and less costly procedures. Surgeons, if they are to remain involved in the diagnostic and therapeutic management of patients with peripheral vascular disease, must become versed in endovascular technology.

REFERENCES

1. Fogarty TJ, Biswas A: Evolution of endovascular therapy: Diagnostics & therapeutics, in White RA, Fogarty TJ (eds): *Peripheral Endovascular Interventions.* St Louis, Mosby, 1996, pp 3–12.

2. Yock PG, Johnson EL, Linker DT: Introvascular ultrasound: Development and clinical potential. *Am J Card Imaging* 2:185–193, 1988.

3. Cavaye DM, White RA: The changing spectrum of cardiovascular interventions; the role of intraluminal ultrasound. *Intravasc Ultrasound Imaging* 1:1–11, 1993.

4. Fogarty T, Cranley J, Krause R, et al: A method for extraction of arterial emboli and thrombi. *Surg Gynecol Obstet* 116:241–244, 1963.

5. Dotter C, Judkins M: Transluminal treatment of arteriosclerotic obstruction: Description of a new technic and a preliminary report of its application. *Circulation* 30:654–670, 1964.

6. Dotter C: Transluminal angioplasty: A long view. *Radiology* 135:561–564, 1980.

7. Gruntzig A, Hopf H: Perkutane Rekanalisation chronischer arterieller Verschlusse mit neuen Dilatationskather: Modification der Dotter-teknik. *Dtsch Med Wochenschr* 99:2502–2510, 1974.

8. Simpson JB, Selmon MR, Robertson GC, et al: Transluminal atherectomy for occlusive peripheral vascular disease. *Am J Cardiol* 61:96G–101G, 1988.

9. Hinohara T, Selmon MR, Robertson GC, et al: Directional atherectomy: New approaches for treatment of obstructive coronary and peripheral vascular disease. *Circulation* 81:79S–91S, 1990.

10. Palmaz J, Sibbitt R, Tio F, et al: Expandable intraluminal graft: Preliminary study. *Radiology* 156:72–77, 1985.

11. Palmaz J, Sibbitt R, Tio F, et al: Expandable intraluminal vascular graft: A feasibility study. *Surgery* 99:199–205, 1986.

12. Volodos NL, Shekhanin VE, Karpovich IP, et al: Self-fixing synthetic prosthesis for endoprosthetics of the vessels. *Vestn Khir* 136:123–125, 1986.

13. Parodi JC: Transfemoral intraluminal graft implantation for abdominal aortic aneurysms. *Ann Vasc Surg* 5:491–499, 1991.

PART II

Aorta

When to Repair Abdominal Aortic Aneurysms

Jack L. Cronenwett, M.D.

Professor of Surgery, Dartmouth Medical School; Chief, Section of Vascular Surgery, Dartmouth-Hitchcock Medical Center, Lebanon, New Hampshire

The decision to repair an abdominal aortic aneurysm (AAA) depends on an assessment of rupture risk vs. elective operative mortality, taken in the context of age and life expectancy. Improvements in surgical technique, anesthetic management, and perioperative care have reduced the mortality of elective AAA repair to less than 5% in most centers that perform an adequate volume of these procedures. This has led to the suggestion that early surgery be performed for smaller, lower-risk AAAs. In fact, Society for Vascular Surgery/International Society for Cardiovascular Surgery practice guidelines recommend repair of AAAs as small as 4 cm in diameter in properly selected patients.[1] This recommendation is underscored by the fact that current clinical practice has not eliminated AAA rupture, which still ranks 15th among all causes of death for men in the United States.

Because AAA repair is designed to prolong life, it is most effective when applied to younger patients with longer life expectancy. The fact that AAAs occur in elderly patients with limited life expectancy results in more difficult decision making. Furthermore, notwithstanding its morbidity and mortality, AAA repair is an expensive procedure. Given the current economic constraints on health care delivery, all procedures must be evaluated not only in terms of their efficacy but also in terms of their cost-effectiveness. Thus AAAs should be repaired only when this therapy is cost-effective in comparison to other common medical practices. To address these issues, we developed a decision analysis model to identify the key variables that determine the cost-effectiveness of AAA repair, which is the subject of this chapter.

DECISION ANALYSIS

Our computerized model simulated a hypothetical group of patients with AAAs in whom an initial decision must be made between early surgery and watchful waiting (ultrasound size surveillance at 6-month intervals and subsequent repair only if a specific size threshold is reached).[2] Probabilities were assigned to the possible outcomes of each decision, and each possible resulting health state was assigned a utility or quality score. The computer model then calculated the projected life expectancy for the initial decision of early surgery vs. watchful waiting, depending on the

Advances in Vascular Surgery®, vol. 4

specific patient variables that were entered for the simulation. Life expectancy is measured in quality-adjusted life years (QALYs), which reduces the value of survival in the presence of morbidity. For example, dialysis-dependent renal failure after AAA repair is estimated to reduce quality-adjusted survival to 70% of unadjusted survival.

To estimate the probability of different outcomes, we reviewed the literature and selected data from large contemporary series, with an emphasis on population-based data when available. An estimated range was developed for probabilities of elective operative mortality, ruptured AAA mortality, AAA expansion rate, AAA rupture rate, age, compliance with ultrasound follow-up, etc. By examining the outcome of the decision model over the expected range of each of these variables, it is possible to determine whether the decision can be changed by different values of that variable (sensitivity analysis). After performing this analysis, we determined that the choice between early surgery and watchful waiting for a given AAA depended on the following key variables: patient age, elective operative mortality, and AAA rupture risk.[2] Compliance with ultrasound follow-up, threshold size for elective repair, and possible future increase in elective operative risk were also potential key variables that could affect this decision. Other variables, such as operative mortality associated with AAA rupture, did not influence the outcome of this decision when tested over their expected range. It was reassuring to validate the importance of the three commonly used clinical criteria for AAA decision-making, namely, patient age, elective operative mortality, and AAA rupture risk. Thus for appropriate decision-making it is important to understand the variables that influence elective operative risk and AAA rupture risk.

ELECTIVE OPERATIVE RISK

For our decision model, we estimated the average 30-day mortality rate after elective AAA repair to be 4.6% based on a population-based study.[3] This estimate is nearly identical to the elective operative mortality rate of 4.8% reported in the Canadian multicenter trial.[4] In our computer model, however, we tested the influence of elective operative mortality rate over the range of 0% to 26% in order to represent the range of results reported in the literature for patients with different risk factors.

Numerous studies have analyzed the outcome of patients undergoing elective AAA repair and have correlated these results with different patient risk factors. Thus expected operative mortality for patients undergoing elective AAA repair can be estimated quite accurately. Using multivariate analysis, Johnston found that cardiac ischemia, chronic renal insufficiency, and chronic obstructive pulmonary disease (COPD) could stratify expected operative mortality from as low as 2% to as high as 50% if all three of these risk factors were severe.[4] Importantly, chronologic age was not an important risk factor for increased mortality after elective AAA repair (although it does predict worse outcome after ruptured AAA repair). In addition to these patient-specific risk factors, surgeons who performed few AAA repairs (less than 5 per year) experienced an operative mortality rate two to three times higher than normal.[5] Thus the influence of patient-specific variables must be considered in the context of each individual surgeon's results.

Accurate assessment of elective operative risk is essential for appropriate decision making concerning AAA repair. Identification of patients with high operative risk can lead to successful risk reduction in some cases or to foregoing AAA repair in others. Alternatively, identification of low operative risk may allow the repair of lower-risk AAAs with low postoperative morbidity. Implicit in the evaluation of operative risk is a careful assessment of life expectancy after AAA repair. The potential benefit of AAA surgery to improve life expectancy is predictably minimal in very elderly patients, those with incurable malignancy, or those with other factors that would limit survival to only several years. If early postoperative mortality can be avoided after AAA surgery, however, life expectancy is comparable to that of similar patients without AAAs.[6] Not surprisingly, coronary artery disease (CAD) is the largest cause of both early and late mortality in these atherosclerotic patients.

Clinical criteria are useful for stratifying cardiac risk preoperatively.[7] Angina, history of myocardial infarction (MI), Q wave on ECG, ventricular arrhythmia, congestive heart failure (CHF), diabetes, and age greater than 75 years have been found to increase the risk of postoperative cardiac events (unstable angina, MI, ischemic CHF, or death). Combinations of these risk factors can be used to develop an algorithm to predict postoperative cardiac morbidity. These estimates may be further refined by more sophisticated preoperative testing such as cardiac stress imaging, echocardiography, or continuous Holter monitoring.[8] Although these studies may refine the risk estimate for AAA surgery, they are expensive and thus should be used only in borderline cases where their outcome is likely to change the recommendation for AAA repair vs. watchful waiting. This also applies to preoperative coronary angiography, which can precisely delineate coronary lesions but is even more expensive.

Identification of significant CAD (or other cardiac risk factors such as valvular disease or CHF) preoperatively may lead to a decision to (1) delay or avoid AAA repair, (2) perform AAA repair with more intensive perioperative monitoring and management, or (3) reduce cardiac risk before AAA surgery with coronary artery bypass grafting (CABG) or coronary angioplasty. The first choice is most applicable to patients with small, low-risk AAAs or elderly patients in whom the added benefit of AAA surgery is marginal. The choice between options 2 and 3 is the subject of considerable current controversy. Proponents of strategy 2 point to the very low (less than 5%) postoperative AAA mortality without aggressive preoperative cardiac evaluation and treatment, as reported by several centers specializing in vascular surgery.[9] In addition, the added mortality from cardiac intervention must be considered, which is at least 5%. These arguments suggest that only patients with very severe CAD should undergo CABG or coronary angioplasty before AAA surgery. In contrast, proponents of strategy 3 (aggressive preoperative CAD evaluation and treatment) point to the necessity of ensuring long-term survival in these patients in order to receive the benefit of AAA repair.[10] Late survival after AAA repair is improved in patients with CAD corrected by preoperative CABG.[10] However, it may be possible to delay treatment of

CAD for years after AAA repair because in only certain patients do the more traditional indications for CABG develop during follow-up. This question must currently be addressed in each center by analyzing the outcomes and ultimate cost-effectiveness of these preoperative strategies.

It is important to individualize application of the aforementioned principles to the preoperative evaluation of heart disease in patients with AAAs. For patients with no clinical indicators of CAD, it is unlikely that further cardiac evaluation will alter the planned AAA repair. For patients with known or strongly suspected CAD, preoperative stress imaging will further stratify cardiac risk.[11] Coronary arteriography (and possible CABG) should be reserved for patients with two or more major cardiac regions of reversible ischemia on stress imaging—patients in whom a perioperative MI associated with AAA surgery is likely to cause death or significant morbidity from substantial reduction in cardiac function. More extensive evaluation of cardiac risk is appropriate for patients with smaller, lower-risk AAAs because a very low elective operative mortality rate must be ensured if they are to receive benefit from AAA repair. Conversely, patients with large, high-risk AAAs are likely to benefit from AAA repair even in the presence of known cardiac disease, unless they are experiencing unstable angina or have extensive multisegment cardiac ischemia.[11]

RISK OF ABDOMINAL AORTIC ANEURYSM RUPTURE

Although the natural history of AAAs is to expand and rupture, individual AAAs show considerable variation in expansion rate and rupture risk, which makes surgical decision-making more difficult for individual patients. A more precise knowledge of the natural history of AAAs is also thwarted by effective treatment; for example, most large and many small AAAs are selectively repaired, which leads to an underestimate of rupture risk in most "natural history" studies. Despite these constraints, individual patient decisions must be made, and our decision analysis model demonstrated that rupture risk is the key variable that affects this decision. Thus it is important to consider the factors that influence AAA rupture risk to make accurate estimates for individual patients.

Size, measured by diameter, is the best predictor of AAA rupture, especially for large AAAs.[12] The increased rupture risk of larger AAAs has been demonstrated by numerous clinical and autopsy series.[12-16] Although the precise risk at any given size is not known, there is general agreement that AAA rupture risk increases exponentially with size (Fig 1). Several recent studies have demonstrated an abrupt increase in rupture risk for AAAs 5 cm or larger in diameter. Nevitt et al. found the annual rupture risk of AAAs 5 cm or larger to be 6.3% per year, whereas Limet et al. estimated this annual rupture risk to be 15.8% per year despite the fact that approximately one third of the patients in these studies underwent elective AAA repair during follow-up.[13, 14] Thus it is generally agreed that the annual rupture risk for AAAs 5 cm or larger in diameter is at least 5% per year. Furthermore, there is uniform agreement that the rupture risk for AAAs less than 4 cm diameter is negligible. For AAAs in the 4- to 5-cm-diameter range, however, there is less agreement

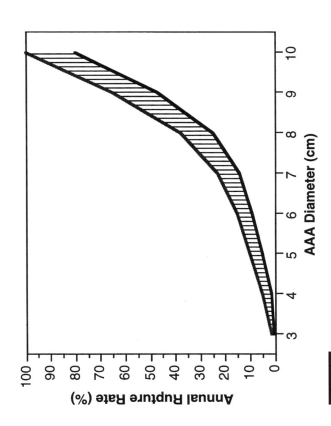

AAA Diameter (cm)

Annual Rupture Rate (%)

FIGURE 1.

Estimated annual rupture rate based on abdominal aortic aneurysm *(AAA)* diameter. The range at each size is based on different published estimates and likely reflects other variables that also influence rupture risk such as hypertension and chronic obstructive pulmonary disease. (Courtesy of Sampson LN, Cronenwett JL: Abdominal aortic aneurysms, in Zelenock GB (ed): *Problems in General Surgery,* vol 2, *Vascular Surgery.* Philadelphia, JB Lippincott, 1995, pp 385–417.)

concerning rupture risk. In a population-based study of selective AAA management in Canada, Brown et al. found that none of the AAAs less than 5 cm in diameter ruptured but that 60% expanded to greater than 5 cm and required elective surgery during the 3.5-year average follow-up.[15] In contrast, Limet et al. found that 5.4% of 4- to 5-cm-diameter AAAs ruptured each year during watchful waiting, even though 38% underwent elective repair during a 2-year follow-up.[14] In our study of patients with small AAAs managed nonoperatively, we calculated the rupture risk to be 3.3% per year for AAAs that remained 4 to 5 cm in diameter.[2, 16] These contrasting results indicate that the natural history of 4- to 5-cm AAAs is unclear, which has stimulated two currently ongoing randomized clinical trials comparing watchful waiting and early surgery for 4- to 5.5-cm-diameter AAAs. This range of estimates for AAA rupture risk also suggests that factors other than size probably influence AAA rupture.

In a multivariate analysis of patients with small AAAs, we found that initial AAA size ($P < 0.01$), hypertension ($P < 0.02$), and COPD ($P < 0.001$) were independent predictors of future AAA rupture.[16] Absolute AAA diameter was a more accurate predictor than the ratio of the AAA diameter to the more proximal aortic diameter. Furthermore, diastolic blood pressure was a more accurate predictor than systolic blood pressure. Chronic obstructive pulmonary disease was the most influential risk factor, which we attributed to a possible increase in systemic proteinase activity affecting both pulmonary and aortic connective tissue. These same three risk factors were found to be independently associated with AAA rupture risk in an autopsy study by Sterpetti et al.[17] These investigators found that patients with ruptured AAAs had significantly larger aneurysms (8.0 vs. 5.1 cm), more frequently had hypertension (54% vs. 28%), and more frequently had both emphysema (67% vs. 42%) and bronchiectasis (29% vs. 15%). These results also suggested a generalized connective tissue defect as the unifying hypothesis to explain the association of COPD and AAA rupture.

The potential interaction between smoking, COPD, and AAA rupture risk is not settled. Based on a large epidemiologic study of male civil servants in England, Strachan found that the relative risk of death from AAA rupture increased 2.4-fold for pipe/cigar smokers, 4.6-fold for cigarette smokers, and fully 14.6-fold for smokers of hand-rolled cigarettes.[18] However, in this large epidemiologic study it was impossible to separate the potentially confounding influence of COPD or other factors that might have been more prevalent among cigarette smokers. In our study, we did not find that smoking history or current smoking status was predictive of AAA rupture despite the important impact of COPD.[16] Similarly, Sterpetti et al. found that COPD, but not smoking, appeared to be the important causative factor influencing rupture.[17] However, from a case management standpoint, the nearly 5-fold increase in AAA rupture for cigarette smokers reported by Strachan cannot be overlooked.

Although a positive family history of AAA has been demonstrated to increase the prevalence of AAAs in other first-degree relatives (FDRs), it is less clear whether familial AAAs have a higher rupture risk. In one study of 86 families with 209 FDRs with AAAs, Darling et al. found that the frequency of rupture increased with the number of FDRs with AAAs: 14.8% rupture rate with 2 FDRs, 29% rupture rate with 3 FDRs, and 36% rupture rate with 4 or more FDRs.[19] Furthermore, these investigators found that women with familial aneurysms had a 30% incidence of rupture whereas men with familial AAAs had only a 17% incidence of rupture. These results suggest that patients with a strong family history of AAAs may have an individually higher risk of rupture, especially if they are female. However, this study was also unable to consider the many potential confounding factors, such as AAA size, that might have been different in the familial group.

Several other factors have been suggested to predict AAA rupture risk but have not been confirmed. By analyzing CT scans of patients undergoing elective and ruptured AAA repair, Ouriel et al. concluded that AAAs smaller than the transverse diameter of the L3 vertebral body did not rupture in their experience.[20] However, this aortic-vertebral ratio was only slightly more accurate (68%) than absolute AAA diameter alone (60%) in discriminating the potential for AAA rupture. The shape of an AAA is another variable that might contribute to rupture risk, and clinical opinion holds that eccentric, saccular aneurysms have a greater rupture risk than do diffuse cylindric aneurysms. This could not be proven, however, and requires further examination.[21] Similarly, the potential of contained thrombus to alter rupture risk has been speculated but not proven. One recent study suggested that thrombus thickness was less (9 mm) in patients with ruptured AAAs than in patients with nonruptured AAAs (19-mm thickness).[22]

Finally, a rapid AAA expansion rate is presumed to increase rupture risk, but it is difficult to separate this effect from the influence of expansion rate on absolute diameter, which alone could influence rupture. In our multivariate analysis we found that absolute AAA size rather than expansion rate was a better predictor of rupture.[16] Nevitt et al. also found that absolute size, but not expansion rate, was associated with increased rupture.[13] Other studies, however, have found that the expansion rate was greater in patients with ruptured than with nonruptured AAAs.[14,23] However, these AAAs with more rapid expansion were also larger, thus making it impossible to separate these confounding effects.

Regardless of whether the AAA expansion rate per se affects rupture or not, it clearly influences subsequent AAA size, an important factor to consider during follow-up. Several studies have now determined that AAAs expand as an exponential function of their initial size. We determined that 3- to 6-cm AAAs expand by 10% of their diameter per year.[24] Thus in 1 year the average 3-cm-diameter AAA would be expected to expand 0.3 cm, whereas a 6-cm-diameter AAA would be expected to expand 0.6 cm. This is nearly identical to a more sophisticated mathematical analysis by Limet et al. in which it was determined that AAAs expand at an exponential rate equivalent to an 11% diameter increase per year for small AAAs.[14] In considering other variables that influence the expansion rate, we determined that increased pulse pressure (largely influenced by systolic hypertension) increased the expansion rate and should be considered when predicting future aneurysm size (Fig 2).[24] Others have demonstrated the importance of hypertension in general on increasing the AAA expansion rate.[23] Furthermore, increased thrombus

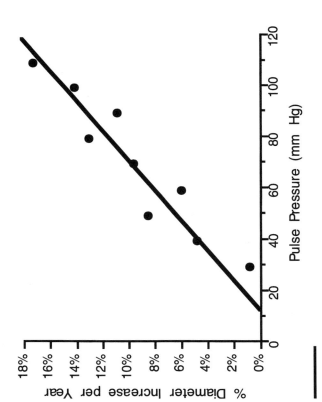

FIGURE 2.

Predicted annual increase in abdominal aortic aneurysm diameter based on varying pulse pressure. (Courtesy of Cronenwett JL: Variables that affect the expansion rate and rupture of abdominal aortic aneurysms. *Ann NY Acad Sci* 1996, in press.)

content within an aneurysm increases the expansion rate, possibly because of thrombus-derived plasmin activation of metalloproteinases in the AAA wall.[21] Finally, cigarette smoking appears to increase the AAA expansion rate.[25]

In summary, the best currently available information indicates that the annual rupture risk for AAAs 4- to 5-cm in diameter ranges from 0.5% to 5% per year, whereas for AAAs greater than 5 cm in diameter, this rupture risk increases to 5% to 15% per year. The precise rupture risk for an individual patient within these ranges is probably influenced by other risk factors, including hypertension, COPD, and family history. By considering these variables it is possible to estimate the rupture risk for individual patients and to estimate the expansion rate in order to predict future increases in rupture risk if watchful waiting is contemplated.

COST-EFFECTIVENESS ANALYSIS

The cost-effectiveness of a procedure that improves life expectancy depends on the incremental cost and improved survival associated with that procedure relative to the alternative strategy. The measure of cost-effectiveness is the ratio of this incremental cost divided by the improved survival, the latter measured in QALYs. Thus a strategy is considered to be more "cost-effective" as the cost-effectiveness ratio decreases. To perform cost-effectiveness analysis it is necessary to determine the specific cost of each outcome, such as elective AAA repair or ultrasound follow-up. The costs of these outcomes are then included in a decision analysis model, after which the preferred strategy can be determined. If a given strategy improves survival and costs *less* than the alternative strategy, it is regarded as dominant and cost saving. If a given strategy improves survival but costs *more* than the alternative strategy, the cost-effectiveness ratio of the preferred strategy can be calculated (incremental cost [$] per year of improved survival [QALYs]).

Confusion sometimes arises in the literature between "costs" and "charges." Charges represent the amount billed for a specific service and are influenced by profit, cost shifting between more and less profitable services, and differential third-party reimbursement. Actual costs are more difficult to determine but represent the real value of specific services based on estimates of factors such as labor, supplies, and overhead. Specific strategies have been developed to estimate hospital costs, but especially agreed formula for estimating physician costs is more problematic. Because there is no generally agreed formula for estimating physician costs, we performed our cost-effectiveness calculations with hospital costs alone (but repeated the analysis for total charges of both the physician and hospital).[26]

To determine the hospital costs at our medical center, we analyzed the detailed financial records of consecutive patients who underwent ruptured and elective AAA repair during fiscal year 1992.[26] Examples of the costs that were used in our model include elective AAA surgery, $33,614; ruptured AAA surgery, $43,208; and expanding AAA surgery, $24,020; abdominal ultrasound, $261. Thus hospital costs for ruptured AAA repair were nearly double those for elective AAA repair, as has previously been reported by others.[27] The ultimate model included all direct costs of early surgery (e.g., elective AAA repair plus morbidity) and watchful waiting (e.g., ultrasound follow-up and eventual elective AAA repair for some patients, plus ruptured AAA repair for some patients). All cost data were adjusted to 1992 dollars, and a discount rate of 5% was used throughout the analysis to adjust costs (and health benefits) to their present value. The rationale for such discounting is that a dollar (or QALY) is considered to be worth more today than at some point in the future.

For purposes of demonstration, we considered the outcome of cost-effectiveness analysis for a 60-year-old man who has an AAA with an estimated annual rupture risk of 3.3% and an elective operative mortality rate of 4.6%.[26] This would correspond to a 4- to 5-cm-diameter AAA in a patient with some additional risk for rupture such as COPD or hypertension. For this patient, early repair of this AAA when it is 4 cm in diameter would provide an average survival benefit of 0.34 QALYs at an additional cost of $5,858 as compared with watchful waiting and elective repair only if the AAA reached 5 cm in diameter. This yields an incremental cost-effectiveness ratio of $17,404 per QALY saved by early surgery when compared with the strategy of watchful waiting. In this scenario the upfront cost of early surgery for all patients makes this strategy more expensive than watchful waiting, in which only 70% of the patients are ultimately predicted to undergo elective surgery because 22% of these patients are predicted to die of other causes before their AAA reaches the 5-cm-diameter threshold for elective repair. However, the additional cost of elective AAA repair is narrowed by the increased cost of treating the 8% of patients whose AAAs rupture during watchful waiting and by the higher cost and greater incidence of chronic complications after ruptured AAA surgery, such as stroke and renal failure. The impact of this significantly greater cost for ruptured AAA repair and its complications results in a relatively low incremental cost of early surgery, approximately $17,000 per QALY saved.

The cost-effectiveness of early surgery for a given aneurysm is critically dependent on the key variables of elective operative mortality—AAA rupture risk and patient age. Importantly, the cost-effectiveness ratio of early surgery is not a linear function, but increases (worsens) markedly above a certain threshold value of each key variable. A conservative definition of "cost-effective" health care is health care that has a cost-effectiveness ratio of $40,000/QALY or less.[28] With this criterion it can be seen that if the annual rupture risk of a 4-cm-diameter AAA is estimated to be 3.3% per year, early AAA repair (vs. waiting until 5 cm) remains cost-effective for patients younger than approximately 70 years of age but, above this age threshold, the cost of early repair increases exponentially (Fig 3). This is not surprising given the shorter life expectancy of older patients and thus the lower opportunity to increase life expectancy with AAA repair. In the same patient with a larger aneurysm, where the estimated rupture risk is 5.5% per year, early repair would remain cost-effective until approximately age 80 (see Fig 3). For patients older than age 80 years, however, AAA repair would not become cost-effective unless the rupture risk were even higher, such as for an AAA greater than 6 cm in diameter or when multiple other risk factors for rupture are also present.

The same nonlinear influence on cost-effectiveness is observed for the

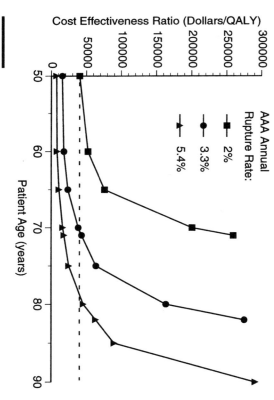

Cost Effectiveness Ratio (Dollars/QALY)

AAA Annual
Rupture Rate:
■ 2%
● 3.3%
▶ 5.4%

Patient Age (years)

FIGURE 3.

Cost-effectiveness of early surgery vs. watchful waiting as a function of initial patient age for three different abdominal aortic aneurysm (AAA) annual rupture rates. The *dotted line* indicates the cost-effectiveness ratio of $40,000 per quality-adjusted life year (*QALY*), below which health care interventions are generally regarded as "cost-effective." (Courtesy of Katz DA, Cronenwett JL: The cost-effectiveness of early surgery versus watchful waiting in the management of small abdominal aortic aneurysms. *J Vasc Surg* 19:980–991, 1994.)

key variables of elective operative mortality and annual rupture rate. For a 70-year-old patient, early repair of a 4-cm-diameter AAA with a 3.3% annual rupture risk remains cost-effective until the elective operative mortality rate exceeds 6% (Fig 4). In a younger, 60-year-old patient, early surgery remains cost-effective if the elective operative mortality rate is less than 12% (see Fig 4). Finally, the effect of rupture risk on cost-effectiveness is illustrated in Figure 5. For a 70-year-old patient with an elective operative mortality rate of 5%, early repair remains cost-effective for AAAs with a rupture risk greater than 3% per year. This probably corresponds to any 5-cm-diameter AAA and 4- to 5-cm-diameter AAAs if other risk factors for rupture (such as hypertension, COPD, or family history) are also present. When rupture risk is low (less than 2% per year), such as in 4- to 5-cm AAAs without other risk factors for rupture, early repair is not cost-effective until these AAAs reach 5 cm in diameter.

Several other variables can have an important effect on the cost-effectiveness of early surgery for AAA repair.[26] As the threshold size for elective AAA repair during watchful waiting increases, early surgery becomes more cost-effective. For example, if the threshold for elective AAA repair is increased from 5 to 6 cm during watchful waiting, the cost-effectiveness ratio of early surgery (at 4 cm) improves from $17,000 to $6,500 per QALY. This is because rupture risk increases substantially beyond 5 cm and is associated with a higher cost. Similarly, if patients are not compliant with ultrasound follow-up, the cost-effectiveness of early surgery is further improved because more AAAs would expand beyond the ideal threshold size and thus rupture during watchful waiting. Two

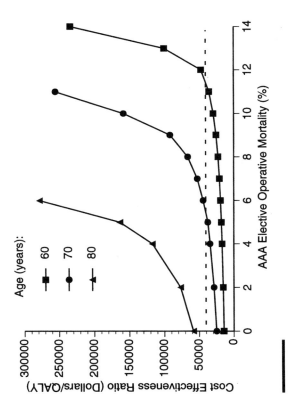

FIGURE 4.

Cost-effectiveness of early surgery *vs.* watchful waiting as a function of elective operative mortality in three age groups. The *dotted line* indicates the cost-effectiveness ratio of $40,000 per quality-adjusted life year (*QALY*), below which health care interventions are generally regarded as "cost-effective." (Courtesy of Katz DA, Cronenwett JL: The cost-effectiveness of early surgery versus watchful waiting in the management of small abdominal aortic aneurysms. *J Vasc Surg* 19:980–991, 1994.)

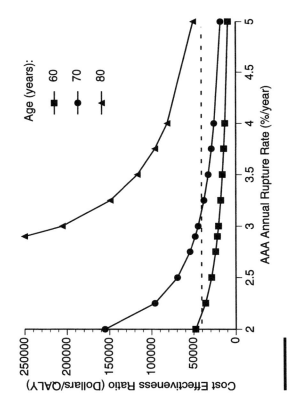

FIGURE 5.

Cost-effectiveness of early surgery *vs.* watchful waiting as a function of the average annual rate of abdominal aortic aneurysm *(AAA)* rupture or acute expansion in three age groups. The *dotted line* indicates the cost-effectiveness ratio of $40,000 per quality-adjusted life year (*QALY*), below which health care interventions are generally regarded as "cost-effective." (Courtesy of Katz DA, Cronenwett JL: The cost-effectiveness of early surgery versus watchful waiting in the management of small abdominal aortic aneurysms. *J Vasc Surg* 19:980–991, 1994.)

other variables have an impact on cost-effectiveness but are more diffi-cult to calculate. These include future anticipated changes in operative risk and patient risk aversion. For patients who are currently at low op-erative risk but in whom a higher operative risk subsequently develops during watchful waiting (such as from MI), the cost-effectiveness of early initial surgery improves. Unfortunately, such future changes are difficult to predict. Patient risk aversion also influences cost-effectiveness, de-pending on whether patients are more fearful of early surgery or more fearful of AAA rupture during watchful waiting. Thus for an elderly pa-tient who fears an operation and values current life, early surgery is less cost-effective. In contrast, for a younger patient who fears subsequent AAA rupture and values subsequent life years comparable to present life years, early surgery becomes more cost-effective.

Depending on the values of the key variables that influence outcome in our decision model, the cost-effectiveness ratio for early surgery for a 60-year-old man varies from $8,085/QALY (at 2% elective operative mor-tality and 5.5% annual rupture rates) to as high as $23,706/QALY (for 10% elective operative mortality and 3.3% annual rupture rates). For AAA rup-tures rates less than 3% per year, cost-effectiveness ratios increase expo-nentially. At these very low rupture rates, watchful waiting is the pre-ferred (dominant) strategy, and thus the cost-effectiveness of early sur-gery cannot be calculated.

To put these calculations into perspective, it is necessary to compare them with the cost-effectiveness of generally accepted preventive health measures. In this regard, our analysis shows that the incremental cost-effectiveness of early surgery compares favorably with the cost-effectiveness of screening for cervical cancer,[29] screening and therapy for hypertension,[30] and the use of β-blockade after acute myocardial infarc-tion.[31] It is also similar to the cost-effectiveness of coronary artery by-pass surgery[32] (Table 1). The price that Americans are willing to pay for health care that improves life expectancy is the focus of considerable de-bate. However, using the criterion of $40,000/QALY, our analysis suggests

TABLE 1.

Comparison of Cost-Effectiveness Ratios for Different Health Care Measures

Early surgery for 4-cm AAA*	$8,085–$23,706/QALY
Screening for cervical cancer[29]	$3,200–$46,200/QALY
Screening and treating hypertension[30]	$13,600–$69,300/QALY
β-Blockade after acute MI[31]	$5,300–$34,200/QALY
Coronary artery bypass[32]	
Single vessel	$51,000/QALY
Left main	$6,500/QALY

*Sixty-year-old man with a 4-cm AAA at an annual rupture rate of 3% to 5.4% and elective operative mortality rate of 2% to 10%.[26]
Abbreviations: AAA, abdominal aortic aneurysm; QALY, quality-adjusted life year; MI, myocardial infarction.

that repair of AAAs is cost-effective when the annual rupture risk is judged to be 3% or greater per year and the elective operative mortality rate is 5% or less per year in patients who are 70 years of age or younger. For older patients or those at higher operative risk, AAA repair is not cost-effective unless the AAA rupture risk approaches 5% per year.

CONCLUSION

It is difficult for physicians who are not accustomed to putting economic consideration above their patient's welfare to integrate cost-effectiveness calculations into their practice. However, as the available resources for health care become more limited, it is difficult to ignore the criterion of cost-effectiveness as a guiding principle. Evolution in the standard of care is dependent on the results of clinical trials, practice guidelines developed by specialty organizations, and detailed analyses comparing alternative practice strategies and their outcomes. Although they are not a substitute for clinical judgment, quantitative cost-effectiveness analyses are useful tools that help shape the public policy debate and help physicians focus on the essential trade-offs and uncertainties in patient care. Presently, decision models for prediction of the exact benefit (or loss) from early surgery for small AAAs are limited by the lack of precision in our estimates of AAA rupture risk. The results of ongoing clinical trials may provide better data to quantitate these key variables for individual patients. This would allow for more precise identification of patients for whom early surgery is most effective. Based on our current results, however, we would recommend early repair of 4- to 5-cm-diameter AAAs if a patient has other risk factors that would increase rupture risk, such as COPD, hypertension, or a strong family history. This aggressive approach can only be recommended for patients younger than approximately 70 years who have a long projected life expectancy based on the absence of CAD. For patients without other risks for AAA rupture, an elective AAA size threshold of 5 cm in diameter is usually appropriate provided that the average elective operative risk is 5% or less. For patients older than 80 years of age, AAA repair is probably not cost-effective until AAA size approaches 6 cm in diameter. For patients with a high elective operative risk (greater than 10%), AAA repair is probably also not cost-effective unless a 6-cm-diameter threshold is exceeded. It is important to reiterate that despite our substantial knowledge of the key variables that influence this decision, appropriate decision-making for AAA repair still requires considerable surgical judgment to customize the management strategy for individual patients.

REFERENCES

1. Hollier LH, Taylor LM, Ochsner J: Recommended indications for operative treatment of abdominal aortic aneurysms. Report of a subcommittee of the Joint Council of the Society for Vascular Surgery and the International Society for Cardiovascular Surgery. *J Vasc Surg* 15:1046–1056, 1992.
2. Katz DA, Littenberg BL, Cronenwett JL: Management of small abdominal aortic aneurysm: Early surgery vs watchful waiting. *JAMA* 268:2678–2686, 1992.

3. Roger VL, Ballard DJ, Nallett JW Jr, et al: Influence of coronary artery disease on morbidity and mortality following abdominal aortic aneurysm: A population-based study, 1971–87. *J Am Coll Cardiol* 14:1245–1252, 1989.

4. Johnston KW: Multicenter prospective study of nonruptured abdominal aortic aneurysm. Part II. Variables predicting morbidity and mortality. *J Vasc Surg* 9:437–447, 1989.

5. Veith FJ, Goldsmith J, Leather RP, et al: The need for quality assurance in vascular surgery. *J Vasc Surg* 13:523–526, 1991.

6. Hollier LH, Plate G, O'Brien PC, et al: Late survival after abdominal aortic aneurysm repair: Influence of coronary artery disease. *J Vasc Surg* 1:290, 1984.

7. Wong T, Detsky AS: Preoperative cardiac risk assessment for patients having peripheral vascular surgery. *Ann Intern Med* 116:743, 1992.

8. Eagle KA, Coley CM, Newell JB, et al: Combining clinical and thallium data optimizes preoperative assessment of cardiac risk before major vascular surgery. *Ann Intern Med* 110:859, 1989.

9. Taylor L Jr, Yeager RA, Moneta GL, et al: The incidence of perioperative myocardial infarction in general vascular surgery. *J Vasc Surg* 15:52, 1991.

10. Hertzer NR, Young JR, Beven EG, et al: Late results of coronary bypass in patients with infrarenal aortic aneurysm: The Cleveland Clinic study. *Ann Surg* 205:360, 1987.

11. Levinson JR, Boucher CA, Coley CM, et al: Usefulness of semiquantitative analysis of dipyridamole-thallium-201 redistribution for improving risk stratification before vascular surgery. *Am J Cardiol* 66:406, 1990.

12. Darling RC, Messina CR, Brewster DC, et al: Autopsy study of unoperated abdominal aortic aneurysm: The case for early resection. *Circulation* 56(3):161S–164S, 1977.

13. Nevitt MP, Ballard DJ, Hallett JW Jr: Prognosis of abdominal aortic aneurysms: A population-based study. *N Engl J Med* 321:1009–1013, 1989.

14. Limet R, Sakalihassan N, Albert A: Determination of the expansion rate and incidence of rupture of abdominal aortic aneurysms. *J Vasc Surg* 14:540–548, 1991.

15. Brown PM, Pattenden R, Gutelius JR: The selective management of small abdominal aortic aneurysms: The Kingston study. *J Vasc Surg* 15:21–27, 1992.

16. Cronenwett JL, Murphy TF, Zelenock GB, et al: Actuarial analysis of variables associated with rupture of small abdominal aortic aneurysms. *Surgery* 98:472–483, 1985.

17. Sterpetti AV, Cavallaro A, Cavallari N, et al: Factors influencing the rupture of abdominal aortic aneurysms. *Surg Gynecol Obstet* 173:175–178, 1991.

18. Strachan DP: Predictors of death from aortic aneurysm among middle-aged men: The Whitehall study. *Br J Surg* 78:401–404, 1991.

19. Darling RC III, Brewster DC, Darling RC, et al: Are familial abdominal aortic aneurysms different? *J Vasc Surg* 10:39–43, 1989.

20. Ouriel K, Green RM, Donayre C, et al: An evaluation of new methods of expressing aortic aneurysm size: Relationship to rupture. *J Vasc Surg* 15:12–20, 1992.

21. Wolf YG, Thomas WS, Brennan FG, et al: Computed tomography scanning findings associated with rapid expansion of abdominal aortic aneurysms. *J Vasc Surg* 20:529–538, 1994.

22. Kushihashi T, Munechika H, Matsui S, et al: CT of abdominal aortic aneurysms—aneurysmal size and thickness of intraaneurysmal thrombus as risk factors or rupture. *Nippon Igaku Hoshasen Gakkai Zasshi* 51:219–227, 1991.

23. Schewe CK, Schweikart HP, Hammel G, et al: Influence of selective management on the prognosis and the risk of rupture of abdominal aortic aneurysms. *Clin Invest* 72:585–591, 1994.

24. Cronenwett JL, Sargent SK, Wall MH, et al: Variables that affect the expansion rate and outcome of small abdominal aortic aneurysms. *J Vasc Surg* 11:260–269, 1990.

25. MacSweeney STR, Ellis M, Worrell PC, et al: Smoking and growth rate of small abdominal aortic aneurysms. *Lancet* 344:651–652, 1994.

26. Katz DA, Cronenwett JL: The cost-effectiveness of early surgery versus watchful waiting in the management of small abdominal aortic aneurysms. *J Vasc Surg* 19:980–991, 1994.

27. Brechwoldt WL, Mackey WC, O'Donnell TF Jr: Economic implications of high-risk abdominal aortic aneurysms. *J Vasc Surg* 13:798–804, 1991.

28. Frame PS, Fryback DG, Patterson C: Screening for abdominal aortic aneurysm in men ages 60 to 80 years. *Ann Intern Med* 119:411–416, 1993.

29. Fahs MC, Mandelblatt J, Schechter C, et al: Cost-effectiveness of cervical cancer screening for the elderly. *Ann Intern Med* 117:520–527, 1992.

30. Littenberg B, Garber AM, Sox HC: Screening for hypertension. *Ann Intern Med* 112:192–202, 1990.

31. Goldman L, Sia STB, Cook EF, et al: Costs and effectiveness of routine therapy with long-term beta-adrenergic antagonists after acute myocardial infarction. *N Engl J Med* 319:152–157, 1988.

32. Weinstein MC, Stason WB: Cost-effectiveness of coronary artery bypass surgery. *Circulation* 66:56S–65S, 1982.

Endovascular Repair of Diffuse Aortoiliac Atherosclerotic Occlusive Disease

Michael L. Marin, M.D.

Assistant Professor of Surgery, Division of Vascular Surgery, Department of Surgery, Montefiore Medical Center, The University Hospital for the Albert Einstein College of Medicine, New York, New York

Frank J. Veith, M.D.

Professor and Chief, Vascular Surgical Services, Division of Vascular Surgery, Department of Surgery, Montefiore Medical Center, The University Hospital for the Albert Einstein College of Medicine, New York, New York

Richard E. Parsons, M.D.

Fellow in Vascular Surgery, Division of Vascular Surgery, Department of Surgery, Montefiore Medical Center, The University Hospital for the Albert Einstein College of Medicine, New York, New York

A ortofemoral bypass has demonstrated durability and effectiveness for the treatment of lower-extremity ischemia with good long-term patency and acceptable procedural morbidity and mortality.[1-6] However, graft thrombosis of at least one limb may occur after aortofemoral grafting in as many as 10% to 20% of patients followed for a 10-year period, with a marked increase in the risk of operative complications from required secondary procedures.[2-4] In addition, patients with extensive aortoiliofemoral occlusive disease frequently have co-morbid medical illnesses related to atherosclerotic heart disease or pulmonary or renal insufficiency. Patients seen with limb-threatening ischemia and tissue necrosis commonly have multiple levels of arterial occlusive disease that will necessitate an infrainguinal bypass after the aortoiliac reconstruction to achieve adequate circulation for tissue healing. Such extensive, multilevel revascularizations are associated with significant morbidity and mortality in this often frail population of medically high-risk patients.

Alternative interventions to open aortic procedures have been sought to improve outcome and reduce morbidity and cost. Percutaneous balloon angioplasty of the iliac vessels with or without the insertion of in-

Supported by grants from the U.S. Public Health Service (HL 02990-03), the James Hilton Manning and Emma Austin Manning Foundation, The Anna S. Brown Trust, and the New York Institute for Vascular Studies.

Advances in Vascular Surgery®, vol. 4
© 1996, Mosby–Year Book, Inc.

travascular stents has proven to be an effective technique for treating focal disease in the common iliac artery.[7-14] Unfortunately, when diffuse disease involving multiple segments of the aorta, iliac, and femoral arteries occurs, unsatisfactory results can be expected with percutaneous techniques.[14,15] Recurrent stenoses at the site of the intervention for diffuse disease with return of clinical symptoms have made these endovascular approaches generally suboptimal in the iliac and femoropopliteal arteries.

An alternative technique that extends the potential of existing endovascular modalities for arterial occlusive disease employs angioplasty in combination with endovascular grafts (a combination of intravascular stents and prosthetic grafts) to bridge long, diffuse arterial occlusive disease.[16] Endovascular graft devices were initially conceptualized by Dotter[17] and subsequently tested in a variety of experimental models.[18-21] Variations in endovascular graft designs have resulted in devices for treating simple and complex aortic aneurysms, peripheral artery aneurysms, long, diffuse arterial occlusive disease, and traumatic arterial injuries.[22-32]

This review will analyze the Montefiore Medical Center experience with 42 long-segment aortoiliofemoral artery occlusions.

METHODS

PATIENTS

Since February 1993, 42 patients with limb-threatening ischemia secondary to aortoiliac and femoropopliteal occlusive disease have been treated at the Montefiore Medical Center in New York with endovascular aortoiliofemoral stented grafts. The 20 men and 22 women ranged in age from 45 to 89 years (mean, 65 years). Ten patients had severe ischemic rest pain, whereas the remaining 32 had varying degrees of ischemic tissue necrosis. Most of these patients had one or more coexisting medical problems, including severe coronary artery disease, renal insufficiency, or chronic obstructive pulmonary disease. Pulse volume recordings, ankle brachial indices, and aortography with femoropopliteal and tibial runoff views were performed in all patients before and after each intervention.

ENDOVASCULAR STENTED GRAFT DEVICES

The endovascular stented grafts used for treating aortoiliac occlusive disease comprised Palmaz balloon expandable stents (30 mm) (Johnson & Johnson Interventional Systems, Warren, NJ) and 6-mm polytetrafluoroethylene (PTFE) thin-walled grafts (W.L. Gore and Associates, Flagstaff, Ariz). Each stent was attached to the proximal end of the PTFE graft by 4 CV-6 PTFE sutures (W.L. Gore and Associates) so that one half of the stent protruded from the end of the graft (Fig 1). The stent and graft combination was then mounted onto an 8-mm × 3-cm angioplasty balloon (Blue Max or PMT, Medi-tech, Inc., Watertown, Mass). The entire balloon, stent, and graft complex was then wrapped around a second balloon catheter shaft ("tip balloon") and inserted into a delivery sheath so that the stent portion of the device was 2 cm from the distal delivery sheath tip (Fig 2). The 6-mm × 4-cm tip balloon was adjusted so that one half of the balloon protruded from the distal portion of the delivery sheath. When in-

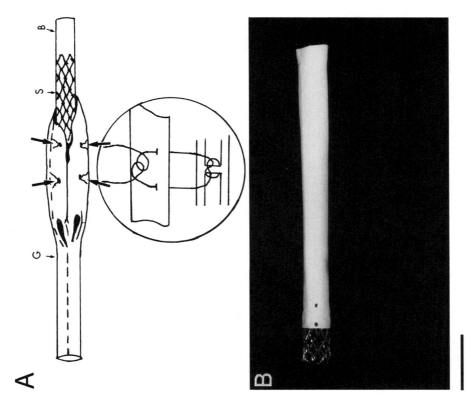

FIGURE 1.

A, schematic representation of an endovascular polytetrafluoroethylene (PTFE) graft similar to that used for aortoiliac reconstruction. A Palmaz balloon expandable stent (*S*) is sutured to a 6-mm PTFE graft (*G*) using four sutures (*small arrows*). The four sutures attach the PTFE graft to the underlying metallic stent as indicated in the **inset. B,** photograph of an endovascular stented graft used for aortoiliac reconstruction. A Palmaz stent is sutured to the overlying PTFE graft with four diametrically opposed PTFE sutures. No distal stent is seen attached to the graft, because in each case the distal end of the endovascular graft was endoluminally suture-anastomosed to an appropriate outflow vessel. *Abbreviation: B,* coaxially loaded balloon angioplasty catheter. (Reprinted with permission from: Marin ML, Veith FJ, Sanchez LA, et al: Endovascular repair of aortoiliac occlusive disease. *World J Surg* 20:679–686, 1996. Copyright Springer-Verlag.)

flated, the tip balloon could then occlude flow from the sheath tip, thus allowing sheath pressurization and providing a smooth, tapered transition point to the end of the delivery sheath. Other variations of this delivery system concept were also used, including a single shaft with two balloons or two balloons linked by a small fenestration in the shaft of the "tip balloon." In every case, the endovascular graft and delivery system were prepared on a separate, sterile table before performing each procedure in the operating room (Fig 3).

OPERATIVE TECHNIQUE

All procedures were performed using an open dissection and exposure of an ipsilateral femoral artery access site. Based on the general medical

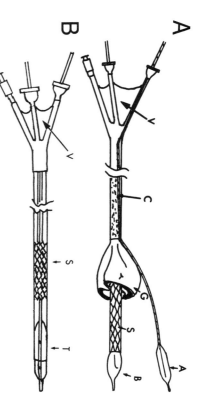

FIGURE 2.

A, introducer/delivery catheter used for delivery and deployment of endovascular stented grafts for aortoiliac reconstruction. Each introducer catheter is equipped with two balloons. Balloon A functions as a mechanism to form a tapered tip to the catheter system. The second balloon (B) functions to deploy the overlying Palmaz stent (S). With balloon expansion of balloon B, the endovascular graft (G) becomes firmly fixed to the underlying arterial wall. B, fully loaded delivery catheter sheath containing a balloon expandable stent and endovascular graft. Abbreviations: C, delivery catheter sheath; V hemostatic valve mechanism; T, tip balloon. (Reprinted with permission from: Marin ML, Veith FJ, Sanchez LA, et al: Endovascular repair of aortoiliac occlusive disease. World J Surg 20:679–686, 1996. Copyright Springer-Verlag.)

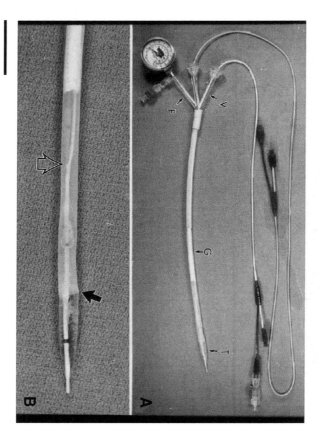

FIGURE 3.

Photograph of the delivery catheter sheath containing a balloon expandable stent and graft used for aortoiliac reconstruction. A, endovascular graft (G) is contained inside the delivery catheter sheath. The tip balloon (T) occludes the tip of the introducer catheter, forming a watertight seal. This balloon tip also functions to taper the distal end of the delivery catheter. The hemostatic valve (V) at the proximal end of the catheter permits individual control of each balloon. The pressurization valve (P) allows pressurization of the introducer catheter, permitting it to have variable pushability and flexibility. B, high magnification of the distal end of the endovascular graft delivery system. Note the smooth, tapered end to the delivery catheter tip (filled arrow). In this configuration of the delivery catheter system, a fenestration in the tip balloon (open arrow) permits coaxial (single wire) integration between the tip balloon and stent graft deployment balloon. (Reprinted with permission from: Marin ML, Veith FJ, Sanchez LA, et al: Endovascular repair of aortoiliac occlusive disease. World J Surg 20:679–686, 1996. Copyright Springer-Verlag.)

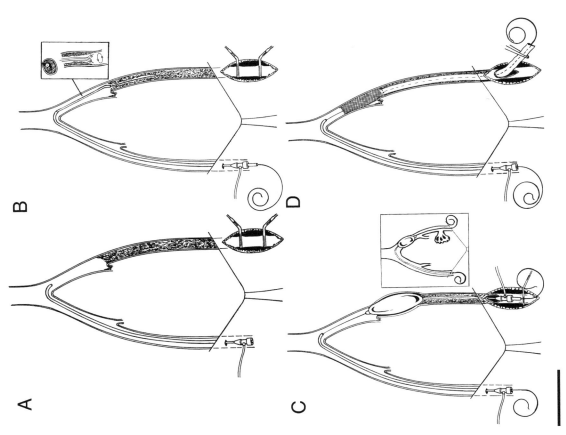

FIGURE 4.

Surgical procedure of endovascular grafting; "up and over" technique. When the contralateral iliac artery is patent, recanalization is carried out by means of a contralateral percutaneously inserted guide wire, up and over the aortic bifurcation, developing a prograde arterial wall dissection plane. This technique allows for maximal control of arterial inflow and ensures that the recanalization process begins within the native arterial lumen. (Reprinted with permission from Marin ML, Veith FJ, Sanchez LA, et al: Endovascular aortoiliac grafts in combination with standard infrainguinal arterial bypasses in the management of limb-threatening ischemia: Preliminary report. *J Vasc Surg* 22:316–25, 1995.)

condition of the patient at the time of the procedure and the complexity of the planned procedure, either general (9 [22%]), epidural (30 [71%]), or local (3 [7%]) anesthesia was selected. Two techniques for arterial recanalization were used to create a wide tract for graft insertion within the diseased iliac artery. When the contralateral iliac artery was patent, recanalization was carried out by means of a contralateral, percutaneously inserted guide wire, "up and over," the aortic bifurcation, developing a

M.L. Marin, F.J. Veith, and R.E. Parsons

prograde dissection plane toward the ipsilateral femoral artery within the occluded arterial wall (Fig 4). This technique allows for maximal, proximal control of arterial inflow (when necessary) and ensures that the recanalization process will begin within the native arterial lumen. When the up-and-over approach was not technically feasible, retrograde recanalization was used (Fig 5). Recanalizations were performed through an occluded artery in 34 patients and through a diffusely stenotic but patent vessel in 8 patients. Arterial recanalization was accomplished with a 0.035-in. hydrophilic guide wire (Glide Wire, Medi-tech Inc.) and an

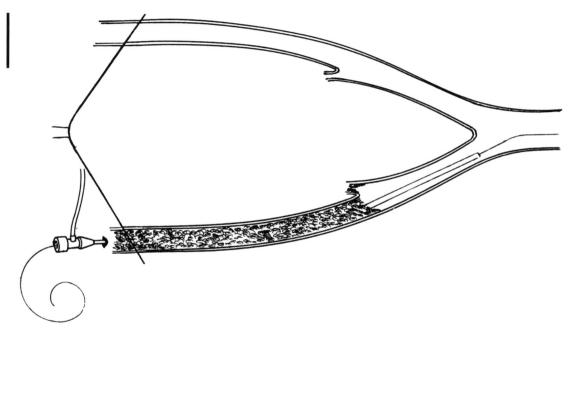

FIGURE 5.

Surgical procedure of endovascular grafting: retrograde technique. When the "up and over" approach was not technically feasible, retrograde recanalization was used. (Reprinted with permission from Marin ML, Veith FJ, Sanchez LA, et al: Endovascular aortoiliac grafts in combination with standard infrainguinal arterial bypasses in the management of limb-threatening ischemia: Preliminary report. *J Vasc Surg* 22:316–25, 1995.)

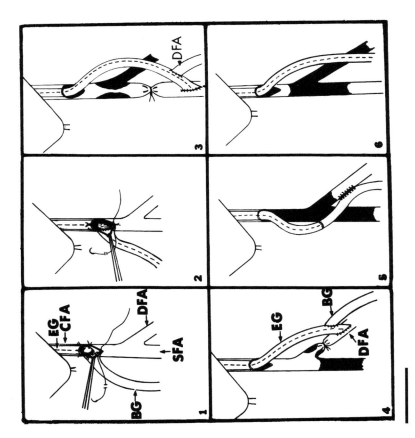

FIGURE 6.

Distal end of the endovascular graft can be anastomosed to the patent distal arterial tree in several ways. *1*, type I, an endoluminal anastomosis to the femoral artery is performed, and a separate proximal anastomosis of the distal extravascular graft is performed to the femoral arteriotomy. *2*, type II, the intravascular anastomosis and proximal anastomosis of the distal extravascular graft are included in a single anastomotic closure. *3*, type III, the stented graft is brought out through the femoral arteriotomy and anastomosed to the patent distal superficial femoral artery *(SFA)*. From this site, a distal extension or a crossover femorofemoral extension can be performed if necessary. *4*, type IV, the endovascular graft *(EG)* is brought out through the femoral arteriotomy and anastomosed to the patent distal profunda femoris artery. An extension to the distal arterial tree or to the contralateral femoral artery can be performed from this graft if necessary. *5*, type V, the end of the endovascular graft is brought out through the femoral arteriotomy and a distal graft extension is anastomosed end to end to this graft, side to side to the patent distal profunda artery, and extended further to the distal arterial tree. *6*, type VI, the endovascular graft is brought out through the femoral arteriotomy and can bypass multiple levels of occlusive disease and be anastomosed distally to the popliteal or tibial arteries if all femoral vessels are occluded. *Abbreviations: BG,* distal bypass graft; *DFA,* deep femoral artery; *CFA,* common femoral artery. (Reprinted with permission from Marin ML, Veith FJ, Sanchez LA, et al: Endovascular aortoiliac grafts in combination with standard infrainguinal arterial bypasses in the management of limb-threatening ischemia: Preliminary report. *J Vasc Surg* 22:316–25, 1995.)

angled directional catheter. Thirty-nine of the 42 patients were successfully recanalized using these techniques. Those patients who were not successfully recanalized underwent successful extra-anatomical bypasses (3 cases). Two additional patients who occluded their grafts within 24 hours were also considered technical failures.

After successful wire passage, the diseased iliac artery was dilated along the entire length of the vessel using an 8-mm diameter angioplasty balloon. The previously prepared endovascular graft system was then inserted over the guide wire into the newly created tract within the arterial wall. Each device was advanced under fluoroscopic guidance to the appropriate predetermined site, and the sheath was partially retracted, exposing the stent and permitting stent expansion and deployment. The introducer sheath was then completely withdrawn, allowing the redundant portion of the endovascular graft to emerge from the access vessel arteriotomy. The distal end of the endovascular graft was then endoluminally or extraluminally anastomosed using one of the techniques illustrated in Figure 6. When foot ischemia was marked or outflow from the femoral region was severely limited because of infrainguinal occlusive disease, an infrainguinal bypass extension (using PTFE or reversed saphenous vein), which originated from the site of the arteriotomy used for the endovascular graft insertion, was performed.

An intraoperative completion angiogram was performed at the conclusion of each endovascular graft procedure. In 8 of the 39 patients (20%), midgraft narrowing from presumed inadequate graft expansion was detected. All these lesions were effectively corrected by balloon dilatation of the narrowed graft segment and, when necessary, the insertion of an additional balloon expandable stent within the graft (4 cases).

Endovascular stented grafts originated from the aorta (5 cases) or the common iliac artery (34 cases) and were inserted into the common femoral or deep femoral artery using endovascular or standard anastomoses. Endovascular stented graft lengths ranged from 16 to 30 cm (mean, 21 cm).

FOLLOW-UP STUDIES

All patients underwent preoperative and postoperative pulse volume recordings and a determination of the ankle brachial index. Additional follow-up pulse volume recordings, ankle brachial indices, and color duplex ultrasonographic evaluations were performed at regular intervals (3 months, 6 months, and every 6 months thereafter). A postoperative follow-up arteriogram was performed in all patients within the first week, with additional arteriographic studies obtained at those intervals when a problem was detected by physical examination or by a noninvasive study.

ANTICOAGULATION

Systemic heparin was administered only during the endovascular graft insertion procedures. Long-term anticoagulation with coumadin was not used, except in those patients treated for a prosthetic tibial graft or those who required anticoagulation for the management of an unrelated medical problem (e.g., a prosthetic heart valve, deep venous thrombosis).

RESULTS

Technical success in arterial recanalization was achieved in 39 of the 42 iliac arteries (93%). Two patients who acutely thrombosed their grafts, which required conversion to a standard operative alternative, were also considered technical failures. Thus, the total technical failure rate was 12%. After endovascular aortoiliofemoral reconstruction and, in some instances, supplementary conventional infrainguinal surgical bypass, ankle brachial indices improved significantly ($P < 0.05$) from a mean of 0.39 to 0.76, and the thigh pulse volume recordings improved from a mean of 9.75 mm to a mean of 37.8 mm. The 18-month primary and secondary cumulative life-table patency rates for endovascular aortoiliofemoral grafts were 89% (± 9 standard error) and 100%, respectively. Limb salvage was achieved in 94% of the patients at 24 months (± 8 standard error).

Minor complications, including lymphocele and groin hematomas, occurred in four instances (10%). One patient sustained an uncomplicated subendocardial myocardial infarction. One patient died of heart failure after an endovascular aortoiliac bypass procedure, resulting in a procedural mortality rate of 2%.

DISCUSSION

Despite the great successes associated with aortoiliac reconstructive surgery, perioperative morbidity and mortality and late graft limb failures may compromise the long-term results of these procedures.[33, 34] In addition, those patients with severe co-morbid medical illnesses, including cardiac and pulmonary and renal insufficiencies, may not be suitable candidates for extensive aortoiliac reconstructive surgery. Moreover, patients who are seen with severe lower-extremity ischemia requiring a multilevel arterial reconstruction for advanced, diffuse atherosclerotic disease may be at an even higher risk for a perioperative complication.

Other less invasive surgical alternatives such as femorofemoral and axillofemoral bypasses may be used to treat patients with severe aortoiliac disease and significant co-morbid medical problems.[35–37] However, these bypasses do not appear to be as durable as direct aortic reconstructions, which have reported patency rates exceeding 80% at 5 years[2, 5, 38, 39] compared with 5-year patency rates of 45% to 65% for femorofemoral and axillofemoral procedures.[40–48] An additional limitation of an extra-anatomical bypass is the need for a surgical intervention on an asymptomatic limb to achieve arterial inflow.

Alternatives to direct surgical repair of the aortoiliac segment include endovascular treatments such as percutaneous transluminal iliac artery angioplasty and, in suitable candidates, insertion of an intravascular stent.[7, 10, 11, 49, 50] Although there have been encouraging results using these minimally invasive techniques in the management of localized common iliac artery occlusive disease, the treatment of long-segment, complex lesions of the aortoiliac segment has not been as promising.[14, 15]

The use of endovascular stented graft technology for the treatment of aortoiliac occlusive disease represents a blending of technologies that include prosthetic grafts, balloon angioplasty catheters, and intravascular stents. Initial clinical experience with endovascular stented grafts for the treatment of arterial occlusive disease at the femoropopliteal and aortoiliac levels has recently been published.[27, 28] In addition, the use of similar technology for the treatment of aneurysmal disease and arterial trauma is also rapidly evolving.[23, 29, 31, 51]

Endovascular stented grafts have several theoretical advantages over standard arterial reconstructions. Direct aortic inflow can be obtained without dissecting an uninvolved artery (i.e., the contralateral femoral or axillary arteries), thus avoiding additional complications and possible arterial compromise to another extremity. These grafts can be inserted through remote access sites, thereby avoiding the need to directly expose an artery for use as an inflow vessel. The use of a remote arterial entrance site permits surgical treatment through small incisions without the need to displace and retract abdominal viscera or to perform an extensive retroperitoneal dissection to expose the aorta or iliac arteries. This is particularly important in those patients who have a scarred operative field as a result of a previous aortic reconstruction. This minimally invasive approach may also allow a wide range of choices for anesthesia.

Endovascular grafting techniques appear to be ideal for long, occluded arterial segments. When other minimally invasive treatments, such as long-segment angioplasty with or without stents, are used for long occlusions, the results have not been good, presumably because of the presence of a highly thrombogenic flow surface with extensive intimal damage created by the diffuse angioplasty.[7, 15] Endovascular stented grafts provide a single, relatively nonthrombogenic flow surface that completely relines the dilated and frequently diffusely fractured and dissected arterial segments. As prosthetic vascular grafts in the aortoiliac segment traditionally have had excellent long-term patency rates,[1, 3] it is anticipated that comparable patency rates will be achieved when similar prosthetic grafts are used in the endoluminal position. Our experience with follow-up to 33 months suggests that this is the case. However, this must be proven with appropriate trials and long-term follow-up.

This clinical experience includes the use of endovascular grafts using a single stent for proximal graft fixation followed by distal suture anastomosis for distal graft fixation. This approach has several distinct advantages over other endovascular grafting techniques. The distal, hand-sewn anastomosis allows the graft to cross the inguinal ligament, which would not be possible with the currently available stented anastomosis. With distal graft tailoring, all aortoiliac grafts can be the same length before insertion and then cut to size before the suture anastomosis is performed. Finally, because the distal end is hand-sewn, standard and often necessary femoral artery procedures can be performed (e.g., endarterectomy, profundoplasty, or distal graft extension).[52, 53] Even the most severely diseased or occluded femoral artery system will not preclude the use of an endovascular graft such as those described in this review.

Endovascular stented grafts have several potential disadvantages. The biological behavior of a prosthetic endovascular graft placed in a diffusely dilated, atherosclerotic artery is unknown. Concern exists regarding the potential for arterial recoil after dilatation, disease progression, and smooth muscle cell proliferation within atheromatous material extrinsic to the endovascular graft. These processes could result in extrinsic compression of the stented graft with subsequent failure. In our series, limited, immediate, early, extrinsic compression of endovascular stented grafts was observed. However, this was eliminated either by intragraft balloon dilatation or by placement of an additional intragraft stent at the site of narrowing. Moreover, our histopathologic analysis of plaque that is located extrinsic to the graft in recovered specimens did not demonstrate the presence of a significant smooth muscle hyperplastic response.[54]

Technical problems may occur during the process of insertion of an endovascular stented graft for occlusive disease. These devices require long-segment balloon angioplasty of the native vessel before insertion. Such procedures could result in arterial rupture with resulting hemorrhage. Local arterial disruption after balloon dilatation occurred in three patients (7%) in our series. Local wire perforation during arterial recanalization may also occur. These perforations and disruptions have been successfully managed by the placement of a proximal occlusion balloon, a technique that is easily accomplished when the up-and-over recanalization procedure is used.

Additional technical limitations relate to the process of arterial recanalization. Because this procedure is performed under fluoroscopic control, the guide wire used for recanalization could only be imaged in two dimensions. This has led to difficulty in directing angiographic wires from a patent vessel, through the occluded arterial segment and back into the patent proximal vessel during retrograde recanalization. The level of difficulty of this portion of the procedure varies from case to case but may be dependent on the chronicity and nature of the arterial occlusion as well as the experience of the operator. The up-and-over technique, when feasible, has facilitated guide wire passage through the occluded segment and avoided unnecessary vessel wall dissection.

Technical success was achieved in 39 (93%) of the recanalization procedures attempted in this study. It is expected that with improved three-dimensional imaging technology (intravascular ultrasound) and improvements in guide wire and catheter instrumentation, guide wire passage success rates will be improved and the process of recanalization will be simplified.

Finally, an open arteriotomy for each endovascular stented graft procedure is necessary because of the diameter of the endovascular stented graft device and its introducer and carrier system. Although it may be possible to reduce this diameter enough to permit percutaneous introduction, as already pointed out, an open, distal anastomosis has several advantages, so we do not believe device diameter reduction is an important priority. The endovascular grafts used in this study were standard thin-walled PTFE grafts. These grafts were designed for extraluminal use and probably have greater burst strength characteristics than will be required for endovascular grafts. It is anticipated that with a better understanding of graft and stent attachment device requirements, a smaller profile device may be developed that would be suitable for percutaneous insertion in selected situations. However, open arteriotomies will always represent a superior alternative for gaining access in those cases that require treatment of extensive disease above and below the inguinal ligament and in those in which a total arterial occlusion exists and introduction of the device must be made through this occluded segment.

We have successfully performed aortoiliac reconstruction by means of inserting an endovascular graft. This technique has proven to be safe and effective for treating multilevel occlusive disease. Increased experience with this method together with an analysis of the results from a larger number of patients over a longer period of time will be required before advocating the widespread use of this technique.

REFERENCES

1. Brewster DC, Darling RC: Optimal methods of aortoiliac reconstruction. *Surgery* 84:739–748, 1978.

2. Szilagyi DE, Elliott JP Jr, Smith RF, et al: A thirty-year survey of the reconstructive surgical treatment of aortoiliac occlusive disease. *J Vasc Surg* 3:421–436, 1986.

3. Brothers TE, Greenfield LJ: Long-term results of aortoiliac reconstruction. *J Vasc Interv Radiol* 1:49–55, 1990.

4. Nevelsteen A, Wouters L, Suy R: Long-term patency of the aortofemoral Dacron graft. A graft limb related study over a 25-year period. *J Cardiovasc Surg (Torino)* 32:174–180, 1991.

5. Poulias GE, Doundoulakis N, Prombonas E, et al: Aorto-femoral bypass and determinants of early success and late favourable outcome. Experience with 1000 consecutive cases. *J Cardiovasc Surg (Torino)* 33:664–678, 1992.

6. Rutherford RB: Aortobifemoral bypass, the gold standard: Technical considerations. *Semin Vasc Surg* 7:11–13, 1994.

7. Johnston KW, Rae M, Hogg-Johnston SA, et al: 5–Year results of a prospective study of percutaneous transluminal angioplasty. *Ann Surg* 206:403–413, 1987.

8. Martin EC: Percutaneous therapy in the management of aortoiliac disease. *Semin Vasc Surg* 7:17–20, 1994.

9. Tegtmeyer CJ, Hartwell GD, Selby JB, et al: Results and complications of angioplasty in aortoiliac disease. *Circulation* 83:53S–60S, 1991.

10. Liermann D, Strecker EP, Peters J: The Strecker stent: Indications and results in iliac and femoropopliteal arteries. *Cardiovasc Intervent Radiol* 15:298–305, 1992.

11. Palmaz JC, Laborde JC, Rivera FJ, et al: Stenting of the iliac arteries with the Palmaz stent: Experience from a multicenter trial. *Cardiovasc Intervent Radiol* 15:291–297, 1992.

12. Hausegger KA, Cragg AH, Lammer J, et al: Iliac artery stent placement: Clinical experience with a Nitinol stent. *Radiology* 190:199–202, 1994.

13. Vorwerk D, Gunther RW: Stent placement in iliac arterial lesions: Three years of clinical experience with the Wallstent. *Cardiovasc Intervent Radiol* 15:285–290, 1992.

14. Johnston KW: Iliac arteries: Reanalysis of results of balloon angioplasty. *Radiology* 186:207–212, 1993.

15. Laborde JC, Palmaz JC, Rivera FJ, et al: Influence of anatomic distribution of atherosclerosis on the outcome of revascularization with iliac stent placement. *J Vasc Interv Radiol* 6:513–520, 1995.

16. Marin ML, Veith FJ, Sanchez LA, et al: Endovascular aortoiliac grafts in combination with standard infrainguinal arterial bypasses in the management of limb-threatening ischemia: Preliminary report. *J Vasc Surg* 22:316–325, 1995.

17. Dotter CT: Transluminally-placed coilspring endarterial tube grafts: Long-term patency in canine popliteal artery. *Invest Radiol* 4:329–332, 1969.

18. Balko A, Piasecki GJ, Shah DM, et al: Transfemoral placement of intraluminal polyurethane prosthesis for abdominal aortic aneurysm. *J Surg Res* 40:305–309, 1986.

19. Mirich D, Wright KC, Wallace S, et al: Percutaneously placed endovascular grafts for aortic aneurysms: Feasibility study. *Radiology* 170:1033–1037, 1989.

20. Laborde JC, Parodi JC, Clem MF, et al: Intraluminal bypass of abdominal aortic aneurysm: Feasibility study. *Radiology* 184:185–190, 1992.

21. Chuter TAM, Green RM, Ouriel K, et al: Transfemoral endovascular aortic graft placement. *J Vasc Surg* 18:185–197, 1993.

22. Marin ML, Veith FJ, Cynamon J, et al: Initial experience with transluminally placed endovascular grafts for the treatment of complex vascular lesions. *Ann Surg* 222:449–469, 1995.

23. Parodi JC, Palmaz JC, Barone HD: Transfemoral intraluminal graft implantation for abdominal aortic aneurysms. *Ann Vasc Surg* 5:491–499, 1991.

24. Parodi JC: Endovascular repair of abdominal aortic aneurysms and other arterial lesions. *J Vasc Surg* 21:549–557, 1995.

25. May J, White G, Waugh R, et al: Treatment of complex abdominal aortic aneurysms by a combination of endoluminal and extraluminal aortofemoral grafts. *J Vasc Surg* 19:924–933, 1994.

26. Scott RAP, Chuter TAM: Clinical endovascular placement of bifurcated graft in abdominal aortic aneurysm without laparotomy. (Letter to the Editor.) *Lancet* 343:413, 1994.

27. Marin ML, Veith FJ, Panetta TF, et al: Transfemoral stented graft treatment of occlusive arterial disease for limb salvage: A preliminary report (abstract). *Circulation* 88:1–11, 1993.

28. Cragg AH, Dake MD: Percutaneous femoropopliteal graft placement. *J Vasc Interv Radiol* 4:455–463, 1993.

29. Marin ML, Veith FJ, Lyon RT, et al: Transfemoral endovascular repair of iliac artery aneurysms. *Am J Surg* 170:179–182, 1995.

30. Marin ML, Veith FJ, Panetta TF, et al: Transfemoral endoluminal stented graft repair of a popliteal artery aneurysm. *J Vasc Surg* 19:754–757, 1994.

31. Marin ML, Veith FJ, Panetta TF, et al: Transluminally placed endovascular stented graft repair for arterial trauma. *J Vasc Surg* 20:466–473, 1994.

32. Volodos NL, Shekhanin VE, Karpovich IP, et al: Self-fixing synthetic prosthesis for endoprosthetics of the vessels. *Vestn Khir* 137:123–125, 1986.

33. Samson RH, Scher LA, Veith FJ: Combined segment arterial disease. *Surgery* 97:385–390, 1985.

34. Veith FJ, Gupta SK, Wengerter KR, et al: Changing arteriosclerotic disease patterns and management strategies in lower-limb-threatening ischemia. *Ann Surg* 212:402–414, 1990.

35. Vetto RM: The treatment of unilateral iliac artery obstruction with a transabdominal, subcutaneous, femorofemoral graft. *Surgery* 52:343–345, 1962.

36. Brief DK, Brener BJ, Alpert J, et al: Crossover femorofemoral grafts followed up five years or more: An analysis. *Arch Surg* 110:1294–1299, 1975.

37. Ascer E, Veith FJ, Gupta SK, et al: Comparison of axillounifemoral and axillobifemoral bypass operations. *Surgery* 97:169–174, 1985.

38. Sladen JG, Gilmour JL, Wong RW: Cumulative patency and actual palliation in patients with claudication after aortofemoral bypass. Prospective long-term follow-up of 100 patients. *Am J Surg* 152:190–195, 1986.

39. Naylor AR, Ah-See AK, Engeset J: Morbidity and mortality after aortofemoral grafting for peripheral limb ischaemia. *J R Coll Surg Edinb* 34:215–218, 1989.

40. Donaldson MC, Louras JC, Bucknam CA: Axillofemoral bypass: A tool with a limited role. *J Vasc Surg* 3:757–763, 1986.

41. Christenson JT, Broome A, Norgren L, et al: The late results after axillofemoral bypass grafts in patients with leg ischaemia. *J Cardiovasc Surg (Torino)* 27:131–133, 1986.

42. Pietri P, Pancrazio F, Adovasio R, et al: Long term results of extra anatomical bypasses. *Int Angiol* 6:429–433, 1987.

43. Rutherford RB, Patt A, Pearce WH: Extra-anatomic bypass: A closer view. *J Vasc Surg* 6:437–446, 1987.

44. Hepp W, de Jonge K, Pallua N: Late results following extra-anatomic bypass procedures for chronic aortoiliac occlusive disease. *J Cardiovasc Surg (Torino)* 29:181–185, 1988.

45. Piotrowski JJ, Pearce WH, Jones DN, et al: Aortobifemoral bypass: The operation of choice for unilateral iliac occlusion? *J Vasc Surg* 8:211–218, 1988.

46. Perler BA, Burdick JF, Williams GM: Femoro-femoral or ilio-femoral bypass for unilateral inflow reconstruction? *Am J Surg* 161:426–430, 1991.

47. Harrington ME, Harrington EB, Haimov M, et al: Iliofemoral versus femoro-femoral bypass: The case for an individualized approach. *J Vasc Surg* 16:841–854, 1992.

48. Brener BJ, Brief DK, Alpert J: Femorofemoral bypass: A twenty-five year experience, in Yao JST, Pearce WH (eds): *Long-term Results in Vascular Surgery*. Norwalk, Conn, Appleton & Lange, 1993, pp 385–393.

49. Dotter CT, Judkins MP: Transluminal treatment of arteriosclerotic obstruction: Description of a new technic and a preliminary report of its application. *Circulation* 30:654–670, 1964.

50. Gruntzig A, Hopff H: Perkutane rekanalisation chronischer arterieller verschlusse mit einem neuen dilatationskatheter modifikation der Dotter-technik. *Dtsch Med Wochenschr* 99:2502–2510, 1974.

51. Marin ML, Veith FJ, Panetta TF, et al: Percutaneous transfemoral insertion of a stented graft to repair a traumatic femoral arteriovenous fistula. *J Vasc Surg* 18:299–302, 1993.

52. Moore WS, Cafferata HT, Hall AD: In defense of grafts across the inguinal ligament: An evaluation of early and late results of aorto-femoral bypass grafts. *Ann Surg* 168:207–214, 1968.

53. Perdue GD, Long WD, Smith RB III: Perspective concerning aorto-femoral arterial reconstruction. *Ann Surg* 173:940–944, 1971.

54. Marin ML, Veith FJ, Cynamon J, et al: Human transluminally placed endovascular stented grafts: Preliminary histopathologic analysis of healing grafts in aortoiliac and femoral artery occlusive disease. *J Vasc Surg* 21:595–604, 1995.

The Bifurcated Endovascular Prosthesis

Timothy A.M. Chuter, M.D.

Assistant Professor of Surgery, University of California, San Francisco

Most patients with abdominal aortic aneurysm lack the cuff of non-dilated aorta between the aneurysm and the bifurcation necessary for insertion of an aortoaortic stent graft.[1] Bifurcated stent grafts overcome this limitation by bringing the distal implantation site down to the iliac arteries. Successful use of bifurcated stent grafts to repair model aneurysms in animals[2] was followed in 1993 by the first clinical application.[3] In this case, the aneurysm was successfully isolated from the circulation, and the patient remains well 2 years later.

This success was not typical, however, of the first 10 cases, 6 of which required conversion to open repair. Since then, the results have improved steadily, despite a concurrent increase in the number of patients with challenging features of arterial anatomy, such as short neck, or tortuous iliac arteries.[4,5] Both trends represent the effects of changing patient selection, apparatus, and technique.

PREOPERATIVE ASSESSMENT

Preoperative arterial imaging forms the primary basis for patient selection and graft sizing. The imaging provided by the referring center sometimes provides a basis for exclusion but rarely provides sufficient information for endovascular repair. Conventional CT and angiography are not intrinsically inadequate for this purpose, but they need to be performed with the needs of endovascular repair in mind. For this reason, patients who initially appear to meet the selection criteria need further imaging. We favor a combination of spiral CT and angiography.

Spiral CT data are acquired in 5-mm-thick cylinders, at 5-mm intervals (5,5,3 mode) after intra-arterial injection of contrast. These data are represented as conventional transaxial slices at 3-mm intervals, multiplanar reconstructions (MPR), or shaded surface display of a three-dimensional construct.

Angiograms are performed by intra-arterial injection of contrast, with intra-arterial markers for calibration. Calibration is needed to compensate for the variable magnification factor and for the apparent foreshortening that occurs when the long axis of the artery is not parallel to the plane of the film.

Despite these precautions, we tend to rely more on CT for measurement of arterial dimensions. Angiography is performed mainly to assess

Advances in Vascular Surgery®, vol. 4

© 1996, Mosby–Year Book, Inc.

the iliac arteries, which are frequently too tortuous and too heavily calcified to be displayed well on any of the CT-based modalities.

PATIENT SELECTION

One of the goals of the early clinical studies was to assess the functional limits of the system and determine the prerequisites of success (how long a neck, how much tortuosity, etc.). While testing the system in this way, the anatomical selection criteria became progressively broader, and the frequency of challenging anatomical features increased. This trend is illustrated by comparing the first 20 patients with the second 20 (Table 1). There was a concurrent change in the size of the aneurysms, most of which exceeded 6 cm in diameter in the recent experience. Indeed, the two trends were related: large aneurysms tended to be associated with more challenging anatomy. In other words, the most difficult patients are often the ones most in need of treatment; hence, the importance of accommodating, rather than avoiding, challenging anatomy.

We currently have no absolute exclusion criteria except the absence of an infrarenal neck. However, relative contraindications for endovascular repair include combinations of the following:

1. Short neck (less than 10 mm).
2. Angulated neck (more than 75 degrees to the long axis of the aneurysm).
3. Conical neck (widening by more than 4 mm from proximal to distal).
4. Thrombus lined neck.
5. Severe iliac artery tortuosity (angulation of more than 90 degrees at any point).
6. Severe iliac artery calcification.
7. Iliac artery dilatation (wider than 16 mm) at, or distal to, the implantation site.
8. Bilaterality of iliac disease.

None of these in isolation would preclude repair, but combinations of 1–4, or 5–7 are avoided. For example, an aneurysm with a short, but otherwise satisfactory, neck would be included (Fig 1).

Improving results also led to liberalization of the physiologic selection criteria. In the early clinical experience, only patients fit enough to withstand conventional operation were included. More recently, as the technique has become more reliable, a number of patients have been in-

---

TABLE 1.
Features of Arterial Anatomy in the First 20 Patients Compared With the Second 20 Patients

	First 20	Second 20
Proximal neck angulation > 60 degrees	1	6
Proximal neck length ≤ 15 mm	1	7
Iliac angulation > 90 degrees	2	8
Aneurysm diameter > 6 cm	4	11

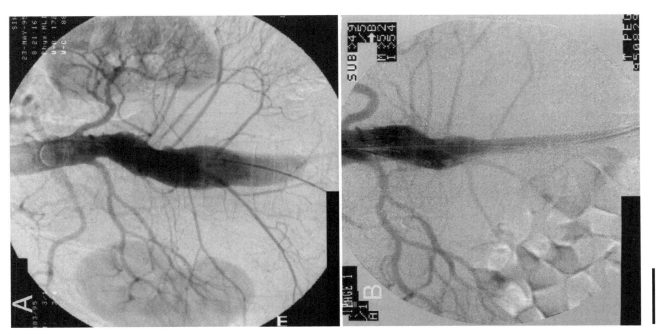

FIGURE 1.

A, preoperative angiogram showing an aneurysm with 9-mm-long neck. **B,** completion angiogram showing an uncovered portion of the proximal stent at the level of the right renal artery.

cluded who were not candidates for conventional repair based on severe cardiopulmonary disease but who were at high risk of rupture from large aneurysms. These patients represent the highest risk, because recourse to conventional surgical repair is not possible, but also the highest potential benefit.

GRAFT SIZING

Each stent graft is constructed for an individual patient, and the size reflects the findings of preoperative imaging.

The proximal diameter of the graft is usually 2–4 mm larger than the luminal diameter of the proximal neck on transaxial CT. When the aorta is tortuous, as it often is, the neck is not parallel to the long axis of the scan, and the profile on the transaxial image is elliptical, even though the neck actually has a circular cross-section. The true diameter is then taken to be the minimum diameter of the ellipse.

The length of the graft is usually calculated from the distance between the slice containing the renal arteries and the slice containing the aortic bifurcation. However, this method is sufficiently accurate only if the interval between slices is less than 5 mm and the aorta is parallel to the long axis of the scan. The length of a tortuous infrarenal aorta is better measured on MPRs, in which the long axis of the aorta is in the plane of the image. Angiograms can also be used for this purpose, but they are unreliable unless a marked catheter or guide wire extends throughout the length of the infrarenal aorta.

Iliac artery dimensions are measured on transaxial CT, MPR spiral CT, or angiograms; each has its advantages and disadvantages. We tend to rely on angiograms but recognize that calibration is sometimes difficult when the vessels are tortuous. Multiple projections should include left and right obliques to minimize the apparent foreshortening that occurs where the common iliac arteries curve posterolaterally along the margin of the pelvis.

One advantage of implanting the distal end of the stent graft in the common iliac artery is the length of the implantation zone, which affords some margin for error in graft length determination. The configuration of the graft can also help to accommodate for errors in iliac artery diameter measurement. The wide bell-bottom at the distal end of the graft limb can be used in vessels measuring between 6 and 16 mm. At the smaller diameters, redundant folds are flattened by the Gianturco Z-stent.

APPARATUS

The stent graft is carried from the femoral artery to the aorta by a system of coaxial catheters, collectively known as the delivery system.

STENT GRAFT

The bifurcated stent graft has one lumen proximally and two lumens distally, each with a stent at its orifice. The graft element is custom-made from Cooley VerisoftR fabric (Meadox Medicals, Inc., Oakland, NJ) based on the dimensions of the infrarenal aorta, as assessed by preoperative imaging. The cut ends of the graft segments are heat-sealed to prevent fraying and are sutured together. The fabric and specific configuration of the graft limbs are the only significant differences between this system and the manufactured system (Cook Critical Care, Inc.; Meadox Medicals, Inc.) currently undergoing European clinical trials.

Gianturco Z-stents are crowns of springy stainless steel in which a loop of wire bends back and forth as though on the curved surface of a cylinder. The proximal stent has eight points at each end connected by the 16 limbs in between. Coils soldered to eight of the limbs provide points of attachment for the graft. Small pairs of barbs are also mounted on four of the proximal stent limbs. One of each pair of barbs extends proximally to the level of the stent angles, where it bends caudally (hook barbs). The other barb extends distally, parallel to the long axis of the stent. The terminal portion of this barb is curved outward, away from the long axis of the stent.

The distal stents are smaller than the proximal stent, measuring 10 mm in length and 10 mm in diameter. They have six bends at each end and no barbs. The proximal stent is attached to the graft so that an 8-mm segment has no fabric covering, whereas the distal stent protrudes only 2 mm beyond the distal end of the graft.

DELIVERY SYSTEM

The stent graft is attached to a "central carrier" by two pairs of suture loops; one pair proximally and another pair distally. These loops pass around the innermost catheter of the carrier and cannot be released while that catheter remains in the carrier. The tension in the suture loops moors the stent graft in a fixed position and fixed orientation relative to the carrier.

The inner diameter of the introducer sheath (18 French) matches the outer diameter of the central carrier at its tip. The resulting smooth transition from one to the other gives the delivery system the external profile necessary for insertion, thereby avoiding the need for preliminary sheath/dilator insertion.

To permit deployment of the contralateral (left) limb of the graft, the two distal stents have to be maintained in a compressed state by their own independent sheaths. The sheath on the left-limb stent is attached to a 2.5-French catheter (the left-limb catheter), which is used during deployment to tow the left limb of the graft out of the aorta into the left common iliac artery. A suture loop runs the length of this catheter and holds the stent within the sheath. The compressed right limb distal stent also has a sheath, which runs along the central carrier to the outside.

BASIC TECHNIQUE

The steps in bifurcated graft insertion are as follows:

1. Bilateral access through the surgically exposed femoral arteries.
2. Heparin, 10,000 units intravenously, before the application of vascular clamps.
3. Placement of a cross femoral catheter. The specific method is not important. The catheter can be passed over a guide wire, which was itself passed through the iliac arteries from one femoral artery to the other, using angulated catheters and standard radiologic techniques. Alternatively, the catheter can be retrieved from the aneurysm using a snare or basket. Whatever the method, it is important to minimize intra-aortic manipulation. We attribute the lack of any detectable microembolism to this policy.
4. Insertion of a stiff guide wire through the right femoral artery. A

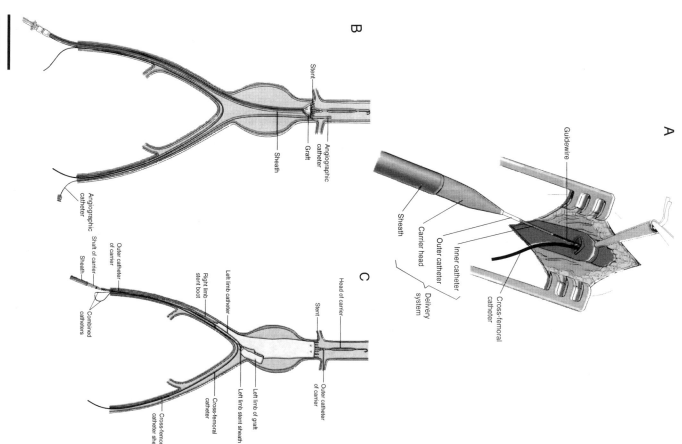

FIGURE 2.
A, delivery system insertion. **B,** sheath withdrawal showing the angiographic catheter necessary for serial angiography. **C,** completion of sheath withdrawal, showing the prosthesis and the associated catheters that were within the delivery system.

(Continued.)

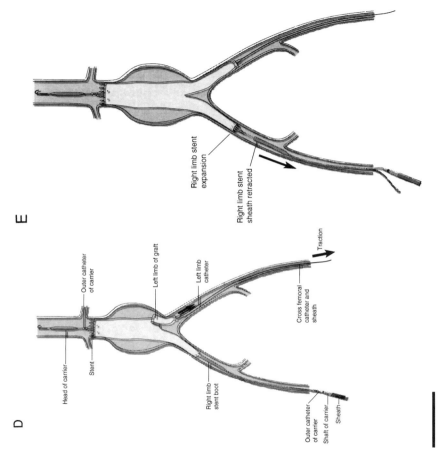

D

E

FIGURE 2 (cont.).

D, left-limb placement. E, right-limb stent deployment.

double-lumen dilator is used to ensure that the guide wire and the cross-femoral catheter do not wind around each other in the right iliac artery.

5. Insertion of an angiographic catheter, from the left femoral artery to the level of the renal arteries.

6. Insertion of the delivery system through the right femoral artery (Fig 2, A).

7. Deployment of the proximal stent by withdrawal of the sheath (Fig 2, B). The proximal stent is usually deployed immediately beneath the renal arteries.

8. Creation of a connection between a small catheter, attached to the left limb of the graft (the left-limb catheter), and the cross-femoral catheter (Fig 2, C). In the past, this connection was made with sutures, but a screw connection has now been developed.

9. Translocation of the left-limb catheter from the right femoral artery to the left, by applying traction to the cross-femoral catheter.

10. Traction on the left-limb catheter at the left groin to pull the left limb of the graft into the left common iliac artery (Fig 2, D).

11. Deployment of the right-limb stent (Fig 2, E).

12. Release of the prosthesis from the core of the delivery system by withdrawing the innermost catheter.

13. Removal of the delivery system.
14. Deployment of the left limb-stent.

TECHNICAL REFINEMENTS

The basic steps in bifurcated graft insertion have changed very little since the procedure was first performed. However, the technique has been refined over this period by the addition of numerous precautions and adjunctive maneuvers. These were developed to eliminate the more common complications and to expand the range of candidates. Each stage in the procedure has its subtleties.

DELIVERY SYSTEM INTRODUCTION

At the time of this writing, all of the bifurcated grafts had been inserted through the right femoral artery and passed through the right iliac system. The main reason was simply the right-handedness of the surgeon, although subsequent review of the data showed that the right rather than the left iliac artery is less prone to severe angulation than the left.[5] The ease of delivery system introduction, often in the presence of a high degree of iliac tortuosity, reflects iliac artery mobility rather than delivery system flexibility. Maneuvers to assist insertion, on the rare occasions when the delivery system does not pass easily, include the application of traction to the partially mobilized external iliac artery (as described by Parodi[6]) or to the common iliac artery through a retroperitoneal approach.

Aortic tortuosity has been a more important impediment to delivery system insertion. The angulated neck of an aneurysm can sometimes be straightened considerably by simply pushing the aneurysm gently to one side with a hand on the abdomen. Alternatively, a guide wire can be passed from the axillary (or brachial) artery to the femoral artery. This guide wire becomes very stable when traction is applied at both ends. The delivery system will then follow the guide wire through the aorta, however tortuous, like a train through a tunnel.

PROXIMAL STENT IMPLANTATION

The main requirements for secure, hemostatic proximal stent implantation are accurate position and alignment. These are easy to achieve when the neck of the aneurysm is long, straight, and cylindrical, but not when the neck is short, angulated, conical, or lined with thrombus. Angulation is a particular problem for two reasons: The delivery system straightens the angulated neck to a variable degree, and straightening of the neck is rarely enough to ensure that it shares a common axis with the delivery system.

Straightening of the aneurysm neck alters the position of the renal arteries. Angiograms that were performed before delivery system insertion cannot be relied on. Therefore, we perform angiograms using a catheter inserted through the contralateral femoral artery. The tip of this catheter remains in the aorta throughout proximal stent deployment, permitting serial angiography.

The disparity between the axial orientation of the tortuous aneurysm neck and the slightly rigid delivery system produces a corresponding disparity between the axes of the aneurysm neck and the proximal stent. The result is perigraft leakage, which, if uncorrected, can lead to aneurysm rupture.[5] The means of correction is a large cardiac valvuloplasty balloon. Inflation of this balloon causes the aorta and stent to rotate into the same axis. We have used this technique in four cases, with cessation of leakage in all four, despite angulation between the aneurysm and the neck of up to 90 degrees.

Another cause of proximal perigraft leakage is malposition of the proximal stent, such that the proximal end of the graft lies not in the neck but in the aneurysm. This consequence of inaccurate proximal stent placement occurred twice early in our bifurcated graft experience, at which time the only available option was conversion to open repair. A better alternative would have been the insertion of a short extension, in the form of a second stent graft. We have not had the opportunity to try this approach with bifurcated grafts, but it provided a successful solution to the problem of low proximal stent placement in three straight graft (two aortoiliac, and one aortoaortic) cases (Fig 3).

Inaccurate proximal stent placement, which results in the stent graft being too high, cannot be corrected except by moving the original stent, to permit perfusion of the renal arteries. Short of open repair and complete proximal stent graft removal, a limited amount of distal displacement can be achieved by applying traction to the stent graft using a large cardiac valvuloplasty, or embolectomy balloon. We have no experience with this technique in bifurcated grafts but have used it successfully on

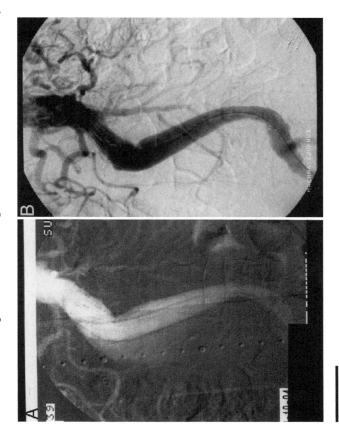

FIGURE 3.

A, intraoperative angiogram after straight aortoiliac graft deployment, showing the conical angulated neck, and proximal perigraft leakage. **B,** angiogram showing that leakage has ceased after insertion of a second, more proximal, stent graft.

two occasions after partial, unilateral renal artery occlusion that occurred in the course of aneurysm exclusion using straight grafts. However, the technique should work as well, if not better, with bifurcated stent grafts because the diameter change at the bifurcation would make it easier to apply the necessary traction.

Concerns for the stability of proximal stent implantation have led us to avoid cases in which the neck was lined with thrombus, had a conical (rather than cylindrical) configuration, or measured more than 26 mm in diameter. All these features were present in the sole case of proximal stent migration. The proximal stent only moved 10 mm distally over the course of a 9-month follow-up, but the patient was converted to open repair for fear of complete stent-graft dislocation and thrombosis.

There are no compelling reasons to think that a proximal stent implanted in a large neck should be unstable in the short- to medium-term. However, we are concerned that the wall of a large (> 30 mm) "neck" may already be structurally compromised and prone to subsequent dilatation, leading to inadequate proximal stent fixation or perigraft leak.

DISTAL STENT IMPLANTATION

The common iliac arteries are usually long enough that the exact location of the distal stents is not critical. This is fortunate, because distal stent position depends mainly on the graft length, which is difficult to modify intraoperatively. An error in distal stent position usually reflects an error in graft sizing, which occurs when the aorta is very tortuous, resulting in the stent graft being too short. It should be possible to identify undersized stent graft before deployment by observing the positions of the proximal and distal stents relative to the renal arteries, as identified angiographically, and the aortic bifurcation, as identified by the position of the cross-femoral catheter. However, if such a graft is deployed, the result is distal perigraft leak into the aneurysm, which leaves the aneurysm still at risk of rupture. The best solution is to insert a second stent graft as a distal extension (Fig 4). Another cause of distal perigraft leak is a mismatch in size between the distal end of the graft limb and the common iliac artery. Possible corrective measures include the addition of a stent graft extension, or the placement of a ligature around the common iliac artery. Both have been found effective.[7]

When the common iliac artery is too dilated for secure, hemostatic distal stent implantation, the distal end of the stent graft may be placed in the external iliac artery, which is rarely aneurysmal. This may prevent leakage around the distal end of the graft but is to be avoided for two reasons: First, the resultant exclusion of the internal iliac artery may compromise perfusion of the colon, the spine, or the buttocks. Second, a patent internal iliac artery may become part of a collateral route for persistent aneurysm perfusion. Both potential problems can be avoided by combining endovascular and open surgical techniques in the manner described by May and colleagues.[8] For example, the graft limb can be brought out through the surgically exposed common iliac artery and sutured directly into the iliac bifurcation. These methods were described

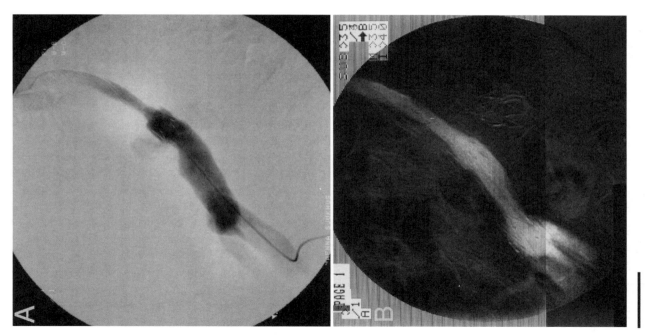

FIGURE 4.

A, angiogram after bifurcated stent graft implantation, showing leakage around the distal end of the right limb of the graft. **B,** angiogram after insertion of a second stent graft distally, showing flow into the distal common iliac, internal iliac, and external iliac arteries and no retrograde perigraft leakage.

for use with aortouniiliac bypass, but they can be applied equally well to aneurysm exclusion with bifurcated aortobiiliac stent grafts.

ADJUNCTIVE STENTING

The noncrimped, woven graft fabric (Cooley VerisoftR, Meadox Medicals, Oakland, NJ), used in most bifurcated grafts to date, is stiff and kinks if it is forced to bend around fixed points in the iliac artery. This kinking was responsible for graft thrombosis in 6 of the first 10 cases,[5] a problem since solved with the insertion of Wallstents. There have been no instances of graft thrombosis in any of the last 35 cases performed during the 2 years since this maneuver was adopted.

EMBOLIZATION OF LUMBAR ARTERIES

Patent lumbar and inferior mesenteric arteries provide a potential route for persistent perfusion of the aneurysm via collaterals. We have seen CT evidence of collateral flow into the aneurysm in six cases; three through a lumbar artery and three through the inferior mesenteric artery.[7] Angiography showed that the offending lumbar arteries received blood from the ileolumbar branch of the internal iliac artery. Perigraft perfusion ceased spontaneously within a month of cessation of anticoagulant therapy in five of the six cases. In the other case, perfusion through a lumber artery persisted by CT and angiography. The ileolumbar artery was catheterized by percutaneous axillary artery puncture, for embolization with Gianturco coils. Follow-up CT showed perigraft perfusion to have ceased.

COST BENEFIT

The cost saving with endovascular repair, compared with that for conventional repair, results from the speed of the recovery. Many patients do not need intensive care, and many are eating and walking on the second postoperative day. As a result, an analysis of cost tends to favor endovascular repair, at least in the short term. However, endovascular repair does involve extra costs, some of which may continue to accumulate for the life of the patient. Systems of endovascular aneurysm repair usually cost nothing while they are still being investigated, but as soon as they become approved for sale, the price will be sure to exceed that of a conventional graft.

The uncertainty that surrounds a new procedure is also a source of additional expense. Until we can be sure that there are no long-term complications, patients will have to be imaged at frequent intervals for signs of some evolving problem such as recurrent aneurysm perfusion, aneurysm enlargement, neck dilatation, or structural failure of the prosthesis. Many patients have long life expectancies after aneurysm repair, and this imaging may become expensive.

PHYSIOLOGIC BENEFIT

Data are accumulating from studies of cardiovascular performance, blood chemistry,[9] colon perfusion, and patients' own assessments of their health[10] that indicate that endovascular aneurysm exclusion is less of a physiologic insult than a conventional repair.

ROLE

The ultimate role of the bifurcated stent graft in treatment of abdominal aortic aneurysm will be determined by several aspects of long-term function, many of which are relevant to all configurations of a stent graft, and all of which are currently unknown. These include the behavior of the artery at the implantation sites, the behavior of the thrombus around the aneurysm, and the behavior of the aneurysm itself. However, it is now clear that the feasibility of aneurysm exclusion, in the short term, depends on the ability of the stent graft and its delivery system to satisfy certain basic prerequisites, one of which is secure, hemostatic stent implantation, both proximally and distally. The lack of a suitable distal implantation site in the aorta limits the alternatives to straight aortouniiliac, and bifurcated aortobiiliac.

A straight aortouniiliac stent graft[6, 8, 11] is easy to implant, but it excludes flow to the contralateral limb and leaves the contralateral common iliac artery open as a potential route of collateral flow into the aneurysm. When a graft of this type is used to exclude an abdominal aortic aneurysm, these problems must be corrected by femorofemoral bypass and contralateral common iliac artery occlusion. The main advantages lie in the simplicity of the delivery system, the speed with which secure hemostatic implantation can be achieved, and the flexibility that results from a choice of iliac arteries for distal implantation. These are particularly important when emergency use necessitates immediate protection of the aneurysm from aortic pressure, while precluding sophisticated preoperative assessment and graft sizing.[12]

In contrast, bifurcated aortobiiliac stent graft insertion requires neither extra-anatomical bypass nor common iliac artery occlusion, because prograde flow to both iliac arteries is maintained through separate graft limbs. However, the initial stent-graft deployment is more complicated, because one limb has to be placed in the contralateral common iliac artery, which lies outside the line of delivery system insertion.

All bifurcated stent grafts currently being investigated fall into one of two categories—unitary or modular—depending on the way they solve the problem of contralateral graft limb placement. Bifurcated stent grafts with a unitary construction are inserted whole; the bifurcation is a preformed part of graft configuration. The contralateral limb of the graft is then pulled into place, and stents are deployed to fix it in position. In contrast, bifurcated stent grafts with a modular construction are built inside the aorta from tubular components. The relative advantages and disadvantages of the two methods are listed in Table 2.

The most significant problem with a modular approach has been leakage through the junction between the component stent grafts. To create a hemostatic seal at this point, the recipient site on the main stent graft and the added limb need to be coaxial. This can be difficult to achieve when the iliac arteries enter the aorta at wide angles, or the axial orientation of the main stent graft is slightly off, because the fully stented com-

TABLE 2.
Differences Between Modular and Unitary Approaches to Bifurcated Stent Graft Reconstruction of the Aorta

Modular	Unitary
Requires catheterization of the recipient site on the main graft.	Requires insertion of a cross-femoral catheter placement.
Simple stent-graft components and delivery systems.	More complex graft construction and delivery system.
Nonidentical limbs easy to customize from stock components.	Customization must be performed at the time of graft manufacture.
Graft-graft junction created within the aneurysm.	Bifurcation sewn, knitted, or woven into the graft.
Easy to deliver in a fully stented form.	Difficult to deliver fully stented: additional stents must be added as needed.

ponents lack flexibility; hence, the high rates of leakage seen with devices of this kind.

The main drawback of the unitary approach is the lack of stent support in the graft limbs. With the current method of delivery, the bifurcated stent graft cannot be delivered in a fully stented form. Additional stents must be added, as needed, once the graft is in place.

CONCLUSION

Endovascular aneurysm exclusion is clearly gentle and effective in a wide range of patients, at least in the short term. However, it remains to be seen whether the long-term results warrant its widespread application.

It is also clear that the use of the iliac artery as the distal implantation site enormously increases the number of candidates. However, the relative advantages and disadvantages of the aortouniiliac, modular aortobiiliac and preformed aortobiiliac stent grafts also remain unknown, and consequently the role of each has yet to be defined.

REFERENCES

1. Chuter TAM, Green RM, Ouriel K, et al: Infrarenal aortic aneurysm morphology: Implications for transfemoral repair. *J Vasc Surg* 20:44–50, 1994.
2. Chuter TAM, Green RM, Ouriel K, et al: Transfemoral aortic aneurysm repair: Straight and bifurcated grafts in dogs. *J Vasc Surg* 17:233, 1993.
3. Chuter TAM, Donayre C, Wendt G: Bifurcated stent-grafts for endovascular repair of abdominal aortic aneurysm: Preliminary case reports. *Surg Endosc* 8:800–802, 1994.
4. Chuter TAM, Wendt G, Hopkinson BR, et al: Transfemoral insertion of a bifurcated endovascular graft for aortic aneurysm repair: The first 22 patients. *Cardiovasc Surg* 3:121–128, 1995.
5. Chuter TAM, Risberg B, Hopkinson BR, et al: Clinical experience with a bifurcated endovascular graft for abdominal aortic aneurysm repair. Presented

at the International Society for Cardiovascular Surgery, New Orleans, La, June 1995.

6. Parodi JC: Limitations of the Parodi device for abdominal aortic aneurysm exclusion based on four years' experience. *J Endovasc Surg* 2:121, 1995.

7. Ivancev K, Chuter TAM, Lindblad B, et al: Endovascular treatment of perigraft perfusion following transfemoral aneurysm repair. *World J Surg*, in press.

8. May J, White G, Waugh R, et al: Treatment of complex abdominal aortic aneurysms by a combination of endoluminal and extraluminal aortofemoral grafts. *J Vasc Surg* 19:924–933, 1994.

9. Baker DM, Viscomi S, Hind R, et al: Metabolic and renal effects of abdominal aortic aneurysm repair using conventional and endovascular techniques. Presented at the 1995 meeting of the ISCVS, Kyoto, Japan.

10. Baker DM: Personal communication.

11. Yusuf SW, Baker DM, Hind RE, et al: Endoluminal transfemoral abdominal aortic aneurysm repair with aorto-uni-iliac graft and femorofemoral bypass. *Br J Surg* 82:916, 1995.

12. Yusuf SW, Whitaker SC, Chuter TAM, et al: Emergency endovascular repair of leaking aortic aneurysm. *Lancet* 344:1645, 1994.

PART III

Carotid Artery Disease

Balloon Angioplasty for Extracranial Carotid Disease

Martin M. Brown, M.D., F.R.C.P.

Reader in Neurology, St. George's Hospital Medical School, London, England

Treatment of carotid stenosis by percutaneous transluminal angioplasty (PTA) has the attraction of avoiding an invasive surgical incision and the general anesthesia usually used for endarterectomy. Angioplasty has become a very common procedure for stenosis of peripheral and coronary vessels, but there has been considerable reluctance to perform PTA for carotid stenosis because of anxiety about the risk of cerebral embolism. However, the published nonrandomized series of carotid PTA suggest that the risks are similar to those of conventional carotid surgery. Expertise in cerebrovascular PTA is rapidly improving, and clinical trials are under way to assess the efficacy of the procedure. Percutaneous transluminal angioplasty already provides a valuable option in experienced centers for the treatment of patients with surgically inaccessible carotid artery stenosis and for patients who are not fit for surgery. If clinical trials confirm the usefulness and comparative safety of carotid PTA, the procedure could become widely used as an alternative to surgery in suitable patients.

DISADVANTAGES OF SURGERY

Carotid endarterectomy has now been convincingly established as beneficial in preventing ipsilateral stroke in recently symptomatic patients with severe internal carotid stenosis.[1,2] However, significant morbidity and mortality are associated with surgery. The combined stroke and death rate within 30 days of surgery was 7.5% in the European Carotid Surgery Trial (ECST) and 5.8% in the North American Symptomatic Carotid Endarterectomy Trial (NASCET). Although death and stroke are the major complications of carotid surgery, other important risks must be considered such as myocardial infarction (which affects between 0.5% and 1.5% of endarterectomy patients). In addition, the systemic effects of the anesthetic and muscle relaxants, the discomfort of intubation, and the risks of pneumonia or deep vein thrombosis are potential complications. Many of these risks cannot be avoided by using a local anesthetic. Local anesthesia may even increase the risk of myocardial problems in patients with ischemic heart disease because of the depressive effect of large doses of local anesthetic and the effects of psychological stress. In addition to systemic risks of surgery and anesthesia, the incision may cause morbidity and discomfort. Hematoma in the neck may require exploration, but wound infection is only an occasional problem. Injury to cutaneous nerves results in numbness around the scar (sometimes extending onto the face), which may be permanent. More disability is caused by injury to the cranial nerves in the neck, most frequently the hypoglossal nerve, damage to which results in ipsilateral weakness of the tongue, and occasionally the glossopharyngeal nerve, although these usually recover. Keloid scar formation may be troublesome in some patients. One of these minor complications affected 10% of the patients after carotid endarterectomy in the ECST and must be considered a disadvantage of surgery, in addition to the risk of stroke and death[3] (Table 1). Carotid surgery is an expensive procedure and requires operating theater time, intensive care, and stay in the hospital of up to a week. Even if discharged after a few days, patients rarely return to full activities until a month after surgery.

Some patients are unable to benefit from carotid surgery because of severe ischemic heart disease, recent myocardial infarction, or uncontrolled hypertension, which are contraindications to the procedure. In the influential study analyzing risk factors for carotid endarterectomy by Sundt et al., the presence of these major medical risk factors increased the risk of surgery sevenfold.[4] These patients were excluded from the recent trials, but even so a recent analysis of risk factors for major surgical complications in the ECST confirmed that hypertension (systolic blood pressure greater than 180 mm Hg) doubled the risk of surgery.[3] Female sex also emerged from the analysis of the ECST data as a risk factor for surgery. This may reflect technical difficulty in operating on the smaller-diameter carotid artery of women. There are also patients who have significant carotid stenosis in arteries supplying the brain at sites that are

TABLE 1.
Complications of Carotid Surgery

Stroke*	Effects of the incision
Cerebral infarction† (7.0%)‡	Wound hematoma§ (3.1%)
Cerebral hemorrhage	Wound infection (0.2%)
Anesthetic complications	Cranial nerve injury (6.3%)
Myocardial infarction (0.5%)	Cutaneous numbness
Unstable angina (0.2%)	
Pulmonary embolus (0.2%)	
Deep vein thrombosis	
Pneumonia	

*The combined death and stroke rate within 30 days of surgery was 7.5%.[1]
†The cerebral infarction rate is that recorded within 30 days of surgery in patients with severe stenosis.
‡The figures in parentheses are the complication rates recorded in the European Carotid Surgery Trial.[3]
§Wound hematoma was defined as hematoma requiring surgery.

not easily or safely accessible to surgeons, such as stenosis beyond the carotid bifurcation.

ADVANTAGES OF PERCUTANEOUS TRANSLUMINAL ANGIOPLASTY

The main advantage of carotid angioplasty is that the procedure is relatively minor and, if all goes well, does not disturb the patient any more than a conventional angiogram. Excellent results can be achieved (Fig 1). Percutaneous transluminal angioplasty is performed with the patient under local anesthesia to avoid the complications of general anesthesia. The discomfort and local neurologic complications of an incision in the neck, particularly cranial and superficial nerve injury, are also avoided, although hematoma can occur in the groin. The discomforts of successful angioplasty are minimal apart from occasional transient pain in the neck and a sore puncture site for a few days. The patient need only stay in the hospital after PTA for the duration of IV heparin therapy (usually 24 hours) and can resume normal activities immediately. Percutaneous transluminal angioplasty consumes fewer financial and hospital resources than surgery in that the angiography suite is required for an hour or less and patients rarely need admission to an ICU. The initial costs are therefore much less than those of surgery, which may be a considerable advantage to health providers, although long-term economic analyses are not yet available. The cost advantage of PTA will be reduced if there is significant requirement for readmission because of symptomatic restenosis, but current data suggest that this will not be as frequent as after coronary PTA. Angioplasty will therefore have considerable advantages over

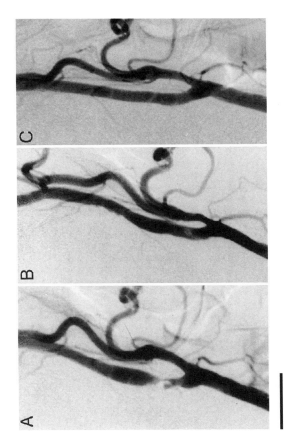

FIGURE 1.

Digital subtraction angiograms showing excellent and long-term immediate results of percutaneous transluminal angioplasty in a patient with severe ulcerated internal carotid stenosis. **A**, immediately before angioplasty. **B**, immediately after angioplasty. **C**, 1 year after angioplasty.

carotid endarterectomy if it can be shown to have a similar or lower complication rate.

CORONARY AND PERIPHERAL PERCUTANEOUS TRANSLUMINAL ANGIOPLASTY

Evidence from studies of the risk of angioplasty at sites other than in cerebrovascular vessels suggests that symptomatic embolization is not more frequent after PTA than after surgery. The National Heart, Lung and Blood Institute's registry of coronary PTA reported an overall risk of nonfatal myocardial infarction of 4%.[5] These figures probably accurately represent the risk of significant embolism resulting from angioplasty because the diagnosis of myocardial infarction is reliably established by ECG and enzyme changes. A similar risk of distal embolization of 5% is quoted for angioplasty of lower limb peripheral vessels. It is only recently that the risks of coronary angioplasty and coronary artery bypass graft surgery have been compared in randomized clinical trials. For example, the Randomised Intervention Treatment of Angina trial found no significant difference in the immediate risk of myocardial infarction or death before discharge from the hospital between patients treated by angioplasty (4.3%) and those treated by surgery (3.6%).[6] During the mean follow-up period of 2 years, there was no significant difference in the incidence of myocardial infarction or death, but angina requiring repeat angioplasty was more common in the group randomized to PTA because of restenosis.

There is no reason to think that the rate of symptomatic emboli after carotid PTA is likely to be any greater than that after coronary or peripheral PTA. The rate of embolization from peripheral and coronary PTA is similar to the stroke and death rate from carotid endarterectomy reported in the ECST and NASCET. The similarity between the major morbidity rates associated with coronary surgery, carotid surgery, and coronary angioplasty strongly suggests that carotid PTA may well have similar risks.

MECHANISMS OF PERCUTANEOUS TRANSLUMINAL ANGIOPLASTY

Experimental studies in animal models have shown that balloon inflation denudes the endothelium, splits atheromatous plaque so that it dehisces from the underlying media, and stretches the media and adventitia. Splitting of the atheromatous plaque appears to be essential for successful angioplasty and is the only way that concentric plaque can be dilated. Compression or redistribution of atheromatous material does not occur, and dilation is achieved by increasing the diameter of the whole vessel and moving the walls outward.[7] A process of repair and remodeling of the artery occurs after successful angioplasty. This continues throughout the first few weeks and possibly months, and the final arterial lumen may become much wider than is apparent immediately after angioplasty (Fig 2). The arterial wall injury caused by angioplasty results in the stimulation of fibroblasts and smooth muscle cells, which may be responsible for the remodeling process but may also result in restenosis. The factors involved in the extent of this reaction are unknown, but im-

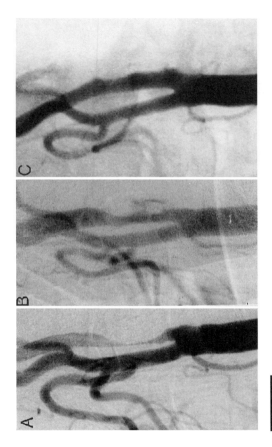

FIGURE 2.

Digital subtraction angiograms showing remodeling of the arterial wall after percutaneous transluminal angioplasty for very severe internal carotid stenosis at the bifurcation. **A,** immediately before angioplasty. **B,** immediately after angioplasty, dilation is suboptimal. Note the line of contrast medium within the atheromatous plaque, indicative of plaque fissuring. **C,** 1 year after angioplasty. Remodeling has resulted in a widely patent lumen.

provement in luminal diameter with time may be related to replacement of proliferative intima and smooth muscle cells by fibrosis.

TECHNIQUE OF CAROTID PERCUTANEOUS TRANSLUMINAL ANGIOPLASTY

The main skill required for successful and safe carotid PTA is the ability to get the guide wire into the internal carotid artery and then negotiate it across a tight stenosis with a minimum of trauma. Experience in using angioplasty balloons in peripheral vessels is helpful in selecting the type of balloon and choosing the technique for stabilizing the balloon catheter across the stenosis. It can be an advantage if carotid PTA is carried out by an experienced interventional neuroradiologist together with an experienced vascular radiologist. Improvements in catheter design over the past few years have included low-profile, rapidly deflating balloons and better guide wire design, which have increased the success rate and safety of the procedure.

Standard balloon angioplasty technique consists of percutaneous insertion under local anesthetic of a sheath into the femoral artery in the groin. Sedation is optional. The femoral artery provides the easiest route to the cervical vessels, but if access through the groin is difficult, a brachial route can be attempted but may be more hazardous. The standard diagnostic catheter for neurologic procedures is then passed through the artery into the common carotid artery and views of the stenosis obtained. The diagnostic catheter is then passed through the stenosis and the guide wire removed. An exchange wire is then inserted through the diagnostic catheter and the latter is withdrawn. An inflatable balloon angioplasty catheter is then passed over the guide wire and maneuvered to straddle the stenosis. The diameter of the balloon is chosen to match the estimated diameter of the vessel, with the aim of avoiding overdilation (usually 5- to 6-mm diameter by 2 cm long for lesions at the carotid bifurcation). The ideal catheter has a low-profile tip and a rapid deflation time. The balloon is inflated across the stenosis up to five times to achieve satisfactory dilation. Although there is no consensus about the pressures required to achieve successful angioplasty, probably less than 2 atm or handheld inflation pressure is adequate. Higher pressures may be hazardous. Inflation time should be less than 10 seconds. This brief total occlusion time considerably limits the risk of hemodynamic ischemia, unless the stenosis is so tight that the guide wire occludes the vessel for a longer time. This is in contrast to carotid endarterectomy, where even if shunts are used it may take several minutes to insert the shunt after the internal carotid artery has been clamped.

CEREBRAL PROTECTION CATHETERS

Theron et al. have suggested that the risk of embolism during carotid PTA may be reduced by using a specially designed cerebral protection catheter.[8] Their technique involves the use of a triple-lumen introducer catheter introduced into the common carotid artery. An occlusion balloon catheter is then passed across the stenosis and inflated beyond the stenosis to occlude the internal carotid artery to prevent emboli from reaching the brain. Next, a balloon dilation catheter is passed over the occlusion balloon catheter and inflated across the stenosis and withdrawn. The third lumen of the introducer catheter is then used to suck blood from below the occluded balloon catheter to remove embolic material. Theron et al. reported finding cholesterol crystals up to 200 µm long in the aspirate.[8] This technique has the disadvantage of using a large introducer catheter, which may not be appropriate for the treatment of very severe stenosis, and the complexity of the procedure is likely to increase the hazard. In particular, the prolonged total occlusion time of over 10 minutes increases the chance of hemodynamic ischemia, and the occlusion balloon adds a risk of thrombosis occurring beyond the occlusion. Doubling the sites of endothelial injury from balloon inflation will also increase the risk of subsequent thrombus formation. Up to now, the majority of experts have therefore not favored use of the occlusive balloon technique, instead preferring the simplicity of single-balloon methods. However, it is possible that advances in technology may make this approach more attractive, and a trial of this technique in carotid stenosis is currently being planned in France.

ARTERIAL STENTS

The recent introduction of stenting, in which a wire mesh is introduced in a collapsed state over a balloon and is then opened and left behind to maintain dilation of the artery, is transforming the percutaneous transluminal treatment of coronary and peripheral atherosclerosis. Experience in carotid stenting is very limited, but it is possible that stents will also transform the treatment of carotid stenosis. Cardiologists in particular are beginning to carry out primary stenting of carotid stenosis, and controlled series of over 100 patients treated in one unit have very recently been reported at international meetings, with a low complication rate. These investigators argue that primary stenting will avoid the complication of vessel occlusion from dissection and should therefore be the method of choice. However, stenting is not likely to prevent occlusion resulting from attempts to cross a tight stenosis before balloon inflation, which in our experience is a more common complication. In theory, stents might reduce the chance of symptomatic embolization after PTA by providing a barrier between the ruptured plaque and the lumen of the artery, but on the other hand, they may increase the risk of embolization by providing a foreign site for thrombosis. Stents may also have the advantage of reducing the incidence of restenosis, although this has yet to be confirmed. Stents have the disadvantage of extra expense, and there is concern that stents may make subsequent carotid surgery, if required, very difficult. We therefore continue to favor simple balloon angioplasty in most cases, except in the presence of eccentric calcified plaque; inflation of a simple

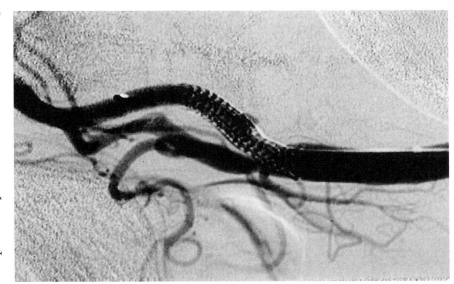

FIGURE 3.

Digital subtraction angiogram immediately after the percutaneous transluminal insertion of a stent across a carotid stenosis at the bifurcation.

angioplasty balloon in this situation usually results in an unsatisfactory result because of recoil of the more normal arterial wall (Fig 3). Calcification may be evident on angiographic films but can also be assessed by ultrasound (where calcified plaque is seen to be heavily echogenic) and by CT. Stenting may also be indicated if initial balloon inflation results in a poor initial result with less than 20% improvement in stenosis or results in dissection with a free flap. Stenting may become the treatment of choice for spontaneous carotid dissection.

COMPLICATIONS OF PERCUTANEOUS TRANSLUMINAL ANGIOPLASTY

Several potential complications of angioplasty have been noted (Table 2). The mechanical complications can be predicted from the consequences of splitting the atheromatous plaque, which is often required for successful angioplasty. Some degree of intimal dissection is inevitable, but this is usually localized to the area of plaque. However, inadvertent subintimal insertion of the guide wire or catheter may result in more extensive dissection, which may lead to vessel occlusion or chronic pseudoaneurysm formation. Irritation of the wall of the artery by the guide wire or catheter causes arterial spasm, but this is usually only symptomatic if severe enough to result in thrombus formation. Vessel rupture is an anxiety-provoking complication that is easily recognized by the sudden onset of very severe pain in the neck associated with extravasation of contrast media outside the vessel. This is a very rare complication. In the single case we have experienced, the extravasation of blood was easily controlled by pressure on the neck, and the rupture sealed spontaneously without intervention or neurologic sequelae. Balloon inflation at the carotid bifurcation results in stimulation of the carotid sinus, which frequently leads to bradycardia and very occasionally to brief periods of asystole. Relative hypotension may be noted for up to 48 hours after the procedure.

The major risks are those of cerebral and carotid occlusion. Risk factors for symptomatic embolism during PTA have not yet been established. In our experience, risk factors for major stroke after PTA have been a combination of very severe stenosis, a history of angina, and "crescendo" transient ischemic attacks. These are factors that have also been shown to be

---

TABLE 2.
Complications of Carotid Angioplasty

Mechanical	Neurologic
Intimal dissection	Hemodynamic ischemia
Aneurysm formation	Emboli during the procedure
Arterial spasm	Vessel thrombosis
Carotid sinus stimulation	Angiographic
Bradycardia and asystole	Contrast reactions
Hypotension	Femoral artery thromboembolism
Vessel rupture	Groin hematoma
Balloon rupture	Hemorrhage from anticoagulation

risk factors for stroke during carotid endarterectomy.[4] To reduce the risk of thromboembolism, patients scheduled for PTA are pretreated with aspirin to reduce the chance of embolism during or immediately after PTA. In some early series, complete anticoagulation was established with warfarin for some weeks before angioplasty to try to remove any thrombus that might have been present within the atheromatous plaque.[9] This is not currently recommended for all patients, but it is a sensible precaution if the patient has had very recent symptoms. Heparin anticoagulation is always instituted during the angiography procedure immediately before angioplasty, and IV heparin is then continued to achieve full anticoagulation for 24 to 48 hours after the procedure. This anticoagulation regimen follows that used after coronary and peripheral PTA and is not yet based on any scientific study. Aspirin therapy is continued during this period and indefinitely thereafter. There is a suggestion that aspirin may reduce restenosis after PTA as well as prevent thrombosis during follow-up.

The risk of hemodynamic stroke from temporary occlusion of the treated artery during the angioplasty procedure is reduced by limiting the duration of balloon inflation to a few seconds. If the stenosis is significantly severe that the guide wire occludes the artery, the procedure can be abandoned if symptoms of cerebral ischemia develop during passage of the guide wire across the stenosis. Hypotension should be avoided during the procedure, and all patients having carotid bifurcation angioplasty are pretreated with atropine to reduce the consequences of baroreceptor stimulation and prevent bradycardia.

Acute occlusion (closure) of the carotid artery can occur as a result of hemorrhage into the plaque or secondary to dissection. It is much less common for occlusion to occur secondary to thrombus on the damaged intima after initially successful dilation. Occlusion is symptomatic in about 50% of patients and has been the main reason for the incidence of major morbidity in most series. If occlusion does occur, options for management include immediate thrombolysis with or without stenting, emergency surgical endarterectomy, or conservative management with continued anticoagulation. Thrombolysis is at present unproven therapy, and if the occlusion is caused by plaque hemorrhage, the situation could be made worse.

An experienced neuroradiologist and the selection of appropriate lesions in which it appears that a guide wire will easily pass across the stenosis are essential to avoid stroke. It is likely that trauma from excessive guide wire manipulation is a major source of complications. The operator should therefore be encouraged to not try too hard and should be prepared to abandon the attempt if it is difficult to cross the stenosis. Excessive inflation pressures above 4 atm and overdilation of the artery by using a balloon diameter greater than the estimated normal should probably be avoided because both of these have been associated with an increased incidence of dissection and may also lead to a higher incidence of restenosis.

Monitoring requirements include pulse and frequent blood pressure measurements because of the risk of carotid sinus stimulation. A frequent simple neurologic examination during the procedure, for example, asking the patient to speak and move all four limbs, is helpful in reassuring the operator that all is well. The ability to carry out a neurologic examination throughout the procedure is one of the advantages of PTA. Heavy sedation is not desirable. Monitoring of intracranial artery blood flow by transcranial Doppler may provide useful information about the adequacy of collateral flow and the occurrence of microemboli, but transcranial Doppler is a research procedure and is not mandatory. If the procedure is near completion when the neurologic symptoms develop, it may be better to complete dilation of the stenosis before rapidly withdrawing the catheter. After angioplasty, the monitoring requirements are those routinely carried out after angiography, namely, regular pulse and blood pressure measurements, examination of the peripheral circulation, and simple neurologic observation for 24 hours. Admission to an ICU after angioplasty is unnecessary unless there have been complications.

About half the patients experience some brief discomfort in the neck at the site of angioplasty, and occasionally this radiates to the eye and forehead or scapula (carotidynia). This pain is usually very short-lived and only lasts a few seconds during balloon inflation, but occasionally it may last up to 48 hours. Groin hematoma may cause problems, particularly if the use of a stent requires a larger introducer sheath.

We have encountered most of the possible complications of carotid PTA at some time or another, but nevertheless, cerebrovascular PTA is very well tolerated by the majority of patients with little discomfort. As for the major complications of stroke and death, in our first consecutive series of 50 patients treated by simple balloon angioplasty, we had 1 nondisabling stroke and 2 major disabling strokes (1 patient died) at the time of the procedure for a stroke and death rate of 6% (Table 3). The majority of these patients had severe internal carotid artery stenosis and were patients who were treated by PTA as an alternative to carotid surgery.

What other evidence is there that carotid angioplasty is relatively

TABLE 3.
Clinical Details of the Author's Personal Series of Carotid Stenosis Treated by Angioplasty

Number attempted		Sites of carotid PTA	
50 stenoses, 49 patients		Internal carotid artery	47
Age and sex		Bifurcation	44
Mean age, 64.0 years (range, 46–82)		High cervical	3
18 females, 31 males		Common carotid artery	1
Symptoms		External carotid artery	2
Amaurosis fugax	7	Strokes during angioplasty	
TIA	22	Nondisabling stroke	1
Retinal infarct	3	Major stroke	2
Stroke	13		
Asymptomatic	5		

Abbreviations: TIA, transient ischemic attack; PTA, percutaneous transluminal angioplasty.

safe? No randomized clinical trials have been reported to date, but small case series describing successful carotid PTA appeared soon after the introduction of balloon inflation catheters. More recently, larger consecutive series of patients with atheromatous internal carotid artery stenosis treated by PTA have accumulated, and over 500 procedures have now been reported in the literature or at international meetings (Brown[10] and data on file). The series all report relatively low complication rates. The mean stroke rate at the time of the procedure for all the published series together is 1.5% for minor or nondisabling stroke and 2.1% for major stroke or death, for an overall rate of 3.6%. The average stroke risk is less than those reported after carotid endarterectomy in the ECST and NASCET in Europe and North America. Caution about these figures must be expressed because the patients and carotid bifurcation lesions included in the series are likely to have been highly selected. Not all of the larger series have been published in full in peer-reviewed journals, and none have been randomized prospective trials. The reported patients may not all have had severe carotid stenosis or have been recently symptomatic. The lesions have been specifically chosen to be suitable for PTA, so ulcerated lesions, for example, have been excluded from some series. Nevertheless, the results provide strong support for further studies of PTA as an alternative to carotid endarterectomy in appropriate patients as part of randomized clinical trials.

INDICATIONS FOR CAROTID PERCUTANEOUS TRANSLUMINAL ANGIOPLASTY

Our current indications for carotid PTA as part of our own ongoing randomized clinical trial, the Carotid and Veretebral Artery Transluminal Angioplasty Study, are similar to those of carotid surgery. Percutaneous transluminal angioplasty should be considered mainly for patients with severe symptomatic internal carotid artery stenosis measuring more than 70% linear diameter reduction according to ECST or NASCET criteria. Selection of atherosclerotic lesions at the carotid bifurcation or proximal internal carotid artery is a matter of experience. We discuss the appropriateness of PTA vs. surgery for individual patients with experienced interventional radiologists and vascular surgeons. The majority of lesions we discuss are suitable for angioplasty. The remainder are referred for surgery or continued medical management. With increasing experience of the technique and the type of lesion appropriate for PTA, the technical success rate for achieving satisfactory dilation has improved at our center to 90% of all attempts. The main consideration for safe PTA is that the residual lumen be in such a position that a guide wire will easily pass through the stenosis. A very tortuous lumen or an acutely angled approach to the stenosis is not suitable because of the risk of the guide wire penetrating the arterial wall. In some cases, severe atheromatous disease of the iliac or femoral arteries prevents access to the cerebrovascular tree through the groin, but a brachial approach may be possible in some of these patients. Allergy to contrast media may be a contraindication to PTA, but in milder cases this may be overcome by pretreating the patient with corticosteroids. The presence of ulceration visible on ultrasound or angiography is not itself a contraindication to PTA, and such lesions can be successfully treated with no complication and excellent results (see Fig 1). The presence of visible thrombus is regarded as a contraindication, although it might be feasible to use local infusions of thrombolytic agents to dissolve the clot before PTA. At present, we do not use PTA for the treatment of acute cerebral infarction, only as prophylactic treatment to prevent cerebral infarction.

If the immediate result after PTA is suboptimal dilation of the artery but the plaque can be seen to be fissured by an outline of contrast media and at least a 20% increase in lumen diameter has been achieved, remodeling is likely to result in a good long-term result (see Fig 2). For example, in our series of ten patients with severe carotid stenosis treated by PTA who were evaluated by angiography at 12 months, eight showed a significant reduction in stenosis by up to 40% between the immediate post-PTA result at the site of the treated stenosis and the diameter at 1 year.[11] Two patients showed an increase in stenosis, indicative of restenosis, but in both cases this was asymptomatic. Both patients with restenosis had an initial reduction of the stenosis of less than 20%. Whether the use of stenting in such a situation of inadequate initial dilation would result in a better long-term result is uncertain.

Very little experience has been accrued in using angioplasty to treat asymptomatic carotid stenosis. Uncertainty remains about the benefit of treating asymptomatic patients with carotid endarterectomy because the risk of surgery is higher than the risk of stroke during the first 2 years or so after asymptomatic stenosis is detected. There is very little experience with angioplasty in asymptomatic patients, but it is quite possible that angioplasty would be safer than surgery in this situation. We have only used angioplasty in patients with severe asymptomatic carotid stenosis who also need coronary artery bypass grafting and in whom the ischemic heart disease is a contraindication to carotid surgery. In this situation, carotid angioplasty may provide a valid alternative to leaving the carotid untreated or carrying out a dual operation of carotid endarterectomy and coronary artery bypass grafting under the same anesthetic. Trials of PTA for aysmptomatic stenosis are needed.

DISTAL INTERNAL CAROTID ARTERY

One of the major potential advantages of PTA is that it can be used to treat stenosis of the distal internal carotid artery high in the neck at sites inaccessible to a surgeon or where it is technically difficult to perform an endarterectomy. Such lesions are uncommon, and replacement of conventional angiography as the screening test for carotid stenosis by Doppler ultrasound or magnetic resonance angiography of the carotid bifurcation has the consequence that distal lesions are rarely detected. Experience in using PTA for distal internal carotid artery lesions is therefore limited, but a few case reports have demonstrated the feasibility of the approach, and we have treated one such patient successfully. The risks of treating distal lesions up to the siphon are probably similar to those of treating stenosis at the carotid bifurcation, but lesions in the siphon or above may be more hazardous to treat.

COMMON AND EXTERNAL CAROTID ARTERY STENOSIS

Although most patients with symptomatic carotid artery disease have internal carotid artery stenosis, common carotid and external carotid artery stenosis is also relatively easily treated by PTA. Experience in treating such lesions is limited because common carotid artery stenosis is rarely severe enough to warrant intervention and external carotid stenosis is rarely relevant. In our series of 50 patients with carotid artery stenosis treated by PTA, only 1 patient had symptomatic common carotid artery stenosis and 2 had relevant external carotid artery stenosis (see Table 3). External carotid artery stenosis only merits prophylactic treatment to prevent stroke if the ipsilateral internal carotid artery is occluded and angiography demonstrates that the external carotid artery provides a significant collateral supply to the ipsilateral hemisphere via the ophthalmic artery.

OUTCOME OF CAROTID PERCUTANEOUS TRANSLUMINAL ANGIOPLASTY

HEMODYNAMIC CONSEQUENCES

Significant improvement in cerebral hemodynamics after PTA can be demonstrated by measurements of cerebrovascular reserve by transcranial Doppler. In our studies we have demonstrated an average improvement over 4 weeks after PTA of about 30% in carbon dioxide reactivity in the hemisphere distal to the treated carotid stenosis, thus implying improved vasodilator capacity secondary to the improvement in perfusion pressure.[12] This improvement was gradual over the first 4 weeks, presumably reflecting the process of remodeling occurring in the days after angioplasty. Marked improvements in carbon dioxide reactivity are only to be expected if there is a relatively poor ipsilateral collateral supply and severe stenosis resulting in a reduction in reactivity before treatment.

EMBOLI DETECTION

Monitoring blood flow in the middle cerebral artery by transcranial Doppler also allows the detection of emboli during and after the procedure. Short-duration, high-intensity signals can be detected by transcranial Doppler monitoring in the middle cerebral artery ipsilateral to severe symptomatic carotid stenosis in about a third of the patients before treatment. It is believed that the majority of these are the result of microemboli that are too small to cause symptoms. Platelet, atheroma, and thrombus emboli have different signal characteristics in laboratory studies, but these characteristics are also affected by the size of the embolus. At present, it is therefore not possible to identify the nature of the material causing the embolic signals in human studies. Embolic signals are detected by transcranial Doppler recording during carotid endarterectomy and are very frequent after clamp removal, which suggests that some of the signals may be the result of air bubbles. Emboli are also seen during arterial dissection before shunt insertion, and these are very likely to be solid material. Numerous high-density signals can also be detected during routine carotid angiography, and these are the result of small bubbles in the contrast medium.[13] In our studies, monitoring during and after PTA has demonstrated that short-duration, high-intensity signals are very frequent during guide wire manipulation and immediately after PTA and then continue at a declining frequency over the next week.[14] The decline in embolic signals after PTA appears to mimic the time course of remodeling demonstrated by measurements of cerebral reactivity. The majority of the embolic signals during and after PTA may be caused by air introduced by the catheter or contrast medium, but this seems unlikely to explain those that occur in the subsequent days. It is likely that at least some result from platelet aggregations.

The emboli detected by transcranial Doppler after PTA are usually asymptomatic, and the duration of the signals suggest that they are very small and unlikely to occlude vessels other than the smallest capillaries. It is remarkable how well the cerebral circulation tolerates the embolism produced by balloon dilation as long as flow is maintained across the artery. It is possible that microembolism may produce subclinical damage to the brain, and studies of cognitive function involving a battery of neuropsychological tests before and after PTA are in progress. Nevertheless, no psychological impairment is evident on routine bedside testing or to the patient or their relatives, and it seems unlikely that the subtle deficits will be revealed. Monitoring for emboli by transcranial Doppler may allow the safety of different techniques to be assessed and the value of different platelet or anticoagulation regimens before PTA to be compared. For example, embolic signals might be less common after the insertion of stents than after simple routine balloon angioplasty. However, it has yet to be demonstrated that the number or frequency of embolic signals detected by transcranial Doppler predicts stroke risk.

LONG-TERM RESULTS

No adequate long-term follow-up data are available to assess the adequacy of cerebrovascular PTA in the prevention of subsequent stroke. The series published to date provide limited data that suggest that successful PTA is effective at preventing stroke, but no data are yet available from randomized trials comparing PTA with surgically or medically treated patients. The available data suggest that the majority of carotid artery lesions in which initial successful dilation is achieved by PTA remain patent. Long-term follow-up data are not available. Restenosis in the cerebrovascular circulation causes symptoms only rarely in comparison to coronary PTA. This is because the cerebrovascular circulation does not suffer from the equivalent of angina, which is a relatively common problem after coronary PTA because of the high demands of the coronary circulation for a hemodynamic increase in flow.

One criticism of PTA in comparison to surgery is that the atheromatous plaque is not removed and the potential for ulceration and thromboembolism remains. The ECST and NASCET findings that the severity of the stenosis is the most important determinant of subsequent stroke in patients with symptomatic carotid stenosis suggest that ulceration after PTA is unlikely to be a significant problem if sufficient dilation is achieved. In any case, the remodeling process that occurs after angioplasty results in new endothelium lining the atheromatous plaque, which will reduce the chance of thrombus formation on the underlying plaque. Full restoration of the normal arterial diameter may not be necessary to prevent stroke. The ECST results[15] showing a low rate of stroke in medically treated patients with stenosis of less than 70% suggest that an improvement in lumen after PTA to below 70% measured by ECST criteria will be enough to prevent the majority of strokes. The same data suggest that restenosis is unlikely to be a problem unless it results in more than 70% stenosis. Even then it is possible that restenosis after PTA resulting from an overgrowth of smooth muscle cells may not be as hazardous as restenosis resulting from irregular atheromatous plaque, particularly if the endothelium remains intact.

THE FUTURE OF CAROTID ANGIOPLASTY

The studies discussed in this chapter all suggest that carotid PTA can be carried out with a risk of stroke or death at the time of the procedure that is similar to that of the conventional surgical approach. At more distal sites inaccessible to surgery, whether the successful angiographic results discussed earlier justify the risk in comparison to conventional medical therapy is uncertain. Long-term studies to establish the effectiveness of PTA at any site in preventing subsequent stroke are lacking. Percutaneous transluminal angioplasty has numerous advantages from the patient's point of view, mainly because of the atraumatic nature of the procedure, the lack of an incision in the neck, and the avoidance of general anesthesia. These argue strongly for more widespread study of PTA as an alternative treatment of cerebrovascular arterial stenosis. Understandably, these arguments have on the whole been rejected by many vascular surgeons. Randomized clinical trials are essential to establish the relative benefits and risks of angioplasty in comparison to surgery and conventional medical management. The Carotid and Vertebral Artery Transluminal Angioplasty Study has centers in Europe, North America, South Africa, and Australia. This is an international multicenter randomized study in which patients with proximal carotid or vertebral artery stenosis are randomized between surgery and angioplasty (if fit for surgery) or between medicine and angioplasty (if not suitable for surgery). The collaborators plan to publish the initial results in 1998. Until the results of randomized trials of sufficient size are published, angioplasty should remain confined to specialist centers participating in ethically approved randomized studies.

The techniques of angioplasty are relatively easily to acquire and are familiar to a cohort of young vascular radiologists and interventional cardiologists. If trials confirm that angioplasty provides a valid alternative to carotid surgery or medical management, there is a large potential market for cerebrovascular PTA. It is essential that radiologists contemplating cerebrovascular PTA have appropriate experience in neuroradiology in addition to skills in balloon angioplasty. Advances in technology are likely to improve the safety and applicability of PTA to the cerebrovascular circulation. In particular, the development of stents of the appropriate size and configuration for the cerebrovascular tree will allow the treatment of eccentric calcified lesions, which were previously inappropriate for balloon angioplasty. Stents may also prove to be safer by reducing the risk of embolism or vessel occlusion from vessel dissection and may also reduce the chance of restenosis. On the other hand, it is possible that the initial risk of the procedure may be greater because of difficulty placing the stent or a greater risk of thrombosis on the stent surface. The added expense of stents means that simple balloon angioplasty is likely to remain the treatment of choice for noncalcified lesions for the time being. Other potential advances in balloon technology include local delivery of anticoagulant agents such as heparin to reduce the chance of thrombosis or other drugs that may inhibit smooth muscle proliferation and limit restenosis.

In conclusion, PTA provides an exciting new advance for the treatment of carotid stenosis and may have advantages over surgery or conventional medical management. Appropriate skills in the neurologic assessment of patients, interventional neuroradiology, and the application of balloon angioplasty techniques are essential to ensure the safety of the procedure. Randomized clinical trials are needed to establish the risks and benefits of PTA for cerebrovascular disease. If these confirm the initial promise of the procedure, carotid PTA will become a useful treatment for the prevention of stroke and will join coronary and peripheral PTA as a major first-line treatment.

REFERENCES

1. European Carotid Surgery Trialists Collaboration Group: MRC European carotid surgery trial: Interim results for symptomatic patients with severe (70–99%) or with mild (0–29%) carotid stenosis. *Lancet* 337:1235–1243, 1991.

2. North American Symptomatic Carotid Endarterectomy Trial Collaborators: Beneficial effect of carotid endarterectomy in symptomatic patients with high-grade carotid stenosis. *N Engl J Med* 325:445–453, 1991.

3. Rothwell P: Morbidity and mortality of carotid endarterectomy in the European Carotid Surgery Trial. *Cerebrovasc Dis* 4:226A, 1995.

4. Sundt TM, Sandok BA, Whisnant JP: Carotid endarterectomy: Complications and preoperative assessment of risk. *Mayo Clin Proc* 50:301–306, 1975.

5. The National Heart, Lung and Blood Institute's Percutaneous Transluminal Coronary Angioplasty Review: Percutaneous transluminal coronary angioplasty in 1985–1986 and 1977–1981. *N Engl J Med* 318:265–270, 1988.

6. Rita Trial Participants: Coronary angioplasty versus coronary artery bypass surgery: The Randomised Intervention Treatment of Angina (RITA) trial. *Lancet* 341:573–580, 1993.

7. Castaneda-Zuniga WR, Formanek A, Tadavarthy M, et al: The mechanisms of balloon angioplasty. *Radiology* 135:565–571, 1980.

8. Theron J, Courtheoux P, Alachkar F, et al: New triple coaxial catheter system for carotid angioplasty with cerebral protection. *Am J Neuroradiol* 11:869–874, 1990.

9. Brown MM, Butler P, Gibbs J, et al: Feasibility of percutaneous angioplasty of atherosclerotic carotid arteries. *J Neurol Neurosurg Psychiatry* 53:238–243, 1990.

10. Brown MM: Balloon angioplasty for cerebrovascular disease. *Neurol Res* 14:159S–173S, 1992.

11. Watts F, Clifton A, Markus HS, et al: Improvement in carotid artery diameter after carotid angioplasty. Submitted for publication, 1996.

12. Markus HS, Clifton A, Brown MM: Carotid angioplasty: Haemodynamic and embolic consequences. *Cerebrovasc Dis* 4:259A, 1994.

13. Markus H, Loh A, Israel D, et al: Microscopic air embolism during cerebral angiography and strategies for its avoidance. *Lancet* 341:784–787, 1993.

14. Markus HS, Clifton A, Buckenham T, et al: Carotid angioplasty: Detection of embolic signals during and after the procedure. *Stroke* 25:2403–2406, 1994.

15. European Carotid Surgery Trialists' Collaborative Group: Endarterectomy for moderate symptomatic carotid stenosis: Interim results from the MRC European Carotid Surgery Trial. *Lancet* 347:1591–1593, 1996.

Thrombolytic Therapy for Acute Stroke

David A. Kumpe, M.D.
Director of Interventional Radiology; Professor of Radiology and Surgery,
University of Colorado School of Medicine, Denver

Richard L. Hughes, M.D.
Assistant Professor of Neurology, University of Colorado School of Medicine,
Denver

Every physician dealing with vascular disease encounters acute stroke on a regular basis. More than 500,000 strokes and more than 150,000 stroke-related deaths occur each year in the United States. Stroke is the third leading cause of death in the United States and remains the leading cause of disability. Despite the magnitude of the problem and the many attempts to develop therapies for acute ischemic stroke, only recently have there been data to support treating stroke with fibrinolysis.

Atherothrombotic and thromboembolic events are responsible for 80% to 90% of ischemic strokes.[1] It was documented as early as 1960 that resolution of carotid-territory occlusions was associated with clinical improvement in selected stroke patients. On the other hand, it was also soon recognized that delayed treatment of completed strokes (greater than 24 hours after symptom onset) does not result in symptomatic benefit, with the added cost of producing intracerebral hemorrhage. The use of thrombolysis to treat stroke in the 1960s was therefore abandoned. With the advent of CT scanning, thrombolysis in the setting of acute stroke was re-evaluated with intervention within 6 hours or less of symptom onset.

The basis of treatment of stroke is the concept of reviving the "ischemic penumbra." When an acute arterial occlusion occurs, the entire brain substance distal to the occlusion is, at a minimum, stunned and on neurologic examination will be dysfunctional. Typically, a small portion of the total ischemic volume actually infarcts in the early postocclusion period. The still viable, but nonfunctioning brain volume is the *"ischemic penumbra."* Within a relatively brief time (1 to 6 hours), this potentially salvageable brain infarcts. The ischemic penumbra decreases in size as the volume of infarction increases. Reversal of acute ischemic stroke depends on restoration of circulation to the ischemic penumbra before irreversible tissue death has occurred and before vascular wall damage distal to the occlusion predisposes to parenchymal hemorrhage. Although the strokes discussed in this chapter are principally of embolic origin and the patients afflicted with them are usually first seen by primary care physicians, internists, and neurologists, it is inevitable that the vascular specialist will be consulted in many cases. The best hope for treating such

Advances in Vascular Surgery®, vol. 4
© 1996, Mosby–Year Book, Inc.

patients lies in rapid institution of thrombolytic therapy after appropriate diagnostic measures. The vascular specialist must be aware of the specific issues that will determine a potentially successful outcome and, conversely, a therapeutic disaster. Providing expeditious therapy in properly selected patients within very proscribed time limits may mean the difference between death or survival with a significant neurologic deficit vs. survival with minimal or no neurologic deficit. One need only see a few patients who lead normal lives after treatment for a proximal middle cerebral occlusion to realize the potential benefit of the approach outlined in this chapter.

The parallels between using fibrinolytic therapy to treat acute ischemic stroke and acute myocardial infarction are instructive. Acute myocardial infarction is associated with an 87% incidence of total occlusion of the infarct-related artery on angiograms performed within 4 hours of the onset of symptoms. Treatment of acute myocardial infarction with IV fibrinolysis is now a mainstay of the management of acute myocardial infarction. Spontaneous reperfusion develops in about 10% of patients in the acute phase of a myocardial infarction. Much higher acute recanalization rates (53% to 72% within 90 minutes) occur when patients are treated systemically with a fibrinolytic agent. Although intracoronary arterial infusion of the lytic agent is more efficacious, the difficulties of getting a catheter into the causative thrombus within a few hours of symptom onset are considerable. Despite the lower percentage of recanalization with systemic infusion of a fibrinolytic drug, the much larger number of patients who can receive such treatment more than compensates for the lower percentage of recanalization because a fibrinolytic agent can be administered before the patient reaches the hospital. In myocardial infarction, the pathologic event is invariably ischemic and caused by an acute thrombus in a coronary artery. In a patient with acute stroke, however, there is a 15% chance that the acute neurologic symptoms are caused by intracranial hemorrhage from an aneurysm or arteriovenous malformation rather than an arterial occlusion producing ischemia. A brain imaging study, usually a CT scan, is necessary to differentiate those patients suffering ischemic stroke from those with intracranial hemorrhage, which may worsen with fibrinolytic treatment. Because the patient will therefore already be in the hospital before treatment is started, intra-arterial catheter-directed treatment is possible if it can be instituted promptly.

Intravenous (systemic) therapy for stroke has recently been shown to be of value in two large randomized, prospective trials.[2,3] In patients who have ischemic symptoms for longer than 180 minutes, the increasing incidence of symptomatic intracranial hemorrhage detracts from the benefit produced by arterial recanalization. There is experimental[4] and clinical[5] evidence that intra-arterial administration of a thrombolytic agent into an intracranial clot produces a higher recanalization rate at a lower dose and yields a better clinical result if there is no delay in treatment.

CLINICAL OUTCOME OF ISCHEMIC STROKE

Overall, mortality associated with stroke (hemorrhagic and ischemic) is about 30%. Patients who have cerebral hemorrhages have a higher mortality rate. The overall mortality rate for ischemic stroke is about 15%. Deaths are attributable to many causes, including transtentorial herniation as a result of cerebral edema in large infarctions and deaths from related disorders that are associated with age and comorbidity (pneumonia, heart failure, etc.).

The clinical outcome of any stroke depends on multiple factors. These include the severity of the initial deficit, the mechanism of stroke, the adequacy of collateral circulation, the patient's age, and a variety of other comorbid factors that affect the stroke population.

The *extent of the initial neurologic deficit* is probably the most important factor in determining outcome. Specific predictors based on an initial deficit are only applicable when the time of onset is known. For example, a hemiplegic deficit at 30 minutes has more potential for reversal than a similar deficit at 24 hours. Similarly, deficits that fluctuate (indicating that there is still sufficient collateralization of the ischemic bed) have more potential for reversal than do fixed deficits.

The *mechanism of stroke* is also important in determining outcome. Patients who suffer a stroke from small-vessel occlusion, which causes a lacunar infarction, often have better recovery and less mortality. A lacunar infarction disrupts only one neurologic system; for example, a pure motor hemiparesis may occur without sensory loss. "Single neurologic system" deficits are better tolerated by the patient. Because most small-vessel strokes occur in white matter, the neurons remain viable and continue to function, but with fewer synaptic connections. Large-vessel strokes (e.g., middle cerebral artery [MCA] occlusions) are predominately caused by embolism, involve multiple neurologic systems (such as motor, sensory, *and* speech), and are prone to both hemorrhage and herniation.

The *location* of a large-vessel occlusion has important ramifications on outcome. Proximal MCA occlusions (M1 and M2) have a 33% 3-month mortality rate, whereas more distal occlusions (M3 segment or branch) have a 14.3% 3-month mortality rate.[6] However, neither mortality nor the final neurologic outcome correlates very well with the anatomic location of the initial occlusion because reperfusion and collateral circulation allow some patients to tolerate occlusions with less permanent residual deficit. Complete occlusion of the internal carotid artery (ICA) or the basilar artery is probably the most devastating anatomic mechanism of stroke. Occlusions of this type cause infarction by *hypoperfusion* (for example, occlusion of the ICA), by *directly blocking penetrating arteries* (for example, penetrating arteries into the pons from basilar artery occlusion), and by *embolization* from the distal end of the occlusion ("tail embolus") causing embolic infarction. Examples include an embolus from the distal ICA that causes an MCA stroke or a basilar occlusion with embolization to the posterior cerebral artery. The prognosis of vertebrobasilar occlusion is extremely poor, with mortality rates of 60% to 100%.

Collateral circulation may be as important as any other factor, but it is unpredictable. Only a small percentage of people have a completely intact circle of Willis without hypoplastic or nonexistent connections at either the anterior or the posterior communicating arteries. The availability of collateral circulation naturally depends on the site of embolic occlusion. For example, an ICA occlusion below the posterior communicating artery may be well tolerated in a patient who has patent anterior and posterior communicating arteries. A patient's *age* correlates with stroke severity and morbidity. The older the patient, the larger the stroke.

Perhaps as damaging for mortality are the extra *comorbid medical conditions* that complicate stroke victims as they get older. Almost any associated illness will hinder recovery from a stroke. Illnesses associated with atherosclerosis, including diabetes and hyperlipidemia, predict a poor outcome. Factors that limit the heart's ability to pump appropriately such as congestive heart failure, dehydration, or valvular heart disease will similarly impede the ability of the collateral circulation to minimize the severity of stroke. Certain blood factors are known to worsen stroke. Patients with a high glucose concentration on initial testing have larger strokes. This may reflect diabetes, viscosity, or other metabolic factors. Patients with high hematocrits similarly have larger strokes, probably because of viscosity.

NATURAL HISTORY—SPONTANEOUS THROMBOLYSIS AND HEMORRHAGE IN ISCHEMIC STROKE

RECANALIZATION

Cerebral arterial occlusions are found in a high percentage of patients when they are studied arteriographically within a short time after symptom onset, with a decreasing frequency as the interval from the onset of symptoms increases.[7]

If it is assumed that at the initial evaluation patients have a 100% incidence of occlusion, data suggest that the rate of spontaneous recanalization in acute ischemic stroke is 20% to 40% by 24 hours and greater than 50% by 7 days. Early recanalization with fibrinolytic therapy must improve on the early spontaneous rate of recanalization if brain infarction is to be minimized.

INTRACRANIAL HEMORRHAGE AND HEMORRHAGIC TRANSFORMATION

The obvious concern with the use of fibrinolytic agents in acute ischemic stroke is the production of intracranial hemorrhage. Two questions then arise: (1) what is the incidence of spontaneous hemorrhage associated with stroke? and (2) what is the risk of intracranial hemorrhage among patients who receive fibrinolytic therapy for indications other than acute stroke?

Two types of intracranial bleeding are associated with strokes. *Parenchymal hematoma formation* is most often symptomatic and refers to the accumulation of a formed blood clot that produces a significant mass effect and compresses adjacent brain parenchyma. This, along with cerebral edema, produces a shift of brain structures detectable on CT. Fatal herniation is common. *Hemorrhagic infarction* is petechial hemorrhage in the region of ischemic injury in 10% to 43% of patients and is not associated with a significant mass effect. The incidence of symptomatic hemorrhagic transformation in ischemic stroke patients approximates 5%.[8]

The incidence of intracranial hemorrhage associated with fibrinolytic therapy given systemically and by local catheter infusion outside the brain is well established. During the treatment of acute myocardial infarction with systemic fibrinolytic agents, symptomatic intracranial hemorrhage occurs in 0.8% of cases (range, 0.3% to 5.0%).[9] For systemic treatment of deep vein thrombosis, rates of intracranial hemorrhage are similar or lower. During the treatment of peripheral arterial ischemia with catheter-directed fibrinolysis using urokinase, rates of intracranial hemorrhage range from 0.1% to 0.5%.

PATIENT SELECTION FOR FIBRINOLYSIS

Patient selection is the most critical question in ensuring a satisfactory (and sometimes spectacular) outcome. Although insufficient information is available to predict which patients will have a good/excellent outcome, there is enough experience to predict which patients will have an unacceptably bad result from intra-arterial fibrinolysis. In simple summary,

- Patients should have lysis of an embolus completed within 6 hours from the onset of ictus. More rapid lysis, e.g., within 4 hours of onset, is optimal.
- The initial CT must show no intracranial hemorrhage and no large hypodense area.
- Intracranial intraluminal thrombus should be present on angiography.

Currently, only 5% to 10% of patients are encountered within the 6-hour interval after having had the initial clinical evaluation, CT, and angiography. If we are to make an impact on stroke, we must reorganize our triage system to treat acute stroke with the same urgency now accorded acute myocardial infarction. This entails a massive education program among physicians and the lay public. *Time is brain!*

INITIAL WORKUP AND MANAGEMENT

CLINICAL EVALUATION

The most important factors in the clinical history used to determine whether thrombolysis should be performed involve making the clinical diagnosis of stroke and determining the time of onset. If the onset of deficit is immediate, painless, and without loss of consciousness, the diagnosis of stroke is fairly easy to confirm. Unusual causes of symptoms and signs should be sought, such as a history of seizures, trauma, infection, or illicit drug use. If the patient is aphasic and the event unwitnessed, the clinician must exclude common mimickers of stroke such as Todd's paralysis after a seizure, complicated migraine, head injury without obvious external injury, multiple sclerosis, and severe metabolic disturbances. Diagnoses that can mimic stroke but are excluded by CT scanning include intracranial hemorrhage, tumor, abscess, and metastasis. Sometimes it is unclear whether a deficit is new or the result of an old stroke that has transiently worsened because of comorbid medical conditions.

Because timing is so crucial to fibrinolytic therapy, every effort should be made to accurately determine the time of onset of the stroke. If the time is uncertain, one should use the last time that the patient was known to be normal. For example, patients who wake up with a hemiplegia must be assumed to have had the stroke at the time they went to bed at night, not at the time of awakening. Patients who have a stroke soon after awakening can usually confirm this by history. In practical experience, the time of stroke can be estimated within 15 minutes in most cases. Beyond that, clinicians must use good judgment and data from CT scanning to identify patients who are within a time window appropriate for thrombolysis. Basic localization is necessary to help interpret subtle CT scan changes and to choose appropriate methods of resuscitation. The physician should be able to identify carotid and basilar syndromes and should recognize those cases with a distal branch MCA occlusion.

A *left cerebral hemisphere* stroke will produce a right-sided hemiplegia (typically the face and arm are affected more than the leg) and aphasia, both expressive and receptive. Language localization to the left hemisphere is nearly universal in right-handed individuals and occurs in more than 50% of left-handed individuals. Because the visual pathways and the fibers from the leg run deeper in the hemisphere, homonymous hemianopsia and complete weakness of the leg indicate ischemia of the *entire* MCA territory. Sparing of the leg and vision indicates a more distal branch embolization with a better overall prognosis. Some patients are seen with complete involvement but improve to a branch occlusion. *Right hemisphere* strokes are similar, but there is no aphasia to help estimate stroke size. However, patients with large-volume right hemisphere strokes will have a complete hemiplegia (including the leg), will neglect or ignore the left side of the body (and sometimes the entire room), and will have a left homonymous hemianopsia.

Theoretically, the more distal *branch occlusions* have a better prognosis and can be treated later with some improvement because they have better collateral compensation. Larger strokes can still respond to thrombolysis but probably need to be reperfused earlier for an equivalent result. The risk of thrombolysis is higher in large-volume, more severe strokes, but then so are the benefits if death or nursing home placement can be avoided.

Basilar artery occlusion is one of the deadliest stroke syndromes. Localization to the basilar artery is based on the presence of bilateral motor involvement in the body or, in the case of a hemipontine infarct, ipsilateral cranial nerve involvement and contralateral weakness in the body. A left pontine infarct, for example, may produce left facial weakness and numbness but right body weakness and numbness. Other clues to basilar or other posterior circulation infarction include diplopia, vertigo, and dysphasia.

Neurovascular examination should include examination of the heart for dysrhythmia, palpation of peripheral and carotid pulses, and auscultation of the neck for bruits. A rapid examination by a neurologist is the most efficient screening test to select patients having an ischemic event that can be corrected with fibrinolytic therapy, as well as to establish the initial degree or deficit. Follow-up neurologic examination is required to establish whether the deficit is increasing or improving.

Initial evaluation should include ECG, chest film, complete blood count, platelet count, prothrombin time, partial thromboplastin time, serum electrolytes, and a blood glucose test. Arterial blood gas measurements, serum alcohol level, and a drug screen are performed as indicated.

COMPUTED TOMOGRAPHY

A noncontrast CT scan should be obtained as rapidly as possible after the initial evaluation. The resuscitation team must assist the emergency department by differentiating those patients who truly need a rapid CT scan before thrombolysis from those who need a CT scan soon but within a few hours. If the clinician has completed a basic examination and has sent blood for appropriate tests, there is time during the CT scan to make preliminary preparations so that the patient can be treated expeditiously with catheter-directed infusion of fibrinolytic agent if appropriate. The interventional neuroradiology team should be made aware of the patient and the angiography suite prepared. Alternatively, if systemic fibrinolytic therapy is anticipated, the thrombolytic drug may be brought to the CT scanning area and systemic administration started as soon as the decision to treat the patient has been made.

The completed CT scan should be reviewed promptly by a physician knowledgeable in stroke resuscitation. Approximately 15% of patients will have hemorrhage on the initial CT that precludes fibrinolysis. Of the patients with acute ischemic stroke, there should be no evidence of a major ischemic infarct as manifested by an area of decreased attenuation occupying the entire distribution of the MCA. If the scan demonstrates a large low-density area appropriate to the clinical deficit, the advisability of proceeding with resuscitation is highly questionable regardless of the time of onset. If the scan findings are normal, a resuscitation plan should already be in place so that therapy can be given without delay. The hyperdense MCA sign, indicative of acute thrombus within the MCA, does not predict whether recanalization will occur after thrombolysis.

For patients with normal CT findings who are clearly within a time window favorable for successful thrombolysis, the decision to proceed is relatively straightforward. Patients who are 4 to 5 hours past onset, yet have subtle early changes on their CT scan are more problematic. If the judgment is made that fibrinolytic therapy is appropriate, rapid institution of treatment is mandatory. Therapy can be catastrophic if the decision to attempt thrombolysis is made and then delayed so that lysis is not achieved until well after 6 hours past onset. In that eventuality, alternate forms of supportive therapy are a better choice.

At the present time, CT is the standard initial noninvasive test. Because of the early time window required for therapy, it is unreasonable to expect other tests such as carotid ultrasound or cardiac echography to be performed before resuscitation. Only on rare occasion is it possible to obtain one or both of these studies while the angiographic suite is being prepared. These tests are typically done after resuscitation efforts have been completed to help understand the overall risk of stroke recurrence.

Undoubtedly, MRI/MR angiography (MRA) will become more important because of increased sensitivity and the ability to visualize the extracranial and intracranial arteries at the same time. At present, however, such imaging technology is not as widely available as CT, nor are MRI/MRA criteria available to determine which patients should be treated.

CEREBRAL ARTERIOGRAPHY

If the noncontrast CT shows no intracerebral hemorrhage and no defect or a small area of hypodensity in the affected distribution and the patient is within a 4-hour interval since the onset of ictus, immediate arteriography should be performed to localize the intracranial thrombus before intra-arterial infusion of a fibrinolytic agent. "Major" occlusive thrombus proximal to the M2 and A2 segments of the middle and anterior cerebral arteries, respectively, and proximal to the P2 segments of the posterior cerebral arteries should be treated. Data that support these contentions are presented in the *Results* section later. In our experience, if no thrombus is seen in these segments, the patient will probably do equally well with supportive care (hypervolemia, blood pressure enhancement, anticoagulation with heparin) because such occlusions intrinsically have a good outcome.

In summary, the highest likelihood of a favorable outcome from fibrinolysis, no matter what the site of arterial occlusion, is associated with two findings: (1) the presence of no defect or only a small hypodensity on the initial CT scan and (2) good collateralization distal to the occlusion on arteriography.[10] These two findings indicate that the brain distal to the acute occlusion is receiving collateral arterial flow and is more likely to remain viable. Unfortunately, these findings do not guarantee a good outcome. On the other hand, *either a large hypodense area with swelling on CT or poor collateral flow beyond the occlusion on angiography portends a grave prognosis. The patient is highly likely to have a poor outcome that will be unaffected or exacerbated with fibrinolysis.*

THROMBOLYSIS: INTRA-ARTERIAL OR INTRAVENOUS?

Appropriate data to guide the selection of either IV or intra-arterial thrombolytic techniques are unavailable, but the most important factor in determining which method to use is time. If a patient must be transferred to another center to receive intra-arterial therapy or if the delay in intra-arterial therapy is too great, then IV therapy given immediately is a better choice. However, in some patients IV thrombolytic therapy is too risky, including those who have a high risk for systemic bleeding, uncontrolled hypertension, or an altered level of consciousness from a seizure or metabolic factors. These patients may be appropriate for intra-arterial thrombolytic therapy after an angiogram has been performed to determine whether a proximal (large artery) intracranial thrombus is present. After the angiogram it is reasonable to initiate intra-arterial thrombolytic therapy, provided that sufficient expertise is available.

Patients in whom IV thrombolytic therapy entails high risk are screened with angiography because there may not be an embolus in an appropriate location for lysis. Similarly, if the entire ICA is occluded or the vertebrobasilar system is involved, IV thrombolysis is unlikely to be of benefit, and although risky, intra-arterial therapy may offer more hope for success.

TECHNIQUES OF THROMBOLYSIS

Unless the patient's arteries are so severely diseased that selective catheterization of all brachiocephalic vessels will require an unacceptable duration, arteriography of both carotid arteries and at least one vertebral artery should be performed. Both the subclavian and vertebral arteries are studied to look for a proximal source for further embolization and cases in which the basilar artery fills from only one vertebral artery. Complete arteriography will also delineate the extent of collateral filling behind the acute occlusion. The presence or absence of significant stenosis(es) in the artery proximal to the intracranial clot will determine whether the infusion is to be administered regionally or locally.

In both experimental and clinical experience, successful recanalization is more frequently achieved with intra-arterial infusion[11, 12] than with systemic IV infusion of the fibrinolytic agent.[1, 4, 10, 13–15] Intra-arterial infusions can be given either *regionally* with a catheter tip placed in the ICA or *locally* by using a coaxial microcatheter with its tip placed directly into the intracranial thrombus. *Regional* infusions are technically simpler but may not deliver the fibrinolytic agent into the intracranial thrombus. The fibrinolytic agent may go only to the perfused arteries and not to the thrombus, especially if the intracranial occlusion is complete. Intracranial techniques are more complicated but reliably deliver the fibrolytic agent into the thrombus. *Local* thrombolysis produces a higher percentage of recanalization and better clinical results than do regional infusions.[5] The added increment of successful recanalization for local thrombolysis has not yet been established in patients who have some flow past the occluding thrombus or in patients who have occlusions of distal MCA branches.

Treating an acute stroke patient with intra-arterial fibrinolysis requires an experienced interventionalist, and an interventional neuroradiologist, if available, will generally perform the procedure. The question arises whether local intracranial thrombolysis should be undertaken by an interventional radiologist in the absence of an interventional neuroradiologist. In our opinion, the answer is a qualified yes. Regional infusion of the fibrinolytic agent, either into the cervical internal carotid or vertebral artery, is within the technical ability of any trained interventional radiologist. To perform a local infusion, however, the interventionalist must be thoroughly familiar both with the use of microcatheter coaxial systems for superselective catheterization and with fibrinolysis principles, including infusion, lacing, and pulse spray techniques. *Patient selection for local infusion should be confined to those patients with acute embolic intracerebral occlusions in whom there are no significant atherosclerotic stenoses at or above the carotid bifurcation.* If at all possible, an interventional radiologist who is contemplating an intracranial infusion yet has limited or no experience with intracranial thrombolysis should consult by telephone with a physician experienced in the intra-arterial treatment of stroke. Even with these stringent qualifications, there are far too many potentially treatable strokes to be managed by the small number of interventional neuroradiologists, and many acute strokes have been successfully managed by general interventional radiologists.

Whichever infusion route for the lytic agent is chosen, the infusion will be short-term (1 to 2 hours). The optimal fibrinolytic agent and its dosage and concentration have not been established. Most investigators have used either urokinase or recombinant tissue-typed plasminogen activator (rt-PA). Our preferred intra-arterial fibrinolytic agent is urokinase, and the following description assumes its use. For urokinase, 250,000 to

TABLE 1.

Summary of Current University of Colorado Health Sciences Center Protocol

Local infusion (intracranial catheter)

UK *preparation* (2 separate solutions, for pulsed spray and infusion)

for the *pulsed spray* portion of treatment

    Concentration of UK, 25,000 IU/mL

    Heparin, 500 U/mL

for the *infusion* portion of treatment

    Concentration, 5,000–10,000 IU of UK/mL

UK administration

    Microcatheter placed beyond the thrombus into patent artery

    Pulsed intraclot administration of concentrated UK while withdrawing catheter: *gentle* pulses of ≤ 0.1 mL every 10–20 sec

    Give ≤ 500,000 IU by pulsed spray until flow re-established (over 30–60 min)

    After flow is present, give infusion at 4,000–10,000 IU/min with the catheter tip just within the proximal residual thrombus (concentration, 5,000–10,000 IU of UK/mL)

    Maximum UK dose, 1.25 million U, including pulse spray and infusion

Systemic heparin

Serial angiograms approximately every 30 min

Serial neurologic exams approximately every 15 min

Halt therapy if clinical or angiographic signs suggest intracranial hemorrhage

Regional infusion (catheter in neck)

UK concentration, 5,000–10,000 IU/mL

UK administered at 250,000–500,000 IU/hr into the ICA or VA

Maximum, 1.25 million IU

Systemic heparin

Serial angiograms approximately every 30 min

Serial neurologic exams approximately every 15 min

Halt therapy if clinical or angiographic signs suggest intracranial hemorrhage

Abbreviations: UK, urokinase; ICA, internal carotid artery; VA, vertebral artery.

750,000 U is commonly used, with a maximum of 1 to 1.5 million units. For rt-PA, dosages range from 20 to 40 mg, [5, 16, 17] with a maximum of 60 mg.[5] Most investigators use full systemic heparinization, and many mix heparin with the urokinase in local infusions. Our current protocol is listed in Table 1.

LOCAL INFUSION

The most commonly encountered intracranial arterial occlusion involves the MCA (Fig 1), which accounts for up to 87% of acute ischemic strokes. Catheterization of the MCA is not technically difficult for an interventional radiologist familiar with superselective catheterization. It is generally more difficult, for example, to selectively catheterize a specific hepatic arterial branch in the liver for a chemotherapy infusion.

If the thrombus/embolus is in the usual MCA location, the microcatheter in most cases will easily pass completely through the thrombus to the M1-M2 junction of the MCA at its entrance into the sylvian fissure. A small injection of contrast will confirm that the catheter tip lies in patient M2 arteries beyond the occluding thrombus. We use urokinase as the fibrinolytic agent, mixed at a concentration of 25,000 IU/mL. Other investigators have used 10,000 to 50,000 IU/mL. Urokinase is injected in *gentle, small* pulsed increments of about 0.1 mL because the urokinase is being injected into a closed system and cerebral arteries have much thinner walls than do peripheral arteries. Several pulses are administered *distal* to the occluding thrombus on the assumption that incipient thrombosis in the distal microcirculation will be minimized. The microcatheter is then withdrawn through the thrombus while delivering pulses of 0.1 mL of concentrated urokinase into the thrombus. After these small pulses have produced sufficient clot lysis to restore flow through the previously obstructed artery, an infusion of urokinase is initiated with the catheter tip placed within the proximal end of the residual (nonoccluding) thrombus. Urokinase is infused at 250,000 U/hr, and serial arteriography is performed through the microcatheter every 30 minutes. The infusion is terminated when thrombus is no longer visible. In some instances a thrombus will migrate distally, in which case the catheter tip is advanced and reinserted into the most proximal portion of the thrombus. If multiple small thrombi are present in the distal branches in or beyond M2, it is not productive (or possible) to place the catheter tip into each occluded segment. It may be valuable to continue the infusion in this circumstance until the maximum intended dose of urokinase is reached. If there is a single occlusion in the M2 segment, the catheter tip can usually be advanced into the thrombus at its new location.

The treatment is illustrated in the following case (see Fig 1).

A 73-year-old female collapsed while playing golf. She was brought emergently to University Hospital, where on physical examination she was obtunded and had right-sided hemiplegia. Computed tomography (Fig 1, A) showed no intracranial hemorrhage and no brain swelling. An increased density was seen in the horizontal (M1) segment of the left MCA, consistent with an acute thrombus ("hyperdense MCA sign"). A diagnosis of acute embolic stroke was made. (In later workup the patient was found to have intermittent atrial fibrillation, previ-

D.A. Kumpe and R.L. Hughes

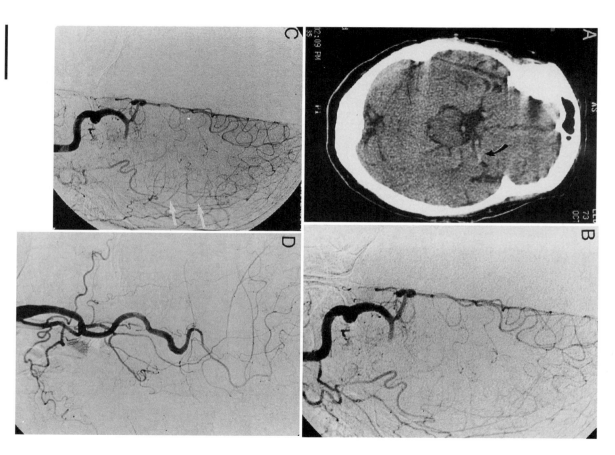

FIGURE 1.

Seventy-three-year-old woman with sudden-onset hemiplegia about 3 hours before the angiogram. **A,** CT scan showing a "hyperdense middle cerebral artery (MCA) sign" (*arrow*) consistent with a thrombus in the M1 segment of the left MCA. No swelling or hypodensity is noted in the parenchymal distribution of the left MCA. **B,** anteroposterior (AP) arteriogram of the left common carotid artery, early phase, showing acute occlusion of the M1 segment of the left MCA. **C,** AP arteriogram of the left common carotid artery, late arterial phase, with visualization of the MCA branches (*arrows*) distal to the occlusion of the proximal MCA and filling via collateral flow. **D,** lateral arteriogram of the left common carotid artery, early phase. Only branches of the anterior cerebral artery are seen.

(Continued.)

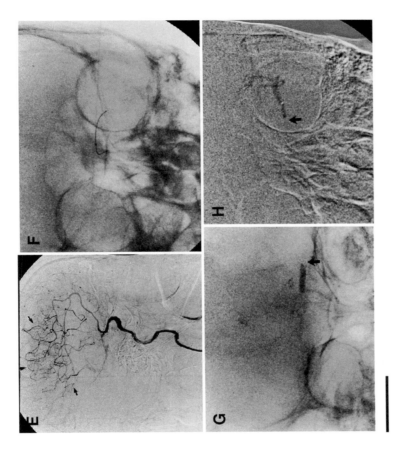

FIGURE 1 (cont.).
___

E, lateral arteriogram of the left common carotid artery, late arterial phase, with filling of distal middle cerebral branches via collateral flow *(arrows).* **F,** passage of the microcatheter into the M1 portion of the left MCA. **G,** injection of contrast through the microcatheter into the proximal M1 segment of the left MCA. Complete occlusion of the midportion of M1 *(arrow)* is noted. **H,** microcatheter passed through the clot (distal end of the clot is at the *arrow*) into the distal M1 segment. Contrast injection confirms patency of the M2 branches distal to the occluding thrombus.

(Continued.)

ously undiagnosed). Cerebral arteriography, performed about 3.5 hours after the onset of ictus, showed the expected occlusion of the proximal M1 segment of the left MCA (Fig 1, B and D). Late-phase images showed filling of MCA branches distal to the occlusion via collateral flow (Fig 1, C and E). The lack of brain swelling/hypodensity on the initial CT scan and collateral filling of branches distal to the occlusion are both indicators favoring a satisfactory outcome of fibrinolysis. Local fibrinolysis was performed. A microcatheter was passed through the occlusion (Fig 1, F and G) and the thrombus treated with pulses of 0.1 mL of concentrated urokinase. After 250,000 IU of urokinase delivered in pulses, the clot had migrated from the proximal M1 segment to the M1-M2 junction of the MCA, and there was flow past the residual clot (Fig 1, H–J). Another 450,000 U of urokinase was administered by continuous infusion at 250,000 IU/hr with the catheter tip just proximal to the thrombus. Arteriographic findings after a total of 700,000 IU of urokinase were normal (Fig 1, K and L). Computed tomography at 24 and 48 hours (Fig 1, M) after infusion showed significant brain edema with some petechial hemorrhage in the basal ganglia, findings that cleared slowly over the next several weeks (Fig

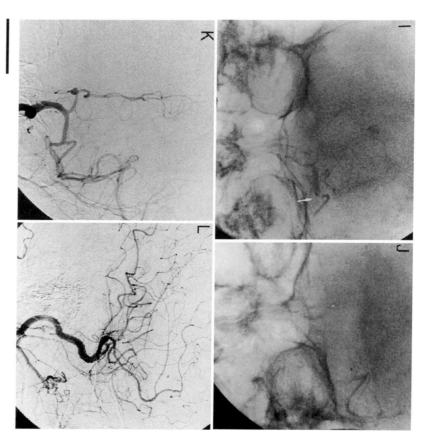

FIGURE 1 (cont.).

I, microcatheter withdrawn through the clot while lacing urokinase in small pulses of approximately 0.1 mL. The clot (*arrow*) has migrated distally and lies in the distal M1 segment at the trifurcation of the MCA. **J,** flow re-established, with persistent thrombus after 250,000 IU of urokinase was administered in pulses of 0.1 mL into the thrombus. At this point, urokinase was infused with the catheter tip immediately proximal to the residual clot. **K,** normal AP angiogram after 700,000 IU of urokinase. **L,** normal lateral angiogram after 700,000 IU of urokinase.

(Continued.)

1, N). Clinically, the patient's hemiparesis had cleared by 24 hours; she had only an expressive aphasia, which gradually improved over the next month. At 15-month follow-up, the patient was neurologically intact with a trivial expressive aphasia.

REGIONAL INFUSION

If intracranial infusion is not possible because of inexperience or intervening stenoses, regional infusion into the appropriate extracranial artery is technically straightforward. The tip of the diagnostic catheter, usually 5 French in diameter, is placed in the cervical internal carotid or vertebral artery. Urokinase is infused at 250,000 to 500,000 IU/hr, with serial arteriography at least every 30 minutes and neurologic examination at least every 15 minutes.

After fibrinolysis, a CT scan is obtained to look for signs of hemorrhage. Patients who do not have hemorrhage are treated with systemic

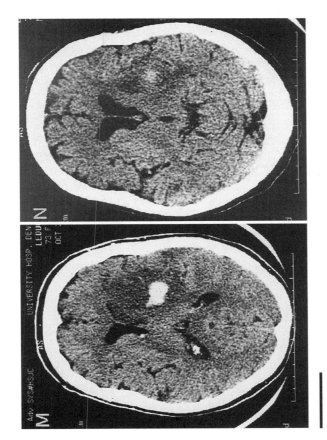

FIGURE 1 (cont.).

M, CT scan 48 hours after urokinase administration. Hypodensity and a mass effect are seen in the right MCA distribution because of brain swelling, with petechial hemorrhage in the posterior basal ganglia. The patient had an expressive aphasia at this time but had normal motor and sensory function of her right side. N, CT scan 14 days after urokinase therapy with improved CT findings. The patient's motor examination was normal; expressive aphasia was persistent but improved. The aphasia cleared nearly completely over a period of several months.

heparin. It is not clear whether patients who have petechial hemorrhage after fibrinolysis should receive anticoagulation or not, but most investigators refrain from using it. Staining from contrast in the brain parenchyma seen on CT scan after fibrinolysis is common[18] and will clear within 24 hours. It is common to have CT findings of infarction (hypodensity, edema), possibly with petechial hemorrhage after fibrinolysis (Fig 1, M).

RESULTS OF THROMBOLYSIS IN ACUTE ISCHEMIC STROKE

The results of local infusion of fibrinolytic agents in the carotid and vertebrobasilar systems are given in Tables 2 and 3. Results of earlier studies are summarized by del Zoppo and Otis.[7] A review of the literature is confusing because of variable patient selection criteria and different outcome measures (recanalization, clinical improvement, intracranial hemorrhage, clinical deterioration).

CAROTID-TERRITORY OCCLUSIONS

Recent studies indicate that the results of thrombolysis will be affected by the site of arterial occlusion, the findings on pretreatment CT scan, and the extent of collateral flow distal to the acute occlusion. Four papers have outlined the neurologic outcome by location of the thrombus.[5, 8, 16, 17]

TABLE 2.
Carotid Territory: Intracranial Superselective Infusions of Fibrinolytic Agent

Author	Agent	N	Patency Rate	Outcome	Intracranial Bleed (Deterioration)
Zeumer,[17] 1993	UK/rt-PA	33	13/33 complete 18/33 partial	Minimal mild deficit, 10; moderate, 7; severe, 8; died, 8	6/33 (18%) (no deterioration)
Barnwell,[19] 1994*	UK	13	10/13 (77%)	9/13 (69%) improved at 48 hr	2/13 (15%) (asymptomatic)
Barr,[18] 1994	UK	11	6/11 complete 4/11 partial	8/11 completely or moderately improved	2/11† (18%)
Higashida,[20] 1994*	UK	27 (45 vascular territories)	37/45 vascular territories	18/27 improved 9/27 deaths long-term	3/27 (11%)
Barnwell,[8] 1995‡	UK	17	13/17	Excellent, 7/17 Improved, significant deficit, 5/17 Death, 5/17 (all outcomes at 3 mo)	3/17 (18%)
Sasaki,[5] 1995	UK, rt-PA	35	Complete, 16/35 Partial, 12/35 No change, 7/35	See Table 5	8/35 (23%) 7/35 (asymptomatic) 1/35 (symptomatic)

*Carotid and basilar artery territories.
†No hemorrhage reported,[18] but two hemorrhages were reported in the same series,[21] also in 1994.
‡Includes patients from an earlier report (above).
Abbreviations: UK, urokinase; *rt-PA,* recombinant tissue-type plasminogen activator.

TABLE 3.
Vertebrobasilar Territory: Local Infusions of Fibrinolytic Agent

Author	Agent	N	Patency Rate	Outcome	Intracranial Bleed
Hacke,[22] 1988	SK/UK	43	19/43	Favorable, 10/43	4/43 (9%) (all 4 died, 2 of hemorrhage)
Möbius,[23] 1991	SK/UK	18	14/18		
Zeumer,[17] 1993	UK, rt-PA	28	Complete, 21/28; Incomplete, 6/28	10/28 survived > 3 mo, 7/10 with minimal/mild deficit	2/28 (7%) (no deterioration)
Barnwell,[8] 1995	UK	7	6/7	Good/excellent, 4/7; Moderate, 2/7; Died, 1/7	1/7 (14%) (no deterioration)
Sasaki,[5] 1995	UK, rt-PA	9	Complete, 7/9; Partial, 2/9	Good, 3/9; Severe deficit, 5/9; Died, 1/9	2/9 (22%) (no deterioration)

Abbreviations: SK, streptokinase; UK, urokinase; rt-PA, recombinant tissue-type plasminogen activator.

Zeumer and colleagues[17] showed that there is significant variability in outcome in treating carotid-territory stroke locally, depending on the initial location of the thrombus within five defined MCA areas and, more importantly, on whether complete recanalization has occurred. Patients with successful recanalization had better outcomes than patients who had incomplete or no recanalization (Table 4).

Barnwell et al.[8] treated 26 patients with acute intracranial occlusions. In 11 patients who had acute M1 MCA occlusions, clinical evaluation at 3 months showed that 5 patients (45%) had significant improvement whereas another 2 patients (18%) had a moderate recovery and 4 patients (36%) ultimately died. None of the deaths were attributed to fibrinolytic therapy.

Sasaki and colleagues[5] compared the results of local high-dose fibrinolytic therapy in 44 patients with results in 51 patients treated with either regional (n = 18) or IV (n = 33) fibrinolysis using either urokinase or rt-PA. Both the carotid and vertebrobasilar territories were infused. Carotid-territory results are listed in Table 5 for the three techniques. The outcomes of patients who have IV and regional infusions were worse than the outcomes of patients undergoing local thrombolysis. No difference could be found in the recanalization rate of urokinase or rt-PA, a finding also reported previously by Zeumer et al.[17] The outcome was good and the size of infarction reduced in patients who had complete recanalization of the affected artery.

Theron and co-workers have a large experience with carotid-territory strokes, unfortunately only reported in abstract form.[16] They treated 118 patients with 20 to 40 mg of rt-PA into the ICA and MCA. Patients who did not have involvement of the lenticulostriate arteries by the occlusion (i.e., occlusion at the distal M1 segment and beyond) had a 75% rate of good results and a 0% rate of bad results for fibrinolysis performed up to 12 hours after the onset of ictus. On the other hand, patients who had involvement of the lenticulostriate arteries had a 57% rate of good results and a 23% rate of bad results. In the latter group the risk of hemorrhage was 16% if they were treated after the sixth hour vs. 1% if they were treated before the sixth hour. There were 7 deaths in this experience, 6

TABLE 4.
Clinical Result According to the Degree of Recanalization

Degree of Recanalization	N	Neurologic Deficit			
		Minimal/Mild	Moderate	Severe	Dead
Complete	13	10 (77%)	2 (15%)	1 (8%)	
Incomplete	18		5 (28%)	5 (28%)	8 (44%)
None	2				2 (100%)

(Data summarized from Zeumer H, Freitag H, Zanella F, et al: Local intra-arterial fibrinolytic therapy in patients with stroke: Urokinase versus recombinant tissue plasminogen activator (r-TPA). *Neuroradiology* 35:159–162, 1993.)

TABLE 5.
Clinical Result of Local, Regional, and Intravenous Infusion According to Thrombus Location

Occlusion Location	N	Neurological Deficit			
		Minimal/Mild	Moderate	Severe	Dead
Local infusion					
M1	13	5 (38%)		7 (54%)	1 (8%)
M2	12	6 (50%)	3 (25%)	3 (25%)	
ICA	10	2 (20%)	3 (30%)	2 (20%)	3 (30%)
Regional infusion					
M1	10	1 (10%)	4 (40%)	4 (40%)	1 (10%)
M2	6	2 (33%)	2 (33%)	2 (33%)	
ICA	2				2 (100%)
Intravenous infusion					
M1	11	2 (18%)	4 (36%)	2 (18%)	3 (27%)
M2	8	4 (50%)	1 (12.5%)	2 (25%)	1 (12.5%)
ICA	8		3 (37.5%)	2 (25%)	3 (37.5%)

Abbreviations: M1, M2, segments of the middle cerebral artery; *ICA,* internal carotid artery.
(Data synthesized from Sasaki O, Takeuchi S, Koike T, et al: Fibrinolytic therapy for acute embolic stroke: intravenous, intracarotid, and intra-arterial local approaches. *Neurosurgery* 36:246–253, 1995.)

because of "inefficient revascularizaiton of the parenchyma with vasogenic edema."

The aforementioned experiences document substantial variability in the clinical outcome of patients with acute occlusions in any of the territories involved, particularly in the proximal MCA: good outcomes occurred in 38% to 60% of the patients treated, and the incidence of severe residual deficit or mortality varied from 10% to 62%. In the reported experience with intra-arterial thrombolysis, no stratification of results has been done regarding patient risk factors, yet it is clear that patients with the same type of occlusion have different risks. A proximal MCA occlusion successfully lysed in timely fashion may well have a different outcome depending on clinical risk factors. A 40-year-old patient with coronary artery disease who sustains a middle cerebral embolus during cardiac catheterization will likely have a better outcome with fibrinolysis than an 85-year-old patient with myocardiopathy who has an acute cardiogenic embolus in the same location treated within the same time frame.

Instead of considering the location of the thrombus, von Kummer and Hacke[10,24] investigated the value of initial CT findings and collateral circulation distal to the occlusion on pretreatment arteriograms as predictors of outcome in 61 patients with acute carotid-territory strokes treated with intra-arterial and IV rt-PA. Clinical outcome was significantly better if CT showed minimal hypodensity or focal brain swelling, angiography demonstrated a patent ICA and adequate collateral filling of arteries distal to the occlusion, and arterial recanalization occurred. The extent of parenchymal hypodensity did not correlate significantly with the site of arterial occlusion. Mortality was high when the prefibrinolysis CT showed a large hypodensity (78%) or brain swelling (63%) and when the arteriogram showed ICA occlusion (55%) or scarce collaterals (55%).

Commensurate with adequate good collateral flow, parts of the ischemic volume of brain (ischemic penumbra) can remain viable beyond the "golden period" of 6 hours, and it may be that fibrinolytic therapy can be successfully applied later than the 6-hour time limit in such patients as one recent experience suggests. Barnwell and colleagues[19] reported clinical improvement in 9 of 13 patients (69%) who were treated with intraarterial urokinase 3.5 to 48 (mean, 12) hours after the onset of ictus. All patients had been excluded from a 6-hour multicenter thrombolytic trial because of duration of symptoms, recent surgery, age, seizure, or myocardial infarction. All patients who improved had normal initial CT scans.

On the other hand, a good clinical outcome is not ensured even when all the criteria outlined and followed. Major cerebral infarctions can result from acute occlusions that are rapidly recanalized if the collateral circulation is poor. A case in our recent experience is illustrative (Fig 2).

A 62-year-old man sustained an embolic occlusion of the right posterior cerebral artery while undergoing diagnostic cerebral arteriography. He had a history of repeated transient ischemic attacks despite aspirin. Doppler studies showed bilateral carotid bifurcation atherosclerosis, with 60% to 80% stenosis of the left ICA origin and 40% narrowing of the right ICA origin. During his arteriogram, hemiparesis and a left homonymous hemianopsia developed shortly after catheterization of the right common carotid artery. Vertebral arteriography revealed an embolus in the proximal right posterior cerebral artery (Fig 2, A). The embolus was completely lysed and a normal angiographic appearance restored within 3.5 hours of the event (Fig 2, B). An infarct nonetheless developed in the entire distribution of the posterior cerebral artery and the patient was left with a complete left visual field cut (Fig 2, C).

A recent case report of Barr et al.[25] is of importance to vascular surgeons.

A 71-year-old patient sustained a middle cerebral occlusion during carotid endarterectomy. The occlusion was detected by a change in the somatosensory evoked potential monitored intraoperatively for the median and peroneal nerves. A single-shot intraoperative arteriogram showed an occlusive thrombus in the proximal MCA. With a portable C-arm fluoroscope moved into the operating room, a microcatheter was introduced through the arteriotomy into the MCA and the thrombus was successfully lysed with urokinase. The patient had no neurologic deficit 8 days after surgery.

INTERNAL CAROTID ARTERY THROMBUS

There are few reports of lysis of a thrombus in the ICA. In the series of 16 patients reported by Maiza and associates,[26] 8 had complete thrombosis of the ICA, 5 had proximal stenoses of the internal carotid with extensive thrombus, 1 had thrombus confined to the carotid siphon, and 2

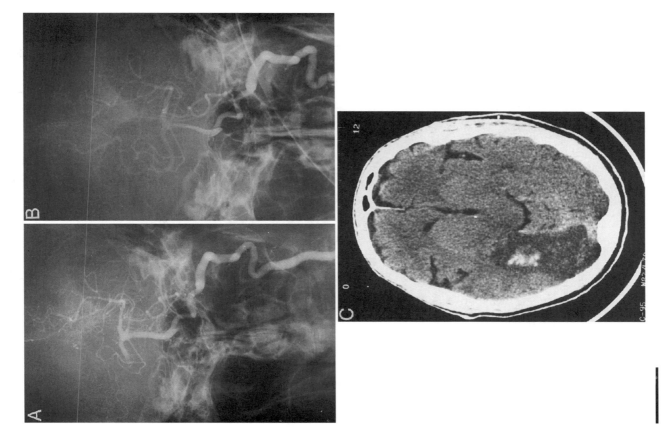

FIGURE 2.

Sixty-two-year-old man undergoing diagnostic arteriographic evaluation of transient ischemic attacks in the distribution of the left carotid artery in whom acute hemiparesis and left homonymous hemianopsia developed. **A**, left vertebral arteriography showing acute occlusion of the proximal right posterior cerebral artery. **B**, after successful thrombolysis with restoration of flow to the entire distribution of the affected artery within 3.5 hours of the embolic event. **C**, CT scan 48 hours after thrombolysis showing infarction of the distribution of the right posterior cerebral artery. The patient had persistent left homonymous hemianopsia that did not clear.

had middle cerebral emboli. Fibrinolytic therapy was given intraoperatively during carotid endarterectomy in 3 and via catheter in 13. Fibrinolysis occurred in all patients. One patient died of a frontal lobe hemorrhage. All other patients survived and had at least some neurologic improvement. Barnwell et al.[8] treated 6 patients with ICA plus MCA occlusions. Flow through the circle of Willis was restored in all 6; 2 patients had residual occlusion of the ICA. Two patients had no residual symptoms, 3 had significant residual deficits, and 1 died. In the Zeumer series,[17] patients who had occlusions of the ICA extending into the proximal middle and anterior cerebral arteries, a configuration they designated as an "M"-type occlusion, had terrible outcomes: of 14 such patients, 2 (14%) had a moderate residual deficit, 4 (29%) had a severe residual deficit, and 8 (57%) died. In the same setting, Sasaki et al.[5] found low rates of recanalization and similar poor clinical results.

When an intraluminal thrombus is free floating and nonocclusive, the role of fibrinolytic therapy is even less clear because the thrombus will often clear spontaneously with simple anticoagulation. In one experience, Combe et al.[27] studied seven patients who had patent ICAs with intraluminal clots identified angiographically. Six thrombi were longer than 1.5 cm. At examination, four patients had had a mild stroke and 3 had suffered a major stroke. Three had had a prior transient ischemic attack. By angiography the seven patients had three severe atherosclerotic stenoses, three ulcerated plaques, and one dissection causing the thrombus. One patient died. The other six patients were treated with anticoagulation without neurologic complication. At 4 weeks, repeat angiography showed that four patients had complete resolution of the thrombus, one had partial lysis, and one had mild extension. Five patients underwent delayed endarterectomy.

In our opinion, a large nonocclusive thrombus adherent to an ICA origin stenosis in a patient who otherwise has no angiographically demonstrable arterial occlusion should be managed with anticoagulation and expeditious surgical thromboendarterectomy. Endovascular treatment in this circumstance should be reserved for patients who cannot tolerate surgery. In addition, acutely symptomatic patients with a small amount of intracranial nonocclusive thrombus in the A1 and/or M1 segments of the anterior and middle cerebral arteries recover satisfactorily with anticoagulation and no fibrinolysis.

VERTEBROBASILAR OCCLUSION

There is a strong correlation between the initial clinical state and the outcome of lysis in patients with vertebrobasilar occlusions. Patients who are comatose and who have lost brain stem reflexes have a poor prognosis no matter what the angiographic outcome.[17]

Although favorable outcomes with recanalization of acute vertebrobasilar occlusions have been reported, the grim prognosis of this disease must be recognized. In the three largest experiences treating vertebrobasilar occlusions with regional or local thrombolysis, mortality rates were 64%,[17] 67%,[22] and 68%.[28] In the Sasaki series there was a 27% mortality rate, but another 53% of the patients had a severe neurologic deficit.

Recanalization rates are high with basilar artery occlusion,[5, 17] and patients who ultimately recover from a vertebrobasilar ischemic stroke almost invariably have recanalization of the occlusion.[5, 17, 22] However, older patients with an occlusion that involves more than a focal area of the basilar artery, with poor collateral filling distal to the occlusion, or with loss of consciousness and brain stem reflexes have a poor prognosis no matter what the angiographic outcome.[17] In their analysis of 40 patients with vertebrobasilar ischemic strokes treated with intra-arterial urokinase ($n = 33$), intra-arterial rt-PA ($n = 1$), and IV rt-PA ($n = 6$), von Kummer[28] found that despite recanalization in 5 of 10 of their patients with "long" occlusions, all the patients died. Among 16 patients with scarce collaterals, despite recanalization in 9, only 2 patients survived with moderate disability. A good clinical outcome correlated significantly with younger age, short occlusions, good collaterals, and recanalization at 24 hours after the onset of ictus.

COMPLICATIONS—HEMORRHAGIC TRANSFORMATION AND PARENCHYMAL HEMATOMA

Inherent in the use of all thrombolytic agents is the risk of intracranial hemorrhage, the mechanisms for which are not yet understood. Hemorrhage in infarcted brain tissue may occur without a mass effect (petechial hemorrhages) or may be accompanied by a mass effect (parenchymal hematoma), frequently with clinical deterioration. The incidence of *symptomatic* hemorrhagic transformation (usually with parenchymal hematoma) is 5% among patients treated with standard means. The incidence of asymptomatic petechial hemorrhage is 15% to 43%. The longer the delay before institution of fibrinolytic therapy, the higher the risk of intracranial hemorrhage. Because the time to reperfusion varies from study to study, direct comparisons are difficult. The National Institutes of Health rt-PA trial[3] found a 6.4% rate of symptomatic intracranial hemorrhage and a 5% rate of asymptomatic hemorrhagic transformation in rt-PA–treated patients (vs. 0.6% and 4%, respectively, in the placebo group). This was an IV trial with the drug administered within 3 hours. The European Cooperative Acute Stroke Study trial[2] compared IV rt-PA with placebo within 6 hours of symptom onset; 39.8% of all patients had some degree of intracranial hemorrhage. No difference could be found in the treatment and control groups in the incidence of intracranial hemorrhage, but the incidence of hemorrhagic infarction was higher in the placebo group than the rt-PA group (30.3% vs. 23.0%, $P < 0.001$), whereas the incidence of parenchymal hematoma was higher in the rt-PA group (6.5% vs 19.8%, $P < 0.001$). The expected rate of hemorrhage for a longer time window, often the case in intra-arterial therapy, will be higher, especially if there is also an adverse selection of cases treated intra-arterially.

In the carotid territory the incidence of parenchymal hematoma formation after intra-arterial infusion of urokinase or streptokinase was 10.6% in four trials.[11, 12, 29, 30] This was similar to a 9.5% rate of parenchymal hematoma found in four earlier prospective trials using IV rt-PA.[1, 10, 13, 14]

SUMMARY

The following conclusions seem appropriate at this time[7]:

1. Symptomatic carotid-territory occlusions can be treated with fibrinolytic agents. Recanalization and clinical improvement in MCA occlusions can be expected when treatment is started within 4 hours of the onset of ictus. In the vertebrobasilar area, recanalizations are also possible, but with less favorable results.

2. Thrombolytic therapy can rescue viable tissue within the "ischemic penumbra," the size of which is related to collateral flow, the location of the arterial occlusion, and the presence and extent of arteriosclerotic cerebrovascular disease.

3. There may be a relation between the location of an embolus and the efficacy of recanalization. Intracranial emboli are more susceptible to thrombolysis than is atheroma-based in situ thrombosis in the cervical portion of the ICA, particularly for systemic thrombolysis.

4. Early partial or complete recanalization of occluded cerebral arteries correlates with a significant reduction in residual infarction volume by CT.

5. The incidence of successful arterial recanalization is greater when the thrombolytic agents are delivered intra-arterially rather than by systemic infusion.

6. The incidence of symptomatic hemorrhagic transformation after intraarterial or IV fibrinolysis initiated within four hours of onset of ictus appears to be similar to that in patients who are not treated with fibrinolysis.

Intra-arterial and IV thrombolysis for acute stroke should be applied only to carefully selected patients. Further trials are clearly necessary to better establish time limits after the onset of ictus for fibrinolytic intervention in the large variety of clinical stroke syndromes, the location of occlusions most likely to be treated successfully with the least risk of complications, the optimal dosage rates and route(s) of administration of fibrinolytic treatment of arterial occlusions in different locations, and the role of metabolic blocking agents. In the meantime, however, an immediate problem is the dissemination of knowledge among the lay public *and physicians* that an incipient stroke may warrant prompt interaction. It is widely known that a patient with crushing chest pain may have an immediate need for administration of a "clot-busting drug." At present, there is no similar awareness of the clinical urgency facing a patient who experiences an acute ictal event. With today's technology, in a properly selected patient a major ischemic stroke can be reversed. Time is brain!

REFERENCES

1. del Zoppo G, Poeck K, Pessin M: Recombinant tissue plasminogen activator in acute thrombotic and embolic stroke. *Ann Neurol* 32:78–86, 1992.
2. Hacke W, Kaste M, Fieschi C, et al: Intravenous thrombolysis with recombinant tissue plasminogen activator for acute hemispheric stroke. The European Cooperative Acute Stroke Study (ECASS). *JAMA* 274:1017–1025, 1995.
3. National Institute of Neurological Disorders and Stroke rt-PA Stroke Study

Group: Tissue plasminogen activator for acute ischemic stroke. *N Engl J Med* 333:1581–1587, 1995.

4. Russell D, Madden K, Clark W, et al: Tissue plasminogen activator cerebrovascular thrombolysis in rabbits is dependent on the rate and route of administration. *Stroke* 23:388–393, 1992.

5. Sasaki O, Takeuchi S, Koike T, et al: Fibrinolytic therapy for acute embolic stroke: Intravenous, intracarotid, and intra-arterial local approaches. *Neurosurgery* 36:246–253, 1995.

6. Caplan L, Hier D, D'Cruz I: Cerebral embolism in the Michael Reese Stroke Registry. *Stroke* 14:450, 1983.

7. del Zoppo G, Otis S: Thrombolytic therapy for acute stroke, in Comerota A (ed): *Thrombolytic Therapy for Peripheral Vascular Disease.* Philadelphia, JB Lippincott, 1995, pp 399–417.

8. Barnwell S, Nesbit G, Clark W: Local thrombolytic therapy for cerebrovascular disease: Current Oregon Health Sciences University experience (July 1991 through April 1995). *J Vasc Interv Radiol* 6:79S–82S, 1995.

9. de Bono DP, More RS: Prevention and management of bleeding complications after thrombolysis. *Int J Cardiol* 38:1–6, 1993.

10. von Kummer R, Hacke W: Safety and efficacy of intravenous tissue plasminogen activator and heparin in acute middle cerebral artery. *Stroke* 23:646, 1992.

11. Mori E, Tabuchi M, Yoshida T, et al: Intracarotid urokinase with thromboembolic occlusion of the middle cerebral artery. *Stroke* 19:802, 1988.

12. Matsumoto K, Satoh K: Topical intraarterial urokinase infusion for acute stroke, in Hacke W, del Zoppo G, Hirschberg M (eds): *Thrombolytic Therapy in Acute Ischemic Stroke.* Heidelberg, Springer-Verlag, 1991, p 207.

13. Mori E, Yoneda Y, Tabuchi M: Intravenous recombinant tissue plasminogen activator in acute carotid artery territory stroke. *Neurology* 42:976, 1992.

14. Yamaguchi T: Intravenous tissue plasminogen activator in acute thromboembolic stroke: A placebo-controlled, double-blind trial, in del Zoppo G, Mori E, Hacke W (eds): *Thrombolytic Therapy in Acute Ischemic Stroke,* ed 2. Heidelberg, Springer-Verlag, 1993.

15. Brott T, Haley E, Levy D: Urgent therapy for stroke: I. Pilot study of tissue plasminogen activator administered within 90 minutes. *Stroke* 23:632, 1992.

16. Theron J, Coskun O, Payelle G, et al: Local intraarterial thrombolysis of ischemic strokes in the carotid territory. *Radiology* 197:206A, 1995.

17. Zeumer H, Freitag H, Zanella F, et al: Local intra-arterial fibrinolytic therapy in patients with stroke: Urokinase versus recombinant tissue plasminogen activator (r-TPA). *Neuroradiology* 35:159–162, 1993.

18. Barr J, Mathis J, Wildenhain S, et al: Acute stroke intervention with intraarterial urokinase infusion. *J Vasc Interv Radiol* 5:705–712, 1994.

19. Barnwell S, Clark W, Nguyen T, et al: Safety and efficacy of delayed intraarterial urokinase therapy with mechanical clot disruption for thromboembolic stroke. *AJNR Am J Neuroradiol* 15:1817–1822, 1994.

20. Higashida R, Halbach V, Barnwell S, et al: Thrombolytic therapy in acute stroke. *J Endovasc Surg* 1:4–15, 1994.

21. Wildenhain C, Jungreis C, Barr J, et al: CT after intracranial intraarterial thrombolysis for acute stroke. *AJNR Am J Neuroradiol* 15:487–492, 1994.

22. Hacke W, Zeumer H, Ferbeert A: Intraarterial thrombolytic therapy improves outcome in patients with acute vertebrobasilar occlusive disease. *Stroke* 19:1216, 1988.

23. Möbius E, Berg-Dammer E, Kühne D, et al: Local thrombolytic therapy in acute basilar artery occlusion: Experience with 18 patients, in Hacke W, del Zoppo G, Hirschberg M (eds): *Thrombolytic Therapy in Acute Ischemic Stroke.* Berlin, Springer-Verlag, 1991, p 213.

24. von Kummer R: Early neuroradiological predictors for clinical outcome in hemispheric stroke caused by MCA occlusion, in *Changing Perspectives in the Management of Stroke*. Denver, Medical Education Collaborative, 1994, pp 26–30.

25. Barr J, Horowitz M, Mathis J, et al: Intraoperative urokinase infusion for embolic stroke during carotid endarterectomy. *Neurosurgery* 36:606–611, 1995.

26. Maiza D, Theron J, Pelouze G, et al: Local fibrinolytic therapy in ischemic carotid pathology. *Ann Vasc Surg* 2:205–214, 1988.

27. Combe J, Poinsard P, Besancenot J, et al: Free-floating thrombus of the extracranial internal carotid artery. *Ann Vasc Surg* 4:558–562, 1990.

28. von Kummer R: Thrombolytic therapy of basilar artery occlusion: Preconditions for recanalization and good clinical outcome, in *Changing Perspectives in the Management of Stroke*. Denver, Medical Education Collaborative, 1994, pp 40–44.

29. del Zoppo G, Ferbert A, Otis S: Local intraarterial fibrinolytic therapy in acute carotid territory stroke: A pilot study. *Stroke* 19:307, 1988.

30. Theron J, Courtheoux P, Casaseo A: Local intraarterial fibrinolysis in the carotid territory. *AJNR Am J Neuroradiol* 10:753–765, 1989.

Spiral Computed Tomographic Angiography in Evaluation of the Carotid Bifurcation

James B. Knox, M.D.

Fellow in Vascular Surgery, Brigham and Women's Hospital, Boston, Massachusetts

Anthony D. Whittemore, M.D.

Professor of Surgery, Harvard Medical School; Chief, Division of Vascular Surgery, Brigham and Women's Hospital, Boston, Massachusetts

With a reported 1% to 2% incidence of stroke associated with conventional cerebral angiography, increasing reliance is being placed on color-assisted duplex scanning in the preoperative evaluation of extracranial carotid disease.[1,2] Although the accuracy of this noninvasive modality has largely obviated the need for routine angiography in many centers, several sources of misinterpretation exist and necessitate further imaging.[3] Duplex scanning may be inadequate for the evaluation of carotid disease if the vessels are particularly tortuous or if the carotid bifurcation is high in the neck or enveloped in heavy circumferential calcification. Duplex scanning may misinterpret a high-grade stenosis or pseudo-occlusion as totally occluded.[3] If a pseudo-occlusion is identified, the duplex scan frequently cannot give an adequate assessment of the quality of the distal extracranial internal carotid artery, i.e., is the vessel of normal caliber or is it sclerotic or hypoplastic.

Although MR angiography (MRA) is frequently recommended and is highly sensitive in diagnosing carotid stenoses, it may result in overestimation of the degree of stenosis or in false positive diagnoses of occlusion.[4,5] Magnetic resonance angiography gives little information regarding the quality of the distal internal carotid in cases of pseudo-occlusion and also lacks efficacy when vessels are tortuous. Motion artifact and patient intolerance further decrease the usefulness of MRA.

Many recommend the use of conventional intra-arterial angiography when confronted with an equivocal duplex scan. An invasive procedure with significant morbidity, angiography may also fail to differentiate occlusion from pseudo-occlusion in the presence of extremely slow flow.[6] Again, only the image from flow of contrast is obtained, and little may be learned regarding the nature of the plaque or the distal internal carotid artery in the presence of a "string sign."

Advances in Vascular Surgery®, vol. 4

Spiral CT angiography is a relatively new noninvasive modality that provides (1) reformatted images of the contrast-enhanced arterial lumen similar to conventional angiography and (2) axial views that yield additional information regarding the vessel itself.[7-13] Spiral CT techniques allow rapid, continuous scanning as the patient is advanced through a rotating gantry. Contrast may be administered intravenously and data acquisition timed to visualize the contrast as it flows through the arterial system. Early attempts with slower, thin-section dynamic CT scanners required a contrast bolus and continuous drip and frequently visualized only a small portion of the carotid artery. The introduction of slip-ring CT technology with rapid imaging and the manipulation of data on three-dimensional workstations has resulted in the present-day spiral CT angiography, which provides images closely resembling those available with conventional angiography. As modifications in technique improve image resolution, this modality may play a significant role in diagnosing disease of the carotid bifurcation.

Spiral CT techniques result in a large volume of rapidly acquired data

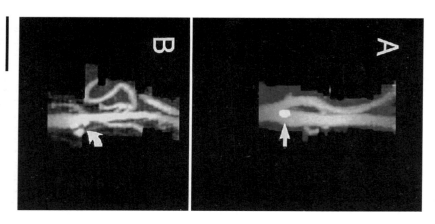

FIGURE 1.

A, three-dimensional reconstruction of spiral CT images of the right carotid artery bifurcation. A small amount of calcium is evident (*arrow*) without significant narrowing of the internal carotid artery. **B,** spiral CT of the contralateral carotid bifurcation demonstrating complete occlusion at the origin of the internal carotid artery (*arrow*).

and a differentiation of soft-tissue densities that is not possible with conventional CT scanning. The images may be displayed as serial cuts in the axial plane perpendicular to the course of the carotid artery to allow precise cross-sectional visualization of the arterial lumen. Three-dimensional reconstructions of the data by using shaded-surface display or a volume-rendering technique using maximal-intensity–projection (MIP) algorithms similar to MR reconstructions permit conventional angiographic-type images that may be viewed from multiple angles. Figure 1, A, shows a typical spiral CT scan of the carotid bifurcation. Note the angiogram-like images and the small amount of calcification seen near the proximal internal carotid artery. Figure 1, B, is an image of the contralateral carotid in the same patient. The internal carotid artery is totally occluded, although the duplex scan could not rule out a pseudo-occlusion.

TECHNIQUE

A lateral topogram of the neck is initially performed to localize the sixth cervical vertebral body. A preliminary run is performed by injecting a small amount of contrast intravenously while images are obtained in the carotid bifurcation region. This allows a determination of the time of peak intra-arterial contrast density and minimizes the contribution of jugular venous filling.

For the actual data acquisition, 75 mL of a nonionic, iodinated contrast is power-injected via an antecubital vein at a rate of 2.5 mL/sec. Spiral CT scanning is initiated approximately 20 seconds after the start of injection. In the initial experience, the CT table was withdrawn through the gantry at a speed of 4 mm/sec during 24 seconds of continuous exposure, which resulted in 9.6 cm of acquired data extending from the middle of the sixth cervical vertebral body to the skull base.[7] Although ensuring visualization of the carotid bifurcation, the higher table speeds and larger beam collimation (4 mm) did not provide optimal resolution. Subsequently, slower table speeds (2 mm/sec) and smaller beam collimation (2 mm) improved z-axis resolution and image quality while still allowing adequate scanning distance.[7] Improvements in CT scanners also permit longer scan acquisition times, which increase the distance that may be scanned.

The gantry angle is positioned parallel to the cervical disk space, although a greater angle is sometimes required to limit artifact in the presence of dental hardware. Patients are asked to breathe quietly and refrain from swallowing during the examination. Various centers report the use of 60–120 mL of contrast for this examination and scan times ranging from 24 to 40 seconds.[7–13] Conventional extracranial cerebral angiography requires 100–120 mL of contrast, although significantly more contrast is required if aortic arch injections are to be used.

Three-dimensional reconstructions are acquired by using shaded-surface display software packages. Briefly, the axial images are viewed and the density of the intraluminal contrast at the most stenotic point of the internal carotid artery is chosen as the lower threshold for data extraction. All less dense structures are erased. Venous structures, bone, and calcified laryngeal cartilage are manually traced, and this region of interest is removed via a semiautomated system. A three-dimensional shaded-surface rendering is created of the remaining contrast-enhanced arterial vasculature and calcified plaque. Reconstruction times are approximately 30 minutes. Additional postprocessing may be desired to separate calcified plaque from enhancing arterial structures. A segmentation program is used to exclude calcifications that do not contact the arterial lumen. This process typically requires an additional 30 minutes per carotid study.

These shaded-surface displays, however, are susceptible to faulty data reconstruction. If the contrast bolus in the stenotic artery is suboptimal or there is loss of contrast density in the distal end of the artery because of low flow, artifact, or partial volume effects, the attenuation in this artery may be reduced. A software program that automatically deletes images below a given threshold may delete pertinent vasculature.[8]

An alternate reconstruction technique is the MIP that is used in MRI displays. Maximal-intensity projection is a volume-rendering method that creates a three-dimensional reconstruction by stacking together the highest intensity regions from a series of two-dimensional images. A preprocessing time is required to exclude bone and calcified plaque, and then the contrast-enhanced vascular structures represent the highest attenuation projected by MIP. Images are produced that closely resemble those of conventional angiography.

Leclerc et al. report that axial sections appear to be the most reliable method of determining the degree of carotid stenosis.[11] Three-dimensional reconstruction techniques, shaded-surface displays, and MIP are susceptible to errors in quantification of carotid disease when extraction of calcified plaque from the contrast-enhanced lumen is required. When atherosclerotic plaques are not heavily calcified, MIP reconstructions may be more accurate in grading carotid stenoses.

CORRELATION WITH CONVENTIONAL ANGIOGRAPHY

An initial report by Castillo in 1993 demonstrated poor correlation between spiral CT and angiography, with agreement in only 50% of cases.[12] Furthermore, six patent arteries identified by angiography were reported as occluded on spiral CT. These results reflected early experience with spiral CT, and subsequent work by Castillo and Wilson supports a positive evolution in image quality and carotid stenosis assessment.[13] In 1994, Castillo and Wilson compared two groups of patients undergoing spiral CT.[13] Group 1 received a smaller dose of IV contrast (60 mL), and the CT data were acquired from 5-mm slices with 3-mm slice reconstruction and a postprocessing MIP algorithm. Only 45% of the spiral CT scans agreed with angiographic results, and six high-grade stenoses on angiograms were misread as occluded on spiral CT. In group 2, a larger dose of contrast was administered (90 mL), the table speed was reduced, and more closely spaced slices were used for data acquisition and reconstruction. These modifications resulted in improved image resolution enabling a 90% correlation between spiral CT and angiography with no patent carotids falsely interpreted as occluded.

Recently, several investigators have compared spiral CT angiography with conventional angiography, and a summary of their results is presented in Table 1.[7-11] In these studies, the carotid stenoses were graded according to North American Symptomatic Carotid Endarterectomy Trial criteria.[14] The site of maximal stenosis was measured with calipers and compared with the more distal, postbulbar normal internal carotid artery. The percent diameter reduction was calculated and graded according to the following categories: mild, 0% to 19% reduction; moderate, 20% to 69%; severe, 70% to 99%; and occlusion, 100%. The degree of correlation in grading stenoses was contrasted between spiral CT and angiography. Particular attention was directed toward discriminating between severe stenoses and occlusions; mention was also made of characterization of plaque morphology.

As can be seen in Table 1, recent experience with refined imaging techniques has demonstrated a high degree of correlation between spiral CT and conventional angiography (82% to 96%). No angiographically demonstrated high-grade stenoses were interpreted as occluded on spiral CT. In one case, a carotid artery was found to be patent on spiral CT and the angiogram revealed it to be occluded.[9] Retrospective review of the angiogram determined that a string sign was probably present and the initial interpretation of the angiogram represented a false positive occlusion. This is consistent with previous concerns that in the presence of slow flow through a severe stenosis, an angiogram may result in a false positive diagnosis of occlusion.[6]

In our own experience, we have occasionally had similar difficulties in differentiating a severe stenosis from an occlusion on angiography. A recent case shown in Figure 2 involved a patient who underwent a carotid duplex scan after being evaluated for transient ischemic attacks. The scan was unable to adequately identify flow in the carotid artery because of heavy concentric calcification. An angiogram was obtained and re-

TABLE 1.
Recent Studies Comparing Spiral Computed Tomography and Conventional Angiography

Author	Year	No. Carotid Arteries Studied	Spiral CT and Angiography Correlation,* %	No. Occluded by Spiral CT	No. Occluded by Angiography
Schwartz	1992	40	92	3	3
Marks	1993	28	89	2	2
Dillon	1993	50	82	7	8†
Cumming	1994	70	92	7	7
Leclerc	1995	28	96	4	4

*Correlations reflect the percentage of carotid arteries examined in which spiral CT and angiography agreed with respect to carotid disease categories defined by the North American Symptomatic Carotid Endarterectomy Trial (see the text).

†Patient with high-grade stenosis by spiral CT in whom angiography was interpreted as carotid occlusion. Subsequent review of the angiogram revealed a string sign suggesting patency.

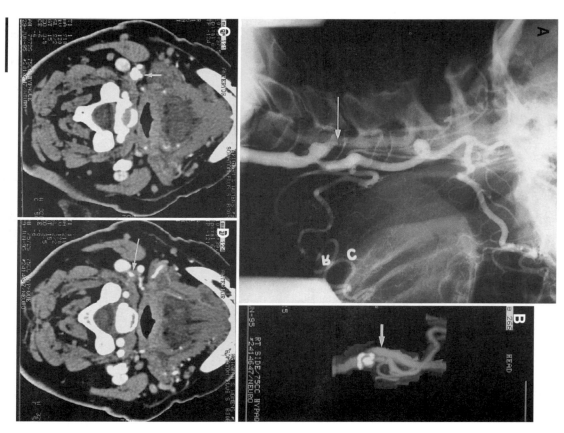

FIGURE 2.

A, intra-arterial angiogram of the right carotid artery demonstrating complete occlusion of the internal carotid artery slightly distal to the bifurcation (arrow). **B,** three-dimensional reconstruction of a spiral CT scan in the same patient demonstrating a patent internal carotid artery (arrow). Note the heavy calcification in the region of the bifurcation. **C,** axial image of a spiral CT scan just distal to the carotid bifurcation. The arrow indicates a patent proximal internal carotid. **D,** axial image of the distal internal carotid, which appeared occluded by conventional angiography. Note the stenotic but patent lumen (arrow) with surrounding arterial wall suggestive of a normal-caliber, nonsclerotic vessel amenable to endarterectomy. Findings were confirmed at surgery.

vealed total occlusion of the internal carotid artery (Fig 2, A). Because of persistent symptoms, a spiral CT with three-dimensional reconstruction was obtained (Fig 2, B) and clearly demonstrated flow through the internal carotid artery. Axial images also demonstrated a patent internal carotid artery. Figure 2, C is an axial image just distal to the bifurcation,

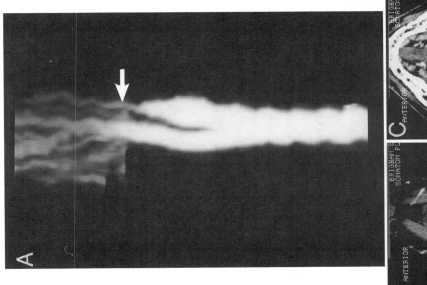

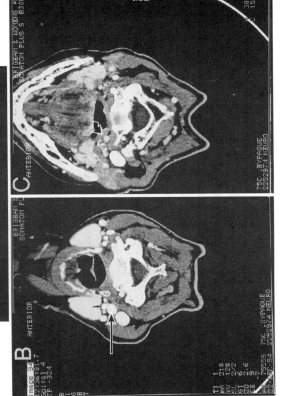

FIGURE 3.

Three-dimensional reconstruction of a spiral CT scan in a patient with a duplex scan indicating total occlusion of the internal carotid artery. Spiral CT demonstrates a pseudo-occlusion of the internal carotid artery *(arrow)*. **B**, axial images of the proximal internal carotid artery *(large arrow)* demonstrating a patent lumen. Note the external carotid artery with a branch vessel *(small arrow)*. **C**, axial images of the distal internal carotid artery *(arrow)* in the same patient revealing a stenotic, atretic vessel without reconstitution of a normal-caliber vessel.

and Figure 2, D, is an axial image at the site of maximal stenosis with a small but clearly patent lumen. The patient underwent an uneventful carotid endarterectomy with resolution of her symptoms.

Spiral CT may not only demonstrate a patent carotid artery in these difficult cases but will also give information regarding the quality of the distal extracranial internal carotid artery. Figure 3 presents a patient whose initial duplex scan suggested carotid occlusion; however, spiral CT revealed a pseudo-occlusion as seen in Figure 3, A. The axial images of the proximal internal carotid artery confirmed patency of the lumen (Fig 3, B), although axial images of the distal internal carotid artery (Fig 3, C) demonstrated a hypoplastic artery without reconstitution of a normal-caliber vessel, therefore precluding routine endarterectomy.

DISCUSSION

Based on current studies, spiral CT angiography generates reliable images of the carotid bifurcation and provides an accurate alternative to conventional angiography.[7-11] Visualization of the carotid from multiple angles, including axial images, may permit greater differentiation of contrast from plaque and result in more precise measurements of carotid stenoses and better assessment of plaque morphology than is currently provided by angiography.[10] Even patients with heavy concentric calcification can undergo effective evaluation of the degree of stenoses from the axial images. Additionally, postprocessing techniques allow removal of the plaque for high-quality three-dimensional reconstructions.

Although not enough information exists at the present time, spiral CT may become the most sensitive modality for identifying ulcerative lesions. Further refinements in techniques (e.g., preshooting to time contrast injection; decreased scanning distance, collimation, and table speed; and increased contrast dose and imaging time) continue to result in improvements in image resolution.

Spiral CT does have certain limitations. Artifacts caused by scattered radiation (e.g., in patients with metallic dental fillings), partial volume effects, or beam hardening may hinder resolution. Spiral CT does require contrast with risks of nephrotoxicity and allergic reactions. Although spiral CT subjects patients to ionizing radiation, the total exposure is actually less than that received during a standard cervical spine series.[7] Because of the limited distance that may be scanned, spiral CT does not provide information regarding tandem lesions outside the field, but it does provide pertinent information regarding anomalies within the carotid bifurcation region such as kinks, aneurysms, or even ulcers.[9]

Duplex scanning remains the most used initial carotid examination, and many surgeons, including ourselves, will perform endarterectomies without any additional studies.[2] Duplex scanning has a reported accuracy in excess of 90%; however, it is frequently unreliable in differentiating high-grade stenoses from occlusions, with a high false positive occlusion rate.[2] Furthermore, heavily calcified plaque will create acoustic shadowing and limit the usefulness of ultrasound. We have been reluctant to resort to conventional angiography in these situations given a small but significant procedure-related risk of stroke (1.2%), as evident in the

Asymptomatic Carotid Atherosclerosis Study trial,[1] and have preferred the use of spiral CT. Figure 4 depicts a patient with a heavily calcified carotid bifurcation precluding effective duplex scanning. The three-dimensional spiral CT reconstruction seen in Figure 4, A, demonstrates the calcified plaque and contrast-enhanced carotid lumen. In Figure 4, B, the image is rotated and the lumen is better visualized. Axial images of the distal common carotid artery (Fig. 4, C) demonstrates the large region of calcified plaque and a narrowed eccentric lumen. The spiral CT findings of high-grade stenosis (95% diameter reduction) were confirmed at surgery.

When duplex scanning is equivocal, many clinicians have turned to another noninvasive method, MRA. Magnetic resonance angiography has an additional advantage of not requiring contrast and a reported sensitivity of 90% in diagnosing severe stenoses.[5, 15] However, because of a tendency to overestimate the degree of stenosis, MRA has a less acceptable positive predictive value, as low as 40% in some series.[4, 5] This is thought to be related to turbulence distal to a severe stenosis causing signal loss.[15] Calcified plaque may result in local field inhomogeneities, which may also result in an overestimation of the stenosis. Figure 5, A, is an MRA in a patient with a tortuous internal carotid artery. Signal loss is evident and could be misinterpreted as a stenosis. Spiral CT of the carotid (Fig 5, B) shows the tortuous, yet nonstenotic carotid artery.

Additional disadvantages of MRA include an inability to study patients with indwelling metallic devices and the long imaging times (10–15

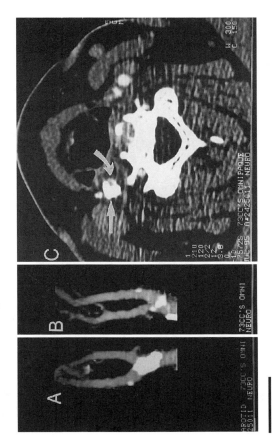

FIGURE 4.

A, three-dimensional reconstruction of a spiral CT scan in a patient with heavy calcification in the region of the carotid bifurcation precluding successful estimation of carotid disease by color-flow duplex scanning. **B,** spiral CT reconstructions may be viewed from multiple angles. Rotation of the three-dimensional carotid artery image from **(A)** enables improved visualization of the carotid bifurcation. **C,** axial image of the distal common carotid artery in the same patient provides excellent visualization of the large calcified plaque (*straight arrow*) and the residual lumen (*curved arrow*) to allow an estimation of the degree of stenosis. The adverse effect of motion artifact is also demonstrated.

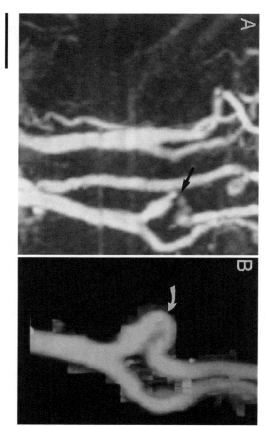

FIGURE 5.

A, MR angiogram of the extracranial carotid vessels. A tortuous internal carotid artery (*arrow*) results in signal loss and an apparent stenosis. **B**, three-dimensional reconstruction of a spiral CT scan in the same patient. Again note the tortuous vessel (*arrow*); however, there is no significant disease in the internal carotid artery.

minutes) and smaller gantry, which are unacceptable to patients who are claustrophobic. Patient intolerance results in a 5% to 7% failure rate in attempts to perform MRA.[5, 15]

CONCLUSION

Spiral CT angiography is a promising technique for noninvasive evaluation of carotid bifurcation disease. The ability to view the stenotic lesion in an axial dimension as well as in a three-dimensional reconstructed form similar to conventional angiographic images is appealing. Furthermore, the images may be viewed from multiple angles and calcified plaque extracted from the contrast-enhanced lumen. These variables may allow an estimation of stenosis and characterization of plaque morphology that are actually superior to that of angiography. At the present time, patients with equivocal carotid duplex scans at our institution, particularly those with possible pseudo-occlusions, are being evaluated with spiral CT in lieu of MRA or angiography. Spiral CT is less expensive than either MRA or angiography, and the quality and reliability of the images provided have been satisfactory. We anticipate further validation of this technique with a potential expansion of the role of spiral CT in diagnosing extracranial carotid disease.

REFERENCES

1. Executive Committee for the Asymptomatic Carotid Atherosclerosis Study: Endarterectomy for asymptomatic carotid artery stenosis. *JAMA* 273:1421–1428, 1995.
2. Moneta GL, Edwards JM, Chitwood RW, et al: Correlation of North American

Symptomatic Carotid Endarterectomy Trial angiographic definition of 70%–99% internal carotid artery stenosis with duplex scanning. *J Vasc Surg* 17:152–159, 1993.

3. Dawson DL, Zierler RE, Strandness DE, et al: The role of duplex scanning and arteriography before carotid endarterectomy: A prospective study. *J Vasc Surg* 18:673–680, 1993.

4. Riles TS, Eidelman EM, Litt AW, et al: Comparison of magnetic resonance angiography, conventional angiography, and duplex scanning. *Stroke* 23:341–346, 1992.

5. Huston J, Lewis BD, Wiebers DO, et al: Carotid artery: Prospective blinded comparison of two-dimensional time-of-flight MR angiography with conventional angiography and duplex US. *Radiology* 186:339–344, 1993.

6. Ammar AD, Turrentine MW, Farha SJ: The importance of arteriographic interpretation in occlusion or pseudo-occlusion of the carotid artery. *Surg Gynecol Obstet* 167:119–123, 1988.

7. Schwartz RB, Jones KM, Chernoff DM, et al: Common carotid artery bifurcation: Evaluation with spiral CT. *Radiology* 185:513–519, 1992.

8. Marks MP, Napel S, Jordan JE, et al: Diagnosis of carotid artery disease: Preliminary experience with maximum-intensity-projection spiral CT angiography. *AJR Am J Roentgenol* 160:1267–1271, 1993.

9. Dillon EH, van Leeuwen MS, Fernandez MA, et al: CT angiography, application to the evaluation of carotid artery stenosis. *Radiology* 189:211–219, 1993.

10. Cumming MJ, Morrow IM: Carotid artery stenosis: A prospective comparison of CT angiography and conventional angiography. *AJR Am J Roentgenol* 163:517–523, 1994.

11. Leclerc X, Godefroy O, Pruvo JP, et al: Computed tomographic angiography for the evaluation of carotid artery stenosis. *Stroke* 26:1577–1581, 1995.

12. Castillo M: Diagnosis of disease of the common carotid artery bifurcation: CT angiography vs catheter angiography. *AJR Am J Roentgenol* 161:395–398, 1993.

13. Castillo M, Wilson JD: CT angiography of the common carotid artery bifurcation: Comparison between two techniques and conventional angiography. *Neuroradiology* 36:602–604, 1994.

14. NASCET Collaborators: Beneficial effect of carotid endarterectomy in symptomatic patients with high-grade carotid stenosis. *N Engl J Med* 325:445–453, 1991.

15. Heiserman JE, Drayer BP, Fram EK, et al: Carotid artery stenosis: Clinical efficacy of two-dimensional time-of-flight MR angiography. *Radiology* 186:339–344, 1992.

PART IV

Mesenteric Occlusive Disease

Chronic Mesenteric Arterial Insufficiency: Bypass or Endarterectomy?

Timothy R.S. Harward, M.D.

Associate Professor of Surgery, Section of Vascular Surgery, Department of Surgery, University of Florida College of Medicine, Gainesville

C hronic mesenteric ischemia is caused by any condition decreasing blood flow to the gastrointestinal tract to a level insufficient to meet the normal physiologic demands generated by postprandial intestinal motility, secretion, and absorption. This diminished blood supply produces visceral pain and/or abnormalities in bowel function analogous to insufficient coronary artery blood flow causing angina pectoris during periods of increased cardiac work.[1] A number of conditions cause this problem, but the most common etiology is atherosclerotic involvement of the mesenteric arteries[1]; therefore, this chapter will focus primarily on the pathophysiology, diagnosis, and treatment of symptomatic chronic mesenteric arterial insufficiency caused by atherosclerotic occlusive disease.

The clinical picture associated with chronic mesenteric arterial insufficiency was first described by Schnitzler[2] in 1901; however, it took 20 more years before the pathophysiology of this problem was understood as evidenced by Klein's proposed descriptive name "mesenteric intermittent claudication."[3] Fifteen years later in 1936, Dunphy suggested that the postprandial pain associated with chronic mesenteric arterial occlusion was a possible predictor of later intestinal infarction.[4] Surgical treatment for this problem was initially proposed in 1957 by Mikkelson[5] and later accomplished in 1958 by Shaw and Maynard.[6] Since that time, numerous clinical studies have described a myriad of surgical reconstructive techniques and examined short- and long-term patient follow-up.[7-16]

Atherosclerotic involvement of the splanchnic arteries is caused by either calcified plaque originating in the aorta and involving the ostia of the three major mesenteric arteries or atherosclerotic plaque developing in the proximal 1 to 2 cm of the artery. The splanchnic arteries most frequently involved are the celiac axis (CA), superior mesenteric artery (SMA), inferior mesenteric artery (IMA), and splenic artery.[1, 17] In reviewing autopsy specimens, Reiner and Jiminez found atherosclerosis involving the splanchnic arteries in 68 of 88 patients (77%). One or more of the major mesenteric arteries (i.e., CA, SMA, IMA) were found to have significant stenosis in 44 patients. This included 15 arteries that were totally occluded. However, review of each patient's clinical history dem-

Advances in Vascular Surgery®, vol. 4

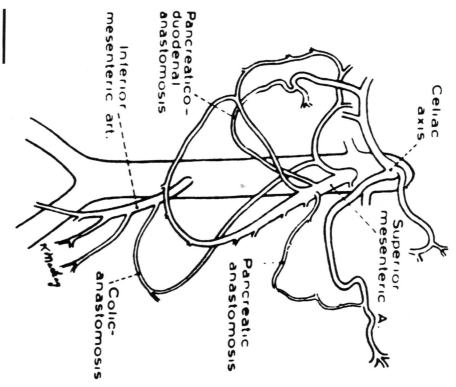

Celiac axis

Superior mesenteric A.

Pancreatico-duodenal anastomosis

Inferior mesenteric art.

Colic-anastomosis

Pancreatic anastomosis

FIGURE 1.

Diagram demonstrating the extensive collateral network between the three major mesenteric arteries. (Courtesy of Perdue GD, Smith R: Intestinal ischemia due to mesenteric arterial disease. Am Surg 36:155, 1970.)

onstrated little correlation between the mesenteric arterial obstruction and the clinical course.[17]

The reason for the poor correlation between arterial stenoses and clinical symptoms is the extensive system of collateral arteries between the various abdominal viscera. The pancreaticoduodenal arcades are the major communication between the CA and the SMA (Fig 1). The major collateral network between the SMA and the IMA is a meandering artery communicating between the middle colic artery originating from the proximal SMA and the ascending branch of the left colic artery off the IMA (Fig 2).[18] These collateral networks are easily visualized during arteriography, and their absence in association with hemodynamically significant proximal mesenteric arterial stenoses is consistent with symptoms of chronic mesenteric arterial insufficiency.[19]

CLINICAL FINDINGS

A variety of postprandial complaints such as a crampy pain, a dull ache, or an indescribable discomfort beginning 10 to 15 minutes after eating and gradually increasing in intensity to a plateau before slowly decreasing over a period of 1 to 3 hours develop in all patients with symptomatic chronic mesenteric arterial insufficiency.[1] Initially, the pain begins only after large meals, but with time, it increases in both frequency and severity. Eventually, the pain may become so intense that patients decrease the size of their meal and develop a true fear of eating known as sitophobia.[1] This is the cause of the weight loss seen in these patients,

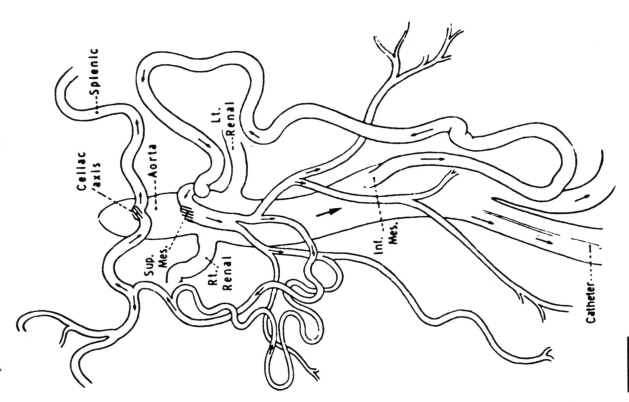

FIGURE 2.

Diagram demonstrating the direction of blood flow and the serpiginous nature of the collateral arteries that develop in the presence of significant chronic mesenteric arterial insufficiency. (Courtesy of Perdue GD, Smith R: Intestinal ischemia due to mesenteric arterial disease. *Am Surg* 36:155, 1970.)

not malabsorption as previously proposed.[20] Other less common symptoms consist of diarrhea or constipation, bloating or nausea, and occasional vomiting caused by problems of abnormal bowel motility.[1]

Unfortunately, signs on physical examination are very nonspecific. Patients are thin and occasionally cachectic. The abdomen is frequently scaphoid with normal bowel sounds. Even during bouts of postprandial pain, the abdomen is soft without guarding or rebound. An epigastric bruit can be heard in approximately 50% of the patients, and it will occasionally radiate into the right lower quadrant if generated by turbulent flow of blood through a severe SMA stenosis.[1]

DIAGNOSIS

Historically, it has been difficult to make a clinical diagnosis of chronic mesenteric ischemia. The classic signs and symptoms are not always present, and several other common problems with similar clinical findings frequently lead physicians to pursue other diagnostic procedures before entertaining the diagnosis of chronic mesenteric ischemia. In the past, the diagnosis was based on clinical findings, arteriographic demonstration of hemodynamically significant mesenteric arterial occlusive disease, and exclusion of other more common intestinal problems. However, physicians are often reluctant to have an elderly, often debilitated patient who commonly has these symptoms undergo arteriography because of the small but real risk of significant complications. As a result, Stoney noted that the average time needed to make the diagnosis of significant mesenteric arterial occlusive disease in patients with chronic mesenteric ischemia was 18 months.[21]

Before seeking surgical consultation, most patients have already undergone upper and lower intestinal endoscopy, multiple CT or MRI scans, as well as conventional upper and lower intestinal barium studies, all with normal findings. More recently, advances in the technology of B-mode ultrasound, pulse-wave Doppler, and computer software have allowed the development of duplex scanners that image mesenteric arteries while providing concomitant Doppler spectral analysis of blood flow in these arteries. Initial reports evaluated both normal baseline and physiologic changes in blood flow in response to feeding.[22–24] These reports were followed by studies comparing the results of duplex scanning with the findings of lateral aortography. Moneta et al. used the velocity of blood flow to determine the degree of stenosis of SMA and CA stenosis in 34 patients. They found that peak systolic velocity of 275 cm/sec or faster and 200 cm/sec or faster defined 70% or greater stenosis of the SMA and CA, respectively. The calculated accuracies of these predictors were 91% and 82%, respectively.[25] Similarly, Bowersox et al. correlated velocity measurements with arterial occlusive disease and found that an end-diastolic velocity greater than 45 cm/sec was 95% accurate in discriminating between less than 50% and 50% or greater stenosis of the SMA; however, they did not identify a velocity parameter that could discriminate various CA stenoses.[26]

Finally, because of intrinsic problems and inaccuracies in estimating blood flow velocity with present-day instrumentation,[27] Harward et al. evaluated 38 patients with Doppler frequency spectral analysis to determine the severity of disease in mesenteric arteries. A peak systolic frequency of 4.5 kHz or greater and 4.0 kHz or greater defined 50% or greater stenosis of the SMA and CA, respectively. The calculated accuracies of these frequency predictors were 95% and 97%, respectively. However, most impressive was the direct, linear relationship seen between changes in peak systolic frequency and arteriographically measured stenoses of 50% to 99%. For the SMA and the CA, the correlation coefficients were 0.89 and 0.86, $P < 0.0001$, respectively (Fig 3). In addition, this technique correctly identified all instances of SMA and CA occlusion.[28]

Despite the exciting results of abdominal duplex scanning, aortography remains the final step in evaluating mesenteric arterial occlusive disease. A complete examination involves both frontal and lateral images. The lateral projection images the proximal 4 to 6 cm of the CA, SMA, and IMA, the segment where the majority of hemodynamically significant stenoses occur. The frontal projection demonstrates the collateral networks between the CA, SMA, and IMA, the extensiveness of which verifies the chronicity of the arterial insufficiency (Fig 4).

Many patients are known to have severe CA and/or SMA stenoses or total occlusions but remain either asymptomatic or complain of atypical gastrointestinal symptoms. Unfortunately, abdominal duplex scanning and arteriography only predict the presence of an anatomical lesion. Neither technique provides information on the physiologic significance that the detected alterations in visceral blood flow have on bowel and/or hepatic function.

Recently, Fiddian-Green et al. introduced the method of intraluminal tonometry by which intestinal mucosal pH is indirectly measured and used as a metabolic marker of adequate blood flow and hence adequate oxygen delivery to the gastrointestinal tract.[29] With this method it was found that mucosal pH remains stable despite declining oxygen delivery (i.e., decreasing blood flow) until a critical threshold is reached. Below this level, any further reduction in blood flow is "accompanied by a precipitous decrease in tissue pH."[30] In addition, this decrease in mucosal pH is accentuated even further during oral feeding.[31]

It seemed only logical to use this method to determine the physiologic significance of CA, SMA, and/or IMA stenoses/occlusions. In fact, Fiddian-Green et al. used tonometry to measure gastric mucosal pH in three patients with abdominal pain and significant mesenteric arterial disease. The initial mean mucosal pH was 7.10 (range, 7.00 to 7.26; normal is 7.32 or greater) and increased to a mean of 7.39 (range, 7.35 to 7.44) after treatment.[32] Although encouraging, more work is needed before this method can be used to assist in deciding when to revascularize the bowel; however, tonometry is a step forward in determining the physiologic significance of mesenteric arterial insufficiency because it measures the adequacy of oxygen delivery related to tissue needs, the true bottom line in defining tissue ischemia.

In summary, whenever an individual experiences both postprandial pain and weight loss, a careful history and physical examination may uncover other findings to suggest chronic mesenteric ischemia (Fig 5). The next step is to obtain an abdominal duplex scan of the mesenteric arteries. If these arteries are free of significant occlusive disease, other meth-

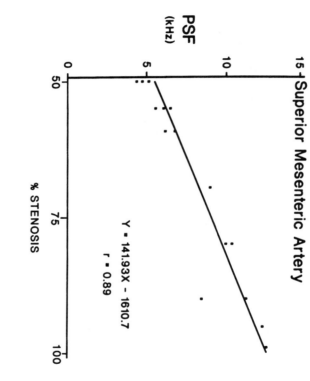

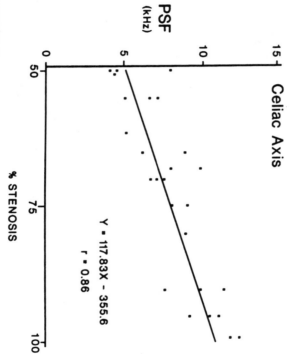

FIGURE 3.

Linear regression analysis of pulsed-wave Doppler peak systolic frequency (*PSF*) values obtained from the superior mesenteric artery (SMA) and celiac axis (CA) compared with percent stenosis when the degree of diameter reduction was greater than 50%; excluded from the analysis are all total SMA and CA occlusions. (Courtesy of Harward TRS, Smith S, Seeger JM: Detection of celiac axis and superior mesenteric artery occlusive disease with use of abdominal duplex scanning. *J Vasc Surg* 17:742, 1993.)

ods of evaluation should be followed (e.g., CT scan, endoscopy); however, if hemodynamically significant mesenteric arterial stenoses are detected, an arteriogram should be obtained. If two or more arteries are diseased, one should consider intervening; however, when less disease is evident, one might consider using intraluminal intestinal tonometry; if the mucosal pH is less than 7.32, consideration is given to intervention, whereas a pH of 7.32 or higher suggests that conservative follow-up is the treatment of choice while other diagnostic studies are pursued.[32a]

The indications for treatment of symptomatic chronic mesenteric arterial insufficiency are difficult to define. Originally, Dunphy suggested that patients with symptomatic mesenteric ischemia were predisposed to acute intestinal infarction.[4] However, this theory has not been supported by recent studies. In fact, the majority of cases (>75%) of acute intestinal

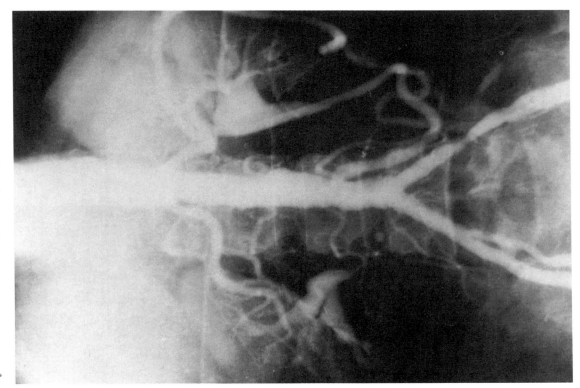

FIGURE 4.

Standard anteroposterior view of an aortogram demonstrating the collateral network that develops between the various mesenteric arteries as chronic mesenteric arterial occlusive disease evolves. Easily seen is the meandering artery that is the collateral between the inferior and superior mesenteric arteries. (Courtesy of Bergan JJ, Yao JST: Chronic intestinal ischemia, in Rutherford RB (ed): *Vascular Surgery*, ed 2. Philadelphia, WB Saunders, 1984, p 968.)

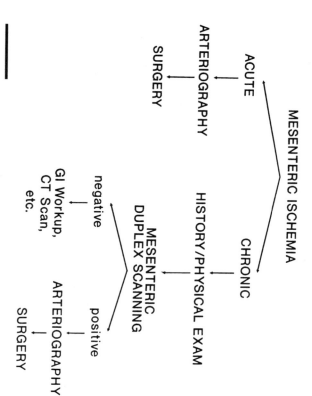

FIGURE 5.

Algorithm for evaluation of a patient with postprandial abdominal pain, weight loss, and changes in bowel habits. *Abbreviation: GI,* gastrointestinal. (Courtesy of Harward TRS: Chronic mesenteric arterial insufficiency: A review of diagnosis and treatment, in Bland KI (ed): *Perspectives in General and Laparoscopic Surgery.* St Louis, Quality Medical Publishing, 1994, p 30.)

infarction are caused by either nonocclusive disease or cardiac emboli.[1] Therefore, the major reason for revascularizing the visceral arteries is to relieve the disturbing symptoms of pain, weight loss, and gastrointestinal motility disturbances, all of which lead to malnutrition and generalized poor health. The only other clear indication for reconstruction of the mesenteric arteries occurs when any type of intra-abdominal operative procedure interferes with the arterial collateral network seen in association with severe CA and SMA occlusive disease. In this situation, the collateral arcade, in particular, the meandering artery, is providing the majority of nutrient blood flow to the small bowel. If this collateral is divided or damaged, acute intestinal ischemia will occur; therefore, to prevent this devastating complication, prophylactic mesenteric arterial revascularization is needed.[33] In contrast, asymptomatic chronic mesenteric arterial occlusive disease should not be repaired. No published data have shown benefit with this approach.

THERAPEUTIC OPTIONS

Methods of therapy are divided into two categories: surgical and radiologic revascularization. There are three different methods of surgical revascularization, and percutaneous balloon angioplasty with or without stent placement remains a new, minimally tested technique.

SURGICAL REVASCULARIZATION

Technique

The initial revascularization procedure was arterial endarterectomy and is still used today. The suprarenal aorta and mesenteric arteries are ex-

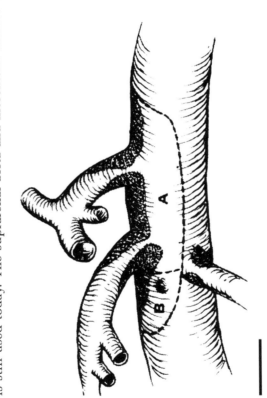

FIGURE 6.

Diagram of the suprarenal aorta demonstrating the "trap-door" technique used for mesenteric artery endarterectomy. **A** and **B** indicate the distal extension of the trap door used, depending upon whether the renal arteries are also to be endarterectomized. (Courtesy of Rapp JH, Reilly LM, Qvarfordt PG, et al: Durability of endarterectomy and antegrade grafts in the treatment of chronic visceral ischemia. *J Vasc Surg* 3:801, 1986.)

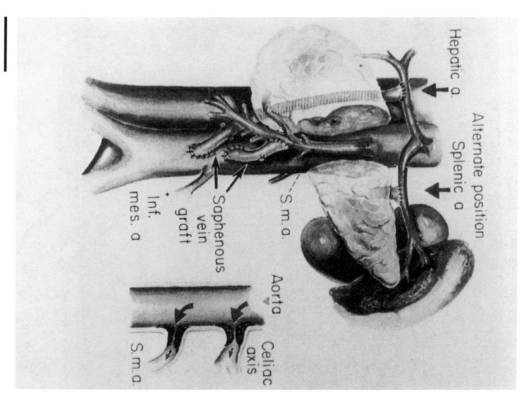

FIGURE 7.

Artist's drawing demonstrating a retrograde saphenous vein bypass from the infrarenal aorta to the superior mesenteric artery (S.m.a.) and the common hepatic or splenic arteries. *Abbreviation: Inf. mes. a.*, inferior mesenteric artery. (Courtesy of Bergan JJ, Yao JST: Chronic intestinal ischemia, in Rutherford RB (ed): *Vascular Surgery*, ed 2. Philadelphia, WB Saunders, 1984, p 968.)

posed via a left eighth-interspace oblique thoracoabdominal incision.[34] Once the aorta is isolated, the CA and SMA are exposed by dividing the dense neural plexus surrounding this area. The SMA can be mobilized distally for 6 to 7 cm. Once all arteries are controlled, systemic anticoagulation is instituted, after which the proximal and distal aorta and the CA, SMA, and renal arteries are occluded. The aorta is opened by using a "trap-door" technique (Fig 6), the anterior aorta and mesenteric arteries are endarterectomized, and then the trap-door aortotomy is closed with sutures. On occasion, the end point of the endarterectomized atherosclerotic plaque cannot be reached through the aortotomy; therefore, the CA or SMA must be opened distally, the endarterectomy completed, and the arteriotomy closed with a vein patch angioplasty.[34]

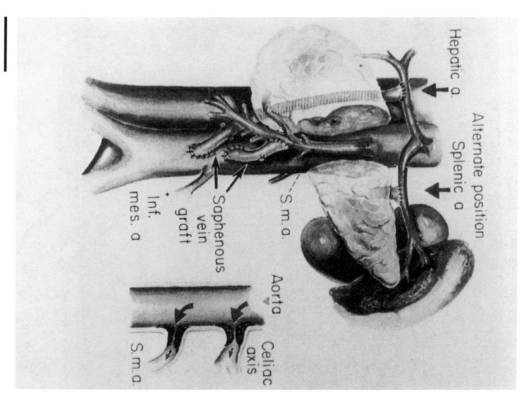

118   T.R.S. Harward

Presently, the most common method of mesenteric arterial revascularization is surgical bypass. Historically, this bypass was done initially with either greater saphenous vein or a Dacron conduit[10, 35–37] and blood flow routed in a retrograde direction from the infrarenal aorta or common iliac arteries to the SMA and the common hepatic or splenic arteries, the latter two arteries being first-order branches of the CA. The conduit to the SMA must be quite short to avoid kinking once the small bowel is returned to the peritoneal cavity, and the conduit supplying the CA is passed parallel to the aorta through a retropancreatic tunnel and anastomosed to the underside of either the common hepatic or splenic artery (Fig 7).

More recently, mesenteric bypass has been done in an antegrade direction from the supraceliac aorta. This procedure is easily performed through a chevron incision with a midline extension.[38] The gastrohepatic ligament is divided, the left lobe of the liver is retracted laterally, and the crus of the diaphragm is split to expose the entire supraceliac aorta below the diaphragm. The CA and its branches are exposed, after which the stomach is retracted inferiorly and the SMA exposed as it exits under the pancreas. The bypass is constructed with a 12 × 6-mm prosthetic graft turned vertically and sutured end-to-side to the aorta. The posterior limb is passed through a retropancreatic tunnel to the SMA, and the anterior limb is anastomosed to the CA with possible extension onto the common hepatic artery (Fig 8). On completion of the bypass, blood flow through each bypass graft limb is quantitated with an electromagnetic flowmeter

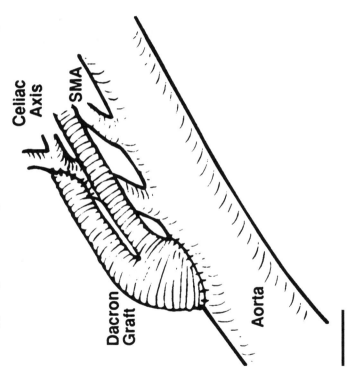

FIGURE 8.

Diagram of an antegrade supraceliac aortomesenteric arterial bypass demonstrating the vertical alignment of a bifurcated Dacron graft. *Abbreviation: SMA,* superior mesenteric artery. (Courtesy of Harward TRS, Brooks D, Flynn TC, et al: Multiple organ dysfunction following mesenteric revascularization. *J Vasc Surg* 18:462, 1993.)

and is adequate when values increase to greater than 500 mL/min after intra-arterial infusion of 30 mg of papaverine.[36]

Numerous variations of these techniques have been proposed. One particular technique suggested by Beebe et al. combines endarterectomy and bypass.[39] The aorta around the CA is exposed and partially occluded. An aortotomy is made and extended into the CA. The CA is endarterectomized and a bypass conduit (Dacron or saphenous vein) is anastomosed to the arteriotomy in the aorta and CA to return normal blood flow to the CA. The bypass conduit is then routed through a retropancreatic tunnel and anastomosed to the SMA (Fig 9).

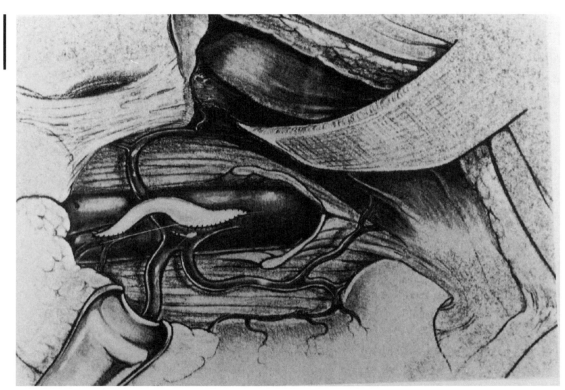

FIGURE 9.
Artist's drawing of an antegrade aortomesenteric bypass graft incorporating the origin of previously endarterectomized celiac axis and anastomosed distally to the superior mesenteric artery. (Courtesy of Beebe HG, MacFarlane S, Raker EJ: Supraceliac aortomesenteric bypass for intestinal ischemia. *J Vasc Surg* 5:751, 1987.)

Perioperative Results

The operative mortality of elective mesenteric revascularization for symptomatic chronic mesenteric arterial insufficiency is reported to be 5% to 17% (Table 1).[7-16] Historically, surgical philosophy has been to reconstruct only one of the major mesenteric arteries[8,11,12] and rely on collateral pathways to supply either intestinal or hepatic blood flow. However, perioperative death from intestinal infarction was found to occur in some patients when only a single bypass was done.[8,11,12,37] On further study, Hollier et al. showed that recurrent symptoms developed in 50% of the patients when one of two or three diseased mesenteric arteries was revascularized whereas they developed in only 11% of the patients when all diseased mesenteric arteries were bypassed.[12] Therefore it is recommended that at least two and, if possible, all three diseased mesenteric arteries be revascularized at the initial operative procedure.

At closer inspection, reports on surgical revascularization reveal that perioperative morbidity/mortality has been due to problems with postoperative bleeding, pulmonary insufficiency, renal failure, etc., not the usual cardiac complications seen after other major arterial reconstructive procedures.[7,9,10,14,15] In the 1963 report by Fry and Kraft, progressive pulmonary insufficiency developed in 1 of 7 patients undergoing bowel revascularization.[7] In Hansen's 1976 report of 12 patients undergoing mesenteric bypass, 1 died of acute renal failure, severe hypovolemia developed in 4 despite adequate fluid resuscitation, and severe coagulopathy developed in 3, leading to death in 2.[9] Similarly, in the 1977 study by Crawford et al., 3 of 40 patients died secondary to "cardiorespiratory and renal disease."[10] More recently, Rapp et al. at the University of California, San Francisco, reported that 5 patients died in the early postoperative period: 2 of severe postoperative bleeding, 2 of multiple systemic failure, and 1 of pulmonary complications.[14] Similarly, Rheudasil et al., reviewing the Emory Clinic experience (41 patients), found that in the early postoperative period, renal failure developed in 3 patients and pulmonary problems requiring mechanical ventilation for more than 24 hours developed in 18.[15] Although they did not directly investigate the problem of multiple organ dysfunction after mesenteric arterial bypass, these studies suggest that the problem of multiple organ dysfunction is significant.

TABLE 1.
Surgical Mortality

Authors	No. Patients	No. Deaths	Mortality, %
Hansen (1976)	12	2	16.6
Crawford et al. (1977)	40	4	10.0
Zelenock et al. (1980)	23	4	17.4
Hollier et al. (1981)	56	5	8.9
Baur et al. (1984)	23	2	8.7
Rapp et al. (1986)	67	5	7.4
Rheudasil et al. (1988)	31	2	6.4

Recently, Harward et al. examined the early postoperative follow-up of 18 patients undergoing mesenteric arterial revascularization.[38] Multiple-vessel antegrade bypass from the supraceliac aorta to the SMA/CA was the surgical procedure performed in 16 of 18 cases, and 2 patients underwent revascularization with saphenous vein in a retrograde fashion.

Immediately after surgery, hepatocellular enzyme elevation was noted: serum glutamic oxaloacetic transaminase (SGOT) increasing 96-fold, serum glutamic pyruvic transaminase (SGPT) increasing 101-fold, and lactate dehydrogenase (LDH) increasing 25-fold (Fig 10). Similarly, the prothrombin and partial thromboplastin times increased significantly, whereas platelet counts dropped from normal to a mean of $38.3 \pm 5.3 \times 1,000/mm^3$. Total bilirubin subsequently increased 13-fold; however, this increase lagged behind the hepatocellular enzyme increase by 2 to 14 days. Between the first and third postoperative days, acute respiratory insufficiency developed in 16 of 18 patients as evidenced by (1) an increase in the pulmonary shunt fraction (Q_s/Q_t) to a mean of $32\% \pm 3\%$ (range, 21% to 60%) (Fig 11), (2) steadily decreasing arterial P_{O_2}, and (3) a chest radiograph showing a diffuse interstitial pattern suggestive of adult respiratory distress syndrome. Overall, this pulmonary failure lasted an average of 8.4 days in surviving patients. Finally, acute anuric renal failure

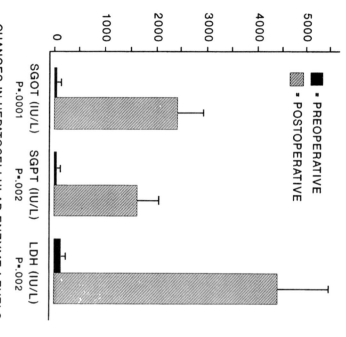

FIGURE 10.
Bar graph demonstrating the increases in serum hepatocellular enzyme levels that occur early after revascularization of a chronically ischemic bowel. *Abbreviations: SGOT,* serum glutamic oxaloacetic transaminase; *SGPT,* serum glutamic pyruvic transaminase; *LDH,* lactate dehydrogenase. (Courtesy of Harward TRS, Brooks D, Flynn TC, et al: Multiple organ dysfunction following mesenteric revascularization. J Vasc Surg 18:464, 1993.)

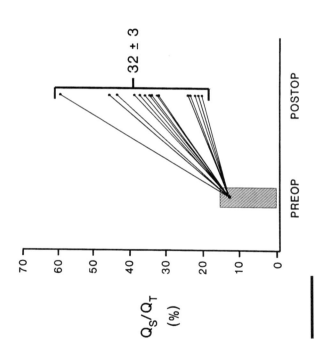

FIGURE 11.

Line graph demonstrating changes in pulmonary shunt fractions (Q_S/Q_T) from the preoperative to the postoperative period. (Courtesy of Harward TRS, Brooks D, Flynn TC et al: Multiple organ dysfunction following mesenteric revascularization. *J Vasc Surg* 18:462, 1993.)

POSSIBLE PATHOPHYSIOLOGY OF I/R INJURY

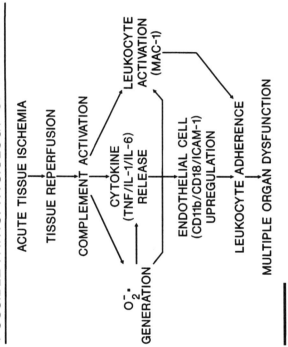

FIGURE 12.

Theoretical cascade of biomolecular events that might occur and cause multiple organ dysfunction after reperfusion of the chronically ischemic bowel. *Abbreviations: I/R,* ischemia/reperfusion; *TNF,* tumor necrosis factor; *IL-1,* interleukin-1; *MAC,* macrophage attack complex; *ICAM,* intercellular adhesion molecule. (Courtesy of Harward TRS: Chronic mesenteric arterial insufficiency: A review of diagnosis and treatment, in Bland KI (ed): *Perspectives in General and Laparoscopic Surgery.* St Louis, Quality Medical Publishing, 1994, p 39.)

FIGURE 13.

Abdominal B-mode ultrasonic image demonstrating the easily visualized proximal anastomosis and limbs of a 12 × 6-mm bifurcated Dacron graft used to construct an antegrade supraceliac aortomesenteric bypass. The distal celiac axis (CA) anastomosis is seen while the limb to the superior mesenteric artery (SMA) passes under the CA and out of the field of view. (Courtesy of Harward TRS: Chronic mesenteric arterial insufficiency: A review of diagnosis and treatment, in Bland KI (ed): *Perspectives in General and Laparoscopic Surgery.* St Louis, Quality Medical Publishing, 1994, p 41.)

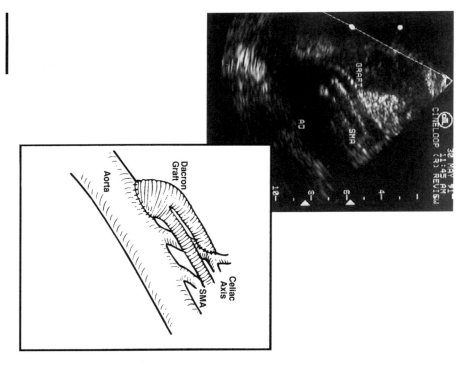

developed in 3 patients within 48 hours of surgery despite aggressive treatment. The only common link observed between these 3 patients was the development of immediate severe postoperative hepatocellular enzyme elevation (LDH, >10,000 IU/L). Overall, all patients exhibited some element of organ failure and 4 died of multiple organ dysfunction during the postoperative period.

The cause of multiple organ dysfunction after reperfusion of chronically ischemic viscera (e.g., intestines, liver) is unclear; however, review of the literature concerning reperfusion of acutely ischemic tissue reveals distant organ injury to be a very well described entity.[40–43] From this work, several intertwining mechanisms have been identified that could lead to multiple organ injury after reperfusion of chronically ischemic viscera (Fig 12). This injury cascade could possibly be initiated by complement activation, which then leads to vascular endothelial cell injury. This complement activation and subsequent cell injury then leads to the generation of reactive oxygen intermediates (ROIs), release of proinflammatory cytokines (e.g., tumor necrosis factor-α, interleukin-1, interleukin-6), and activation of leukocytes. Once liberated, cytokines and ROIs cause upregulation of both endothelial cell membrane glycoprotein receptors CD11b/CD18 and intracellular adhesion molecule type 1 (ICAM-1). The specific affinity of ICAM-1 for the leukocyte receptor (MAC-1) leads to the adherence of leukocytes to the postcapillary venule wall and eventual emigration into the surrounding tissue. Simultaneously, this same cascade of events occurs in distant organs (e.g., lung, kidney) and causes multiple organ injury and dysfunction. It is unclear at this time but quite possible that this or a similar cascade of injurious events occurs after revascularization of chronically ischemic abdominal viscera.

Long-Term Results

Until recently, the long-term natural history of patients undergoing surgical revascularization for symptomatic chronic mesenteric arterial insufficiency was sketchy. Previous reports used only the return of symptoms to evaluate long-term function of the bypass procedure. Rapp et al. at the University of California, San Francisco, observed 69 patients for a mean duration of 52.7 months. Recurrent visceral ischemia developed in 4 patients (7%), leading to death in 2 and reoperation in 2, whereas the remaining 56 patients (93%) remained free of visceral ischemic symptoms.[14]

In the 18 patients seen at the University of Florida, 13 have been observed for a duration of 41.4 months (range, 24 to 63). All patients resumed a regular diet and gained weight. During this follow-up, patency of the bypass graft was monitored and verified with color-flow duplex scanning in 12 patients (Fig 13). 1 patient being lost to follow-up after 2 months. There have been no bypass graft conduit occlusions or anastomotic stenoses, and all patients continue to thrive without exception.

ENDOVASCULAR REVASCULARIZATION

Endovascular revascularization is an accepted standard of treatment for symptomatic arterial stenoses in a variety of locations. Although experience with balloon dilatation of the CA and SMA is limited, it should be considered a first-line therapeutic option in many patients.

The balloon is introduced via the common femoral artery. Once a wire is passed across the arterial stenosis or through a complete occlusion, complete anticoagulation is achieved with heparin. The balloon is then exchanged over a heavy-duty guide wire. Next, an appropriate balloon catheter size and balloon diameter are chosen depending on the arterial diameter measured on the lateral aortogram.[44] Once balloon dilatation is accomplished, the decision of whether to insert an intra-arterial wall stent is made. Although still anecdotal, the theory is that the stent will prevent early recurrent stenosis in the ostia of the mesenteric arteries. Once this procedure is completed, the patient receives 24 hours of systemic heparin before hospital discharge.

Several authors have reported their experience with percutaneous transluminal angioplasty (PTA) for symptomatic chronic mesenteric arterial insufficiency; however, until recently, these reports have been more anecdotal than scientific.[44–46] Golden et al. performed PTA in the SMA in 7 patients and achieved subjective success in 6; however, only 3 patients returned for follow-up and 4 were never seen again.[45] O'Durny et al. performed PTA in 19 SMA and/or CA vessels in 10 patients; however, only 5 patients had typical symptoms of intestinal angina.[44] The average pressure gradient across the stenoses before PTA was 83 mm Hg, and this decreased to only 40 mm Hg after PTA. The authors stated that the stenoses were successfully dilated with initial relief of symptoms in 8 patients; however, in view of the aforementioned postprocedure pressure gradients, this initial success rate is difficult to justify. In addition, of these initial successes, recurrent symptoms developed in 5 and were relieved after a second PTA; however, it is unclear whether these patients had classic or atypical symptoms, and the time course of follow-up and recurrence of symptoms/restenoses was not given.

More recently, Allen et al. from the Baylor University Medical Center presented a 10-year experience with PTA for chronic intestinal ischemia. Twenty-five stenoses in 19 patients were treated with PTA. The initial success rate was 98% (24/25), with total relief of symptoms in 15 patients over a mean follow-up of 51 months. Recurrent symptoms developed in 4 patients, 2 of whom were successfully treated with a second PTA.[47] During the discussion of this paper, the subject of stent placement in the mesenteric artery was addressed, and this topic is considered in Allen's chapter in this book. However, the technique of PTA with primary stent placement for symptomatic mesenteric ischemia has been used in 5 patients at the University of Florida, with immediate relief of symptoms in all cases. In addition, there has been no evidence of postprocedure reperfusion injury with multiple organ dysfunction after PTA! Unfortunately, follow-up is too short at this time to make any definitive conclusion, but no restenoses have occurred within the last 10 months.

SUMMARY

The incidence of chronic mesenteric arterial insufficiency appears to be slowly increasing as the general population grows older. However, the onset of symptoms in these patients is related to the presence or absence of collateral development between the three major mesenteric arteries. At present, whenever this problem is suspected, the initial diagnostic procedure should be a duplex scan, which has quite good accuracy in detecting mesenteric artery stenoses or occlusions. If this examination is positive, a verifying lateral aortogram should be done before proceeding with therapy. Endovascular techniques are in their infancy and appear to be technically successful both initially and long-term if stents are used. However, surgical repair remains the gold standard therapy, with antegrade supraceliac aortomesenteric bypass of at least two major visceral arteries being the optimal treatment. Transaortic endarterectomy, although more demanding technically, provides an equally good outcome.

Finally, in the immediate postoperative period, varying degrees of multiple organ dysfunction appear to develop; however, once recovery is complete, it seems that the long-term outlook for this population of patients is excellent.

REFERENCES

1. Boley SJ, Brandt LJ, Veith FJ: Ischemic disorders of the intestines. *Curr Probl Surg* 15:2–85, 1978.
2. Schnitzler J: Zur Symptomatologie des Sarmarterienverschlusses. *Med Wochenschr* 51:506, 1901.
3. Klein E: Embolism and thrombosis of the superior mesenteric artery. *Surg Gynecol Obstet* 33:385–405, 1921.
4. Dunphy JE: Abdominal pain of vascular origin. *Am J Med Sci* 192:109–113, 1936.
5. Mikkelson WP: Intestinal angina: Its surgical significance. *Am J Surg* 94:262–269, 1957.
6. Shaw RS, Maynard EP: Acute and chronic thrombosis of mesenteric arteries associated with malabsorption: Report of two cases successfully treated by thromboendarterectomy. *N Engl J Med* 258:874–878, 1958.
7. Fry WJ, Kraft RO: Visceral angina. *Surg Gynecol Obstet* 117:414–424, 1963.
8. Reul GJ, Wadasch DC, Sandiford FM, et al: Surgical treatment of abdominal angina: Review of 25 patients. *Surgery* 75:682–689, 1974.
9. Hansen HJB: Abdominal angina. *Acta Chir Scand* 142:319–325, 1976.
10. Crawford ES, Morris GC, Myhre HO, et al: Celiac axis, superior mesenteric artery, and inferior mesenteric artery occlusion: Surgical considerations. *Surgery* 82:856–866, 1977.
11. Zelenock GB, Graham LM, Whitehouse WM, et al: Splanchnic arteriosclerotic disease and intestinal angina. *Arch Surg* 115:497–501, 1980.
12. Hollier LH, Bernatz PE, Pairolero PC, et al: Surgical management of chronic intestinal ischemia: A reappraisal. *Surgery* 90:940–946, 1981.
13. Baur GM, Millay DJ, Taylor LM, et al: Treatment of chronic visceral ischemia. *Am J Surg* 148:138–144, 1984.
14. Rapp JH, Rielly LM, Qvarfordt PG, et al: Durability of endarterectomy and antegrade grafts in the treatment of chronic visceral ischemia. *J Vasc Surg* 3:799–806, 1986.
15. Rheudasil JM, Stewart MT, Schellack JV, et al: Surgical treatment of chronic mesenteric arterial insufficiency. *J Vasc Surg* 8:495–500, 1988.
16. Cormier JM, Fichelle JM, Vennin J, et al: Atherosclerotic occlusive disease of the superior mesenteric artery: Late results of reconstructive surgery. *Ann Vasc Surg* 5:510–518, 1991.
17. Reiner L, Jiminez FA: Anatomic aspects of mesenteric arteriosclerosis, in Boley SJ, Schwartz SS, Williams LF (eds): *Vascular Disorders of the Intestine*, ed 1. New York, Appleton-Century-Crofts, 1971, pp 41–56.
18. Perdue GD, Smith RB: Intestinal ischemia due to mesenteric arterial disease. *Am Surg* 36:152–156, 1970.
19. Connolly JE, Abrams HL, Kieraldo JH: Observations on the diagnosis and treatment of obliterative disease of the visceral branches of the abdominal aorta. *Arch Surg* 90:596–606, 1965.
20. Finlay JM, Hogarth J, Wrightman KJ: Clinical evaluation of the D-xylose tolerance test. *Ann Intern Med* 61:411–419, 1964.
21. Stoney RJ: In discussion of manuscript by Moneta GL, Yeager RA, Kalman R, et al: Duplex ultrasound criteria for diagnosis of splanchnic artery stenosis or occlusion. *J Vasc Surg* 14:519, 1991.

22. Jager K, Bollinger A, Valli C, et al: Measurement of mesenteric blood flow by duplex scanning. *J Vasc Surg* 3:462–469, 1986.

23. Lilly MP, Harward TRS, Flinn WR, et al: Duplex ultrasound measurement of changes in mesenteric flow velocity with pharmacologic and physiologic alterations of intestinal blood flow in man. *J Vasc Surg* 9:18–25, 1989.

24. Moneta GL, Taylor DC, Helton WS, et al: Duplex ultrasound measurement of postprandial intestinal blood flow: Effect of meal composition. *Gastroenterology* 95:1294–1301, 1988.

25. Moneta GL, Yeager RA, Dalman R, et al: Duplex ultrasound criteria for diagnosis of splanchnic artery stenosis or occlusion. *J Vasc Surg* 14:511–520, 1991.

26. Bowersox JC, Zwolak R, Walsh BD, et al: Duplex ultrasonography in the diagnosis of celiac and mesenteric artery occlusive disease. *J Vasc Surg* 14:780–789, 1991.

27. Phillips DJ, Beach KW, Primozich J, et al: Should results of ultrasound Doppler studies be reported in units of frequency or velocity? *Ultrasound Med Biol* 15:205–212, 1989.

28. Harward TRS, Smith S, Seeger JM: Detection of celiac axis and superior mesenteric artery occlusive disease using abdominal duplex scanning. *J Vasc Surg* 17:738–745, 1993.

29. Fiddian-Green RG, Amelin PM, Hermann JB, et al: Prediction of the development of sigmoid ischemia on the day of aortic operation. *Arch Surg* 121:654–660, 1986.

30. Grum CM, Fiddian-Green RG, Pitenger GL, et al: Adequacy of tissue oxygenation in the intact dog intestine. *J Appl Physiol* 5:1065–1069, 1984.

31. Poole JW, Sammartano RJ, Boley SJ: Hemodynamic basis of the pain of chronic mesenteric ischemia. *Am J Surg* 153:171–176, 1987.

32. Fiddian-Green RG, Stanley JC, Nostrant T, et al: Chronic gastric ischemia: A cause of abdominal pain or bleeding identified from the presence of gastric mucosal acidosis. *J Cardiovasc Surg* 30:852–859, 1989.

32a. Harward TRS: Chronic mesenteric arterial insufficiency: A review of diagnosis and treatment, in Bland KI (ed): *Perspectives in General and Laparoscopic Surgery.* St Louis, Quality Medical Publishing, 1994, pp 22–44.

33. Connolly JE, Kwaan JHM: Prophylactic revascularization of the gut. *Ann Surg* 190:514–522, 1979.

34. Stoney RJ, Wylie EJ: Surgical management of arterial lesions of the thoracoabdominal aorta. *Am J Surg* 126:157–164, 1973.

35. Bergan JJ, Dry L, Conn J, et al: Intestinal ischemic syndromes. *Ann Surg* 169:120–126, 1969.

36. Bergan JJ, Yao JST: Chronic intestinal ischemia, in Rutherford RB (ed): *Vascular Surgery,* ed 2. Philadelphia, WB Saunders, 1984, pp 964–971.

37. McCollum CH, Graham JM, DeBakey ME: Chronic mesenteric arterial insufficiency: Results of revascularization in 33 cases. *South Med J* 69:1266–1268, 1976.

38. Harward TRS, Brooks D, Flynn TC, et al: Multiple organ dysfunction following mesenteric revascularization. *J Vasc Surg* 18:459–469, 1993.

39. Beebe HG, MacFarlane S, Raker EJ: Supraceliac aortomesenteric bypass for intestinal ischemia. *J Vasc Surg* 5:749–754, 1987.

40. Schmeling DJ, Caty MG, Oldham KT, et al: Evidence for neutrophil-related acute lung injury after intestinal ischemia-reperfusion. *Surgery* 106:195–202, 1989.

41. Turnage RH, Bagnasco J, Berger J, et al: Hepatocellular oxidant stress following intestinal ischemic-reperfusion injury. *J Surg Res* 51:467–471, 1991.

42. Klausner JM, Paterson IS, Kobzik L, et al: Oxygen free radicals mediate ischemia-induced lung injury. *Surgery* 105:192–199, 1989.

43. Paterson IS, Klausner JM, Goldman G, et al: Pulmonary edema after aneurysm surgery is modified by mannitol. *Ann Surg* 210:796–801, 1989.

44. O'Durny A, Sniderman KW, Colapinto RF: Intestinal angina: Percutaneous transluminal angioplasty of the celiac and superior mesenteric arteries. *Radiology* 167:59–62, 1988.

45. Golden DA, Ring EJ, McLean GK, et al: Percutaneous transluminal angioplasty in the treatment of abdominal angina. *AJR Am J Roentgenol* 139:247–249, 1982.

46. Robert L, Wertman DA, Mills SR, et al: Transluminal angioplasty of the superior mesenteric artery: An alternative to surgical revascularization. *AJR Am J Roentgenol* 141:1039–1042, 1983.

47. Allen RC, Martin GH, Talkington CM, et al: Mesenteric angioplasty in the treatment of chronic intestinal ischemia. *J Vasc Surg*, in press.

Percutaneous Mesenteric Angioplasty in the Treatment of Chronic Intestinal Ischemia

Robert C. Allen, M.D.

Assistant Professor of Surgery, Assistant Director of Surgical Education, Department of General Surgery, Section of Vascular Surgery, Baylor University Medical Center, Dallas, Texas

Treatment of chronic mesenteric ischemia (CMI) has traditionally been surgical, with multiple series reporting high morbidity and mortality as a result of multiple patient comorbidities. Surgical management has included aortomesenteric grafting and transaortic endarterectomy in the majority of patients with morbidity predominantly cardiac in origin. However, CMI is an uncommon clinical manifestation of atherosclerotic disease caused by the extensive collateral circulation between the mesenteric vessels. Therefore, correlation between the symptoms of CMI and the degree of angiographic obstruction of the visceral vessels is poor.[1] The classic symptoms of CMI are postprandial abdominal pain with weight loss and "food fear." Goodman in 1918 first described abdominal angina,[2] and CMI became a recognized entity after the writings of Dunphy in 1936.[3] The etiology of this abdominal pain must be recognized and then followed with elective surgical revascularization to prevent the development of acute mesenteric ischemia and consequent higher surgical mortality rate.

The reported high morbidity and mortality rates associated with the surgical management of CMI have prompted several investigators to attempt percutaneous transluminal angioplasty (PTA) as the primary treatment modality in patients with CMI caused by focal atherosclerotic disease of the visceral arteries.[4, 5] Dotter and Judkins first described PTA in 1964,[6] and Furrer et al. reported the first successful mesenteric PTA of a superior mesenteric artery (SMA) stenosis in 1980.[7] The reports to date have been of small series with limited follow-up.[8–12] Our experience with PTA for CMI has been limited to patients considered to be extremely poor surgical candidates because of multiple comorbidities.

PATIENT EVALUATION

All patients undergo an exhaustive evaluation to rule out other potential causes of their abdominal pain. This may include upper and lower gas-

Advances in Vascular Surgery®, vol. 4
© 1996, Mosby–Year Book, Inc.

trointestinal contrast studies, as well as endoscopy of the esophagus, stomach, duodenum, and colon. The diagnosis of CMI is made only after the exclusion of other gastrointestinal pathology. All patients must have a complete diagnostic abdominal aortogram with selective celiac, SMA, and inferior mesenteric artery (IMA) evaluation. The study should demonstrate the proximal mesenteric arteries, collateral flow, and distal mesenteric vasculature. Stenoses are measured by using cut-film biplanar aortography with supplemental digital subtraction angiograms. Mesenteric artery occlusions and celiac lesions in the presence of median arcuate ligament syndrome are not considered for PTA. No patients believed to have acute mesenteric artery ischemia should undergo PTA.

TECHNIQUE

The mesenteric stenoses are localized and measured with a preprocedural diagnostic lateral aortogram. A luminal diameter stenosis of greater than 70% and a systolic pressure gradient across the stenosis of 10 to 15 mm Hg are considered to be significant. The luminal diameter of the normal mesenteric artery is measured and used to select an angioplasty balloon of appropriate size. The stenosis is defined as ostial or nonostial, with an ostial stenosis located less than 5 mm from the aortic lumen. All angioplasty procedures are performed with the patients fully prepared for emergency operative intervention and the surgical team available for possible complications. The mesenteric PTA is performed by standard technique over a guide wire. The procedure can be performed by the axillary approach or the femoral approach. To minimize patient risk, angioplasty is performed on only a single vessel when possible, with preferential SMA dilatation to maximally perfuse the small intestine. Multiple vessels may undergo PTA if both vessels have extremely high-grade lesions. This usually involves concomitant celiac and SMA PTA. Balloon diameters are chosen with the intent to overdilate by 10% to 20% (1 to 2 mm). The balloon size in our experience is therefore 7 to 8 mm for the celiac artery, 4 to 10 mm for the SMA, 6 to 7 mm for a mesenteric vein graft, and 3 mm for the IMA. Heparin is given during each procedure, and each patient receives aspirin after the procedure. Other adjuncts may include nitroglycerin and nifedipine to reduce arterial spasm. Technical success is defined as a luminal diameter stenosis of less than 50% after angioplasty, and clinical patency is determined by the relief of symptoms after PTA. Each patient has an immediate on-table angiogram to assess the PTA result.

RESULTS

We have treated 24 focal atherosclerotic mesenteric stenoses in 19 patients by PTA. Dilated vessels have included the SMA (18), celiac artery (3), IMA (1), aorto-SMA vein graft (1), and aortosplenic artery vein graft (1). The cohort included 16 females and 3 males with a mean age of 71 years (range, 54 to 88 years). All 19 patients were very high risk and considered to be poor surgical candidates. Comorbidities were peripheral vascular disease in 14 (74%), hypertension in 12 (63%), heavy smoking history in 10 (53%), coronary artery disease in 9 (47%), chronic obstructive pulmonary disease in 4 (21%), diabetes mellitus in 2 (11%), chronic renal insufficiency in 2 (11%), and hyperlipidemia in 2 (11%). In addition, 9 patients had undergone prior abdominal aortic surgery, including 3 mesenteric artery bypasses and 1 mesenteric endarterectomy. Seventeen patients had classic symptoms of CMI: postprandial abdominal pain and weight loss (mean, 24 lb). Two patients had atypical courses, 1 of whom had vague abdominal pain, diarrhea, and heme-positive stool. Finally, 1 patient who had undergone a previous aorto-SMA bypass complained of nondescript abdominal discomfort and had an epigastric bruit. Her arteriogram showed a marked focal stenosis of the aorto-SMA graft and a celiac artery stenosis. There were 18 nonostial stenoses and 6 ostial stenoses.

Initial technical success was achieved in 18 of 19 patients (95%) and 23 of 24 stenoses (96%). The lone technical failure resulted in SMA dissection with thrombosis and bowel infarction. The patient died despite emergency laparotomy with bowel resection and mesenteric revascularization (mortality, 5%). After the initial angioplasty procedure, 15 of the 19 patients (79%) had complete relief of their symptoms. Follow-up revealed continued relief of symptoms for a mean of 39 months (range, 4 to 101 months). Recurrent symptoms developed in 3 of the 15 patients (20%) who initially had complete relief of symptoms at a mean of 28 months after the procedure (range, 9 to 43 months). No correlation could be found between residual percent diameter stenosis and recurrence of symptoms. One patient was treated with repeat PTA of the SMA and had a good technical and clinical result. She remained asymptomatic until her death of a myocardial infarction 15 months later. One of the other 2 patients in this subset was treated with IMA reimplantation and had a good result, and the patient remains asymptomatic. The last patient remains symptomatic and refuses further intervention. Three patients who had classic CMI complaints attained only partial symptomatic relief after PTA despite technically excellent results. The reason for the lack of complete relief of symptoms is unclear; however, 1 patient had a long history of irritable bowel syndrome and the other patients were being treated for ongoing depression. One patient, who had only partial symptomatic relief after the initial PTA and increasing abdominal complaints at 3 months, underwent repeat PTA. The PTA produced substantial pain relief, but symptomatic improvement was incomplete despite an excellent technical result. Recurrent and increasing abdominal complaints developed at 6 months, and surgical revascularization was performed and provided complete relief of symptoms. Both patients who had atypical symptoms on the initial evaluation attained complete symptomatic relief after PTA, and no recurrence was noted during the available follow-up (37 and 83 months). The small sample size resulted in no significant differences in outcome when patients with classic symptoms were compared with those with atypical symptoms.

Fifteen patients initially underwent lone dilatation of the SMA, with good technical results in 14 stenoses and complete symptomatic relief in 12 patients. Recurrent abdominal symptoms developed in 1 patient at 43 months; repeat PTA of the SMA resulted in good dilatation and complete

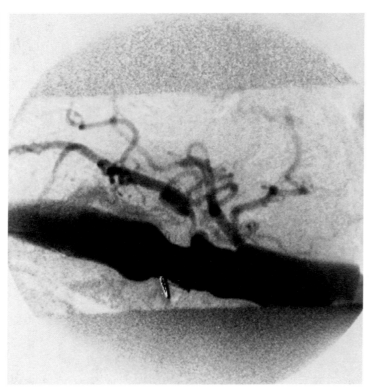

FIGURE 1.
Nonostial high-grade stenosis of the superior mesenteric artery before percutaneous transluminal angioplasty.

relief of symptoms. All 3 celiac artery stenoses underwent PTA in conjunction with concomitant PTA of the SMA (2) or SMA vein graft (1) stenosis in the setting of very high-grade lesions in both vessels. The technical result was good in the 3 celiac stenoses, but only 1 patient achieved full relief of symptoms. The other 2 patients had partial relief. One IMA stenosis was treated by angioplasty; a good technical result and full relief of symptoms for 32 months were obtained. Two aortomesenteric vein grafts were dilated, with good technical results and complete relief of abdominal symptoms. The patients had no recurrent symptoms during the available follow-up (17 and 83 months). There were no significant differences between the technical and clinical results based on the vessels undergoing PTA.

The stenoses consisted of 18 nonostial and 6 ostial lesions. The SMA stenoses included 16 nonostial and 2 ostial lesions. Percutaneous transluminal angioplasty of both ostial SMA lesions produced good technical results and relief of abdominal symptoms. Of the 16 nonostial SMA stenoses, PTA achieved technical success in 15 lesions (Figs 1 and 2): 11 patients had full relief of symptoms and 4 patients had partial symptom relief. All 3 celiac stenoses that underwent PTA were ostial and technically successful; complete symptom relief was achieved in 1 patient and partial relief in 2 patients. The lone IMA stenosis was ostial, and PTA produced complete relief of symptoms and a good technical result. The 2 aortomesenteric vein graft stenoses were nonostial in nature; PTA was

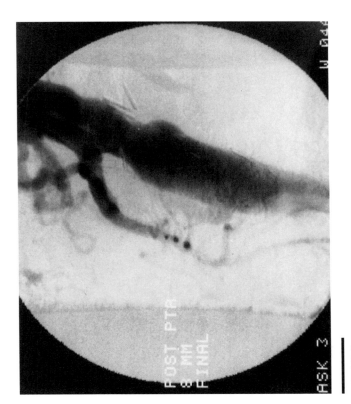

FIGURE 2.
Superior mesenteric artery after angioplasty with no residual stenosis.

technically successful with symptomatic relief in both patients. When comparing ostial and nonostial stenoses, we found no significant difference in technical success or clinical patency as determined by relief of symptoms.

Surgical revascularization was required in 2 patients who achieved only partial relief of abdominal symptoms and had recurrence of abdominal complaints after failure of mesenteric PTA. One patient had twice undergone combined PTA of the celiac artery and SMA, with substantial but incomplete relief of the clinical symptoms and early recurrence of CMI complaints. She eventually had surgical mesenteric revascularization that completely relieved her abdominal complaints, and she had no recurrence on available follow-up. The second patient, who had undergone an aorto-SMA vein bypass approximately 20 years earlier, had classic complaints of CMI. His arteriogram revealed complete occlusion of the celiac, SMA, and SMA vein graft, with a 95% stenosis of the origin of the IMA. Inferior mesenteric artery angioplasty was successful, and the patient remained asymptomatic for 32 months. Recurrent symptoms then prompted mesenteric revascularization by reimplantation of the IMA, with full relief of clinical symptoms and no recurrence on available follow-up.

One mortality was caused by dissection of the SMA at the time of PTA resulting in SMA thrombosis and bowel infarction. The patient was taken emergently to the operating room for mesenteric revascularization and bowel resection. Her postoperative course was complicated by continued sepsis and multiple organ system failure. A symptomatic axillary sheath hematoma developed in one patient and required operative decompression and repair. One conversion from a femoral to an axillary approach was made because of an inability to cannulate the SMA from the femoral approach.

Complete follow-up was available in 17 of the 18 surviving patients (94%). One patient was lost to follow-up 17 months after PTA of an aortosplenic artery vein graft. At that time she was free of symptoms. Four arteriograms were obtained during the follow-up (mean, 22 months) for vague complaints or unrelated pathology; none showed evidence of restenosis involving the mesenteric vessels after PTA. Four patients died during the follow-up period, and myocardial infarction was the most common etiology.

DISCUSSION

Chronic mesenteric ischemia with intestinal angina is an infrequent manifestation of atherosclerosis that usually occurs in elderly patients who have diffuse vascular disease. The clinical picture may be characterized by postprandial abdominal pain and weight loss, but the symptoms can vary widely. Most authors agree that in the majority of patients who have symptomatic CMI, at least two of the three mesenteric vessels have significant stenoses. Surgical management should involve revascularization of all stenotic vessels.[13] Mikkelson in 1957 first recommended surgical management.[14] Shaw and Maynard in 1958 first reported mesenteric revascularization with an SMA endarterectomy.[15] Early series on the surgical treatment of CMI reported significant morbidity and mortality rates in high-risk patients. However, more recent studies report much more acceptable risks, with the operative mortality ranging from 3% to 8%.[13, 16–20]

The improved morbidity and mortality rates are encouraging but still significant, especially in an elderly population with many comorbidities. Percutaneous transluminal angioplasty is quickly becoming an attractive therapeutic option for a variety of vascular procedures because it is minimally invasive and avoids a major operative procedure and general anesthesia. Furrer et al. first reported on mesenteric PTA in a 1980 paper on PTA of the SMA.[7] The early reports that followed had small numbers of patients with limited follow-up.[8–12] Matsumoto et al. and Hallisey and colleagues have recently published larger series that have better follow-up data.[4,5] Meta-analysis of the series of mesenteric PTA shows the efficacy and safety of the procedure.[4] Technical success was achieved in 79% to 100% (mean, 88%), with an initial clinical success rate of 80% to 100% (mean, 88%).[4] The mean long-term, primary clinical success rate was 76%, and the mean secondary success rate was 93%.[4] Morbidity rates varied from 0% to 16% (mean, 6%), and mortality rates were 0% to 20% (mean, 2%).[4] By comparison, our results show a technical success rate of 96% and initial clinical success rate of 79% (15 of 19 patients), with continued relief of clinical symptoms for a mean of 39 months. The morbidity rate in our study was 5% (one patient who had an axillary hematoma); there was one death (5%) from dissection and thrombosis of the SMA. Meta-analysis showed a mean recurrence rate of 24%, with 92% responding to repeat PTA.[4] Our recurrence rate was 20% (three patients) at a mean interval of 28 months, and one of these patients had repeat PTA with good technical and clinical results. There was no correlation in this study between percent residual stenosis and recurrence of symptoms. This analysis is, however, limited by the sample size. The results of the most recent series of PTA in the treatment of CMI are summarized in Table 1.

The patients selected for PTA in our series were considered very poor surgical candidates because of multiple comorbidities. In addition, nine patients had prior abdominal aortic surgery, four of whom had undergone prior mesenteric revascularization. Patients who are acceptable operative risks should always undergo surgical revascularization instead of mesenteric PTA. Other patient subsets not considered to be acceptable candidates for mesenteric PTA include those who had acute mesenteric ischemia, mesenteric artery occlusions, or median arcuate ligament syndrome, as well as asymptomatic patients who had high-grade mesenteric artery stenoses before abdominal aortic surgery (prophylactic PTA). These decisions reflect the paucity of data showing the efficacy of mesenteric PTA in acute mesenteric ischemia and mesenteric artery occlusion and the abundant data showing the failure of PTA in median arcuate ligament syndrome.[4, 21, 22] Fibromuscular dysplasia is an accepted indication for mesenteric PTA, with limited series demonstrating good results.[12] Our series included no patients with fibromuscular dysplasia.

The efficacy of PTA in CMI is not well defined regarding which patients, vessels, or lesions are most likely to yield technical and clinical success. Matsumoto et al. found that patients with symptoms of classic CMI were more likely to have good results from mesenteric PTA, but these results were not statistically significant.[4] Our study also showed no significant difference in success based on characteristic vs. atypical clinical symptoms. These results are unfortunately biased by the small number of patients. The SMA is preferentially dilated in our experience to minimize the risk to the patient and to optimize outcome. Analysis, however, showed no significant difference in the success rate based on the vessel undergoing PTA (SMA vs. celiac). This comparison is biased by preferential angioplasty of the SMA and limited by the small number of patients. Early reports on PTA for renal artery stenoses concluded that a higher success rate was achieved on nonostial lesions than on ostial lesions, but this finding has been challenged in recent reports. Sniderman, in his series of mesenteric PTA, found that mesenteric atherosclerotic stenoses differed from renal artery stenoses and ostial lesions were associated with a higher success rate than nonostial lesions.[23] However, Matsumoto et al. compared the results of mesenteric PTA for ostial vs. nonostial lesions and found no significant difference in the success rate.[4] Our study included 18 nonostial and 6 ostial stenoses. The SMA and SMA vein graft stenoses were more likely to be nonostial, and the celiac and IMA stenoses were more likely to be ostial. Our study also revealed no significant difference in the success of PTA for ostial vs. nonostial lesions. The selection process for mesenteric PTA is further complicated by the finding of a small subset of patients who fail to demonstrate resolution of clinical symptoms despite a technically excellent result. This occurred in 3 patients in our series and has also been reported by other authors.

A particularly difficult problem is recurrent CMI caused by stenosis

TABLE 1.

Summary of Series Results—Percutaneous Transluminal Angioplasty for Chronic Mesenteric Ischemia

Series	Year	No. Patients	Technical Success, %	Clinical Success, %	Morbidity/ Mortality, %	Recurrence, %	Success of Repeat PTA
Sniderman[23]	1994	13	85	100	0/0	45	3 of 3
Hallisey et al.[5]	1995	16	88	75	6/6	25	3 of 3
Matsumoto et al.[4]	1995	19	79	80	16/0	17	1 of 2
Allen	1996	19	95	79	5/5	20	1 of 1

Abbreviation: PTA, percutaneous transluminal angioplasty.

of an aortomesenteric graft. Reoperation increases the risk of complications and patient morbidity. The majority of the stenoses are nonostial and involve the distal anastomosis. Mesenteric PTA is an ideal option in these patients, with several series reporting high technical and clinical success rates.[10, 24] Two patients in our study underwent PTA of mesenteric vein grafts and both had initial technical and clinical success (Figs 3 and 4). Follow-up revealed continued short-term symptomatic relief.

The primary weakness of most studies (surgical or interventional) on mesenteric revascularization is the reliance on symptomatic follow-up without an objective measurement of patency rates. McMillan et al. have documented a 33% sensitivity of symptomatic follow-up in detecting graft thrombosis as compared with mesenteric duplex ultrasound scanning after surgical mesenteric revascularization.[25] This finding is very important if PTA is being considered as a primary therapy for CMI. Several

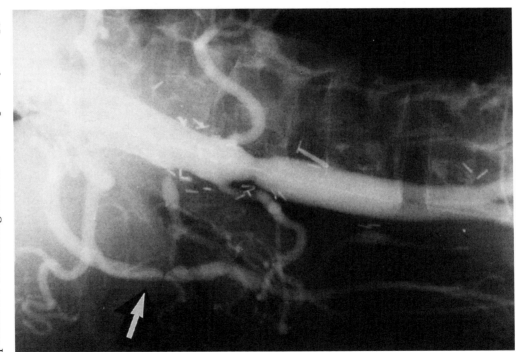

FIGURE 3.

Focal stenosis of a superior mesenteric artery vein bypass graft in a patient with a prior aortobifemoral bypass graft.

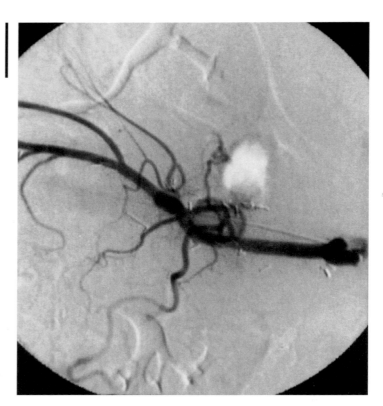

FIGURE 4.

Selective injection of the superior mesenteric artery vein bypass graft after percutaneous transluminal angioplasty with no residual stenosis.

authors have documented a significant restenosis rate after PTA for CMI,[8, 10, 11, 23] which is especially pertinent because surgical mesenteric revascularization has primary patency rates of 90% at long-term follow-up.[18, 25] Mesenteric duplex scanning is a good measure of mesenteric blood flow and can detect celiac and SMA stenoses with high sensitivity and specificity.[26, 27] Duplex scanning has also been used to document patency and stenoses of bypass grafts after mesenteric revascularization.[28] Patients undergoing mesenteric PTA for CMI should be monitored by serial duplex scanning to detect restenosis early and obtain objective documentation of patency rates. The proper interval for duplex scanning is unknown. We suspect that yearly follow-up is appropriate, but our experience is limited and short-term, and therefore we offer no firm recommendation. Duplex criteria for mesenteric stenoses are well documented, but a positive duplex scan should only be followed by a mesenteric angiogram in a symptomatic patient. The duplex scan is a monitor to document patency and restenosis rates after mesenteric PTA in asymptomatic patients. The mesenteric duplex scan is a screening tool in symptomatic patients, with positive studies leading to angiography and repeat PTA.

CONCLUSION

Surgical revascularization is the primary therapeutic option in patients with CMI. Mesenteric PTA is a valuable option in patients who are prohibitive surgical risks because of multiple comorbidities, prior abdominal aortic procedures, or both. The initial technical and clinical success rates are high, with the majority remaining symptom-free at short-term follow-up, but the recurrence rate is significant. Repeat PTA is successful in the majority of cases.

REFERENCES

1. Croft RJ, Menon GP, Marston A: Does intestinal angina exist? A critical study of obstructed visceral arteries. *Br J Surg* 68:316–318, 1981.

2. Goodman GH: Angina abdominis. *Am J Med Sci* 155:524–528, 1918.

3. Dunphy JE: Abdominal pain of vascular origin. *Am J Med Sci* 192:109–112, 1936.

4. Matsumoto AH, Tegtmeyer CJ, Fitzcharles EK, et al: Percutaneous transluminal angioplasty of visceral arterial stenoses: Results and long-term clinical follow-up. *J Vasc Intervent Radiol* 6:165–174, 1995.

5. Hallisey MJ, Deschaine J, Illescas FF, et al: Angioplasty for the treatment of visceral ischemia. *J Vasc Intervent Radiol* 6:785–791, 1995.

6. Dotter CT, Judkins MP: Transluminal treatment of arteriosclerotic obstruction: Description of a new technique and a preliminary report of its application. *Circulation* 30:654–670, 1964.

7. Furrer J, Gruntzig A, Kugelmeier J, et al: Treatment of abdominal angina with percutaneous dilatation of an arteria mesenterica superior stenosis. *Cardiovasc Intervent Radiol* 3:43–44, 1980.

8. McShane MD, Proctor A, Spencer P, et al: Mesenteric angioplasty for chronic intestinal ischaemia. *Eur J Vasc Surg* 6:333–336, 1992.

9. Odurny A, Sniderman KW, Colapinto RF: Intestinal angina: Percutaneous transluminal angioplasty of the celiac and superior mesenteric arteries. *Radiology* 167:59–62, 1988.

10. Levy PJ, Haskell L, Gordon RL: Percutaneous transluminal angioplasty of splanchnic arteries: An alternative method to elective revascularisation in chronic visceral ischaemia. *Eur J Radiol* 7:239–242, 1987.

11. Roberts L, Wertman DA, Mills SR, et al: Transluminal angioplasty of the superior mesenteric artery: An alternative to surgical revascularization. *AJR Am J Roentgenol* 141:1039–1042, 1983.

12. Golden DA, Ring EJ, McLean GK, et al: Percutaneous transluminal angioplasty in the treatment of abdominal angina. *AJR Am J Roentgenol* 139:247–249, 1982.

13. Hollier LH, Bernatz PE, Pairolero PC, et al: Surgical management of chronic intestinal ischemia: A reappraisal. *Surgery* 90:940–946, 1981.

14. Mikkelson WP: Intestinal angina: Its surgical significance. *Am J Surg* 94:262, 1957.

15. Shaw RS, Maynard EP III: Acute and chronic thrombosis of mesenteric arteries associated with malabsorption: Report of two cases successfully treated by thrombo-endarterectomy. *N Engl J Med* 258:874, 1958.

16. Rogers DM, Thompson JE, Garrett WV, et al: Mesenteric vascular problems. *Ann Surg* 195:554–563, 1982.

17. Rheudasil JM, Stewart MT, Schellack JV, et al: Surgical treatment of chronic mesenteric arterial insufficiency. *J Vasc Surg* 8:495–500, 1988.

18. Rapp JH, Reilly LM, Qvarfordt PG, et al: Durability of endarterectomy and antegrade grafts in the treatment of chronic visceral ischemia. *J Vasc Surg* 3:799–806, 1986.

19. Beebe HG, MacFarlane S, Raker EJ: Supraceliac aortomesenteric bypass for intestinal ischemia. *J Vasc Surg* 5:749–754, 1987.

20. Baur GM, Millay DJ, Taylor LM, et al: Treatment of chronic visceral ischemia. *Am J Surg* 148:138–144, 1984.

21. VanDeinse WH, Zawacki JK, Phillips D: Treatment of acute mesenteric ischemia by percutaneous transluminal angioplasty. *Gastroenterology* 91:475–478, 1986.

22. Warnock NG, Gaines PA, Beard JD, et al: Treatment of intestinal angina by percutaneous transluminal angioplasty of a superior mesenteric artery occlusion. *Clin Radiol* 45:18–19, 1992.

23. Sniderman KW: Transluminal angioplasty in the management of chronic intestinal ischemia, in Strandess DE, van Breda A (eds): *Vascular Diseases: Surgical and Interventional Therapy.* New York, Churchill Livingstone, 1994, pp 803–809.

24. Howd A, Loose H, Chamberlain J: Transluminal angioplasty in the treatment of mesenteric vein graft stenosis. *Cardiovasc Intervent Radiol* 10:43–45, 1987.

25. McMillan WD, McCarthy WJ, Bresticker MR, et al: Mesenteric artery bypass: Objective patency determination. *J Vasc Surg* 21:729–741, 1995.

26. Moneta GL, Yeager RA, Dalman R, et al: Duplex ultrasound criteria for diagnosis of splanchnic artery stenosis or occlusion. *J Vasc Surg* 14:511–520, 1991.

27. Moneta GL, Lee RW, Yeager RA, et al: Mesenteric duplex scanning: A blinded prospective study. *J Vasc Surg* 17:79–86, 1993.

28. Flinn WR, Rizzo RJ, Park J, et al: Duplex scanning for assessment of mesenteric ischemia. *Surg Clin North Am* 70:99–107, 1990.

PART V

Infrainguinal Intervention

Thrombolytic Therapy in Peripheral Vascular Disease

Kenneth Ouriel, M.D.

Associate Professor of Surgery, The University of Rochester, Rochester, New York

Thrombolytic therapy has been used for the treatment of occluding processes involving arteries and veins. The thrombolytic drugs comprise a group of agents that can effect dissolution of fibrin thrombi. Some agents are found endogenously in humans, for example, urokinase and tissue-type plasminogen activator. Others, such as vampire bat plasminogen activator, are found in nonhuman mammalian species. Still others, including streptokinase and staphylokinase, comprise exoproducts of prokaryotic organisms. A final group of thrombolytic agents is not found in nature; rather, these compounds, such as recombinant tissue plasminogen activator (rt-PA), recombinant urokinase, and prourokinase, have been synthesized by humans, based on the principles derived from a study of the structure of the naturally occurring agents. Despite the diversity in the origin and structure of thrombolytic agents, each shares a common mechanism of action. All agents bind to plasminogen, activating the compound through a conversion to its active form, plasmin. Plasmin, in turn, converts insoluble fibrin polymer to soluble degradation products, dissolving the thrombus.

Thrombolytic agents have been used clinically since the late 1940s.[1] The early pharmacologic preparations were obtained from the streptococcus bacterium and were impure, containing streptodornase and other foreign proteins in addition to the active agent streptokinase.[2] These contaminants were responsible for a variety of untoward systemic effects and forced Tillet and Sherry[2] to limit the use of thrombolytic agents to nonvascular disease processes, specifically, loculated hemothorax. In 1955, Tillet and his group at New York University reported the results of a clinical trial of intravenous streptokinase in 11 patients. The trial was designed to define the safety of the intravascular administration of the agent.[3] Unfortunately, pyogenic reactions were common, with low-grade fever developing in all of the patients and profound hypotension in four.

In 1956, Cliffton reported successful preliminary results with what was assumed to be the direct thrombolytic agent plasmin.[4] In truth, Cliffton's agent comprised a mixture of plasminogen and streptokinase, which was designed to generate free plasmin. However, it is likely that the observed thrombolytic effects occurred as a result of the streptokinase rather than the free plasmin.[5] Nevertheless, 1 year later, Cliffton reported an experience with 40 patients and documented the beneficial effects of direct

Advances in Vascular Surgery®, vol. 4
© 1996, Mosby–Year Book, Inc.

intra-arterial streptokinase-plasmin infusions in 2 patients with peripheral arterial occlusions.[6] Although Dotter is generally credited with pioneering catheter-directed peripheral arterial thrombolysis in 1974,[7] Cliffton actually documented the use of this technique 17 years earlier.

PHARMACOLOGY OF THROMBOLYTIC AGENTS

All thrombolytic agents represent "plasminogen activators," converting fibrin-bound plasminogen to fibrin-bound plasmin, which subsequently degrades the fibrin thrombus.[8] The administration of exogenous plasmin has very little, if any, thrombolytic activity.[9] In vitro studies have confirmed that free plasmin is ineffective in degrading fibrin, but it does produce degradation of fibrinogen and factors V and VIII.[10] These studies led to the formulation of a scheme of thrombolysis wherein plasminogen exists in two phases: a gel (thrombus) phase where it is bound to fibrin, and a soluble (plasma) phase where it is free.[11] Activation of soluble-phase plasminogen to free plasmin leads to degradation of fibrinogen and other plasma proteins but is ineffective in dissolving fibrin within a thrombus. Free plasmin is also rapidly inactivated by antiplasmins. Gel-phase plasminogen, however, when activated to fibrin-bound plasmin, results in selective fibrinolysis in an environment relatively protected from antiplasmins. This mechanism explains why the degradation of fibrin thrombus is dependent on the concentration of plasminogen activators but independent of the concentration of exogenously administered plasmin.[12]

Four thrombolytic agents currently are approved by the U.S. Food and Drug Administration: streptokinase, urokinase, rt-PA, and acylated plasminogen streptokinase activator complex (APSAC). Streptokinase is a purified isolate from the *Streptococcus* bacterium and is an inactive single-chain 46,000-Dalton protein. It forms a complex with plasminogen or plasmin, and this complex in turn activates additional plasminogen molecules. Urokinase, clinically employed in both high molecular weight (54,000 Dalton) and low molecular weight (31,000 Dalton) forms, is a two-chain compound present in urine. Unlike streptokinase, urokinase directly activates plasminogen without the need for initial binding to an additional plasminogen molecule. Recombinant tissue plasminogen activator is a single-chain molecule, 527 amino acids in length, and contains two kringle structures, one of which is important in the binding of rt-PA to fibrin.[13] Thus, rt-PA has been promoted as an agent with "fibrin specificity" and a low potential for systemic fibrinogen degradation. This contention has not been substantiated in the clinical setting, with similar decreases in plasma fibrinogen concentration after systemic administration of urokinase or rt-PA.[14] Acylated plasminogen streptokinase activator complex consists of an equimolar complex of streptokinase and plasminogen, originally developed to hasten fibrinolysis by eliminating the initial step of plasminogen binding. In practice, the benefits of APSAC may be related to its increased half-life rather than plasminogen supplementation.

The plasminogen activators differ in their relative rate of fibrin dissolution and in their fibrin specificity.[15] An ideal agent would manifest a high degree of fibrinolytic activity with a low potential for systemic fibrinogen degradation. Reputedly, streptokinase has the lowest activity and is not fibrin-specific. Urokinase is intermediate, but rt-PA has been reported to be associated with the highest rate of fibrinolysis and the greatest degree of fibrin specificity. To date, however, few studies have actually documented clinical benefits of any one agent over another.

THROMBOLYSIS FOR PERIPHERAL ARTERIAL OCCLUSION

Before the mid-20th century, the mode of intervention for the ischemic extremity was primary amputation. The advent of surgical revascularization in the late 1940s made salvage of the threatened limb a reality.[16, 17] The subsequent 4 decades witnessed an impressive improvement in technical advances, with the ability to save the vast majority of acutely ischemic limbs. Despite technical advances and decreases in the rate of amputation, limb salvage has been achieved at the cost of an alarmingly high perioperative mortality rate, approaching 25% in the review of Blaisdell[18] and approximately 20% in a later series by Jivegård.[19] More recently, Edwards and colleagues replaced 111 occluded lower-extremity bypass grafts with new autogenous vein conduits and documented a limb salvage rate of 90% at 5 years.[20] However, these results were associated with a mortality rate of 26% at 6 months, and only 12% of patients were alive at 5 years. The observations of these studies suggest that acute limb ischemia develops in a medically compromised subpopulation, a group that may be further jeopardized by invasive reconstructive procedures. The development of thrombolytic techniques provided the potential to restore arterial patency and limb viability in a less invasive manner, with the hope of achieving a lower morbidity than commonly ascribed to surgical revascularization.

TECHNIQUE OF ARTERIAL THROMBOLYSIS

At the outset, the most important caveat of arterial thrombolysis relates to the goal of therapy. One should not expect to replace surgery completely in patients with acute arterial occlusion. Rather, the aim of thrombolysis should be to uncover the anatomical lesion responsible for the occlusive event in most cases. Operation or endovascular interventions must subsequently ensue to correct the unmasked lesion. Only in the minority of cases with arterial thrombosis in the absence of a demonstrable anatomical lesion will thrombolysis not be followed by a remedial invasive intervention. Studies designed to document the effectiveness of thrombolysis are flawed when the primary outcome measure is avoidance of operation. Indeed, the goals of arterial thrombolysis should be to uncover and clearly define the etiologic mechanism of the occlusive event and to lessen the magnitude of subsequent intervention.

Irrespective of the agent used, arterial thrombolysis is best accomplished via a catheter-directed approach, with the delivery of activator agent directly into the substance of the thrombus.[21] In contrast to the setting of acute coronary artery occlusion, IV routes of administration have been entirely unsatisfactory in the periphery. This difference is presumably a result of the larger size of peripheral thrombi and the resultant inability of activator agent to diffuse into the thrombus. Both antegrade and contralateral catheter insertion techniques have been successfully employed. The ipsilateral femoral artery is the insertion site in the antegrade approach, angling the needle in a distal direction. It is frequently difficult to pass the guidewire into an occluded bypass graft using an antegrade approach; the wire preferentially enters the profunda femoris artery, and the close proximity of the graft orifice to the needle insertion site renders catheter manipulation arduous. The contralateral route is safest, especially in inexperienced hands, because failure to accomplish antegrade access may leave the patient with multiple needle-stick holes in the common femoral artery that can bleed during subsequent thrombolytic infusion through a contralateral approach. There is a tendency for thrombus to form on the wall of the catheter during any protracted intra-arterial procedure, and embolization of this "pericatheter thrombus" may occur as the thrombus is sheared off the catheter at the time of removal. The frequency of complications may be lessened through the use of small-bore catheters and concurrent heparin or aspirin therapy.

Several methods of infusion of thrombolytic agents are routinely used. A maximum duration of administration of 48 hours is recommended, as a prime correlate of complications appears to be the duration of infusion. Moreover, if successful lysis has not been accomplished after 48 hours, success is unlikely with continued therapy. Continuous infusions are common, usually beginning with a large dose and tapering thereafter. A "pulse-spray" technique has been used, bolusing the thrombolytic agent through a multiholed catheter along the length of the occlusive thrombus, potentially increasing the rate of dissolution. "Lacing" refers to the infusion of large amounts of agent along the length of the thrombus as the catheter is withdrawn, in an effort to attain even and complete distribution throughout the thrombus. To date, no consistent benefits have been documented with the use of one technique over another.[22]

It is important to follow the progress of thrombolysis with serial arteriographic studies. Catheter manipulation is necessary in most instances, repositioning the infusion holes to keep them within the substance of the undissolved thrombus. Distal embolization is a frequent complication of thrombolysis but is fortunately treatable with an increase in the thrombolytic dose (Table 1). Repositioning of the catheter into the distal emboli is not always necessary, as the material is usually sensitive to upstream administration of thrombolytic agent.

Monitoring of coagulation parameters during thrombolytic therapy remains controversial. Fibrinogen concentration, thrombin time, and other laboratory tests have been advocated as measures with which to gauge the risk of distant bleeding complications, but there is no conclusive evidence in this regard.[8,23] Bleeding complications almost always result from defects in vascular integrity, usually at the site of arterial cannulation. These events were generally thought to bear little correlation with abnormalities in the coagulation tests, but a recent study found a statistical correlation between bleeding and the fibrinogen concentration.[24]

RESULTS OF THROMBOLYSIS IN ACUTE PERIPHERAL ARTERIAL OCCLUSION

Large, retrospective series of patients treated with intra-arterial thrombolytic therapy began to appear in the early 1980s.[25-28] Success was re-

TABLE 1.
Early Complications of Thrombolytic Therapy for Peripheral Arterial Occlusion (1,133 Cases Published in the 1990s)

Author	SK	UK	rt-PA	Hemorrhage	2° Embolization	Limb Loss	Mortality
Graor[49]	200	200	65	75 (16%)	NS	95 (20%)	9 (2%)
McNamara[21]	0	72	0	2 (3%)	11 (15%)	6 (8%)	1 (1%)
Cragg[50]	0	72	0	8 (11%)	NS	5 (7%)	1 (1%)
DeMaioribus[51]	8	76	0	5 (6%)	3 (4%)	5 (6%)	2 (2%)
Faggioli[52]	0	134	0	14 (10%)	2 (1%)	11 (8%)	5 (4%)
Ouriel[33]	0	57	0	6 (11%)	5 (9%)	5 (9%)	7 (12%)
STILE Investigators[24]	0	112	137	14 (6%)	NS	13 (5%)	10 (4%)
Ouriel[34]	0	145	0	15 (10%)	NS	15 (10%)	6 (4%)
Total	208	868	202	139 (11%)	21 (6%)	155 (12%)	41 (3%)

Abbreviations: SK, streptokinase; *UK,* urokinase; *NS,* not specified.

ported in more than 90% of cases over a mean duration of infusion of 6 to 12 hours. Amputation rates averaged less than 10%, with early mortality rates of less than 5% and bleeding complications in 5% to 10% of patients. Urokinase and rt-PA were argued to be safer and more efficacious than streptokinase. There were, however, severe limitations with these studies. Streptokinase was used early in the course of each series, usually at a time when the medical team had little experience in thrombolytic treatment. Patients with acute and chronic limb ischemia were included in many of the studies, precluding meaningful comparison to data on truly threatened extremities. Moreover, outcome measures were frequently subjective, bearing little clinical relevance to limb salvage or mortality.

These early series triggered several contradictory reports, all retrospective and somewhat anecdotal.[29-31] The data generated by these studies argued against the use of thrombolytic agents in acute arterial occlusion, principally on the basis of poor patency rates associated with sole therapy and the frequent need for concurrent operative intervention to achieve an acceptable result. The goal of thrombolysis, however, is not to replace or eliminate surgery. Rather, thrombolytic therapy should be used in an effort to diminish the magnitude of required interventions and thereby decrease the frequency of morbid and mortal events. Studies that failed to tabulate long-term survival and limb salvage as primary end points predictably indicted thrombolysis as a useless therapeutic endeavor.

More recent trials have avoided these limitations by using a randomized, prospective design and objective, clinically relevant end points. There exist four randomized, prospective comparisons of thrombolysis and surgery in the setting of peripheral arterial occlusion. The first study to appear in the literature was a European trial of rt-PA thrombolysis vs. thrombectomy in 20 patients with acute arterial occlusions of fewer than

14 days' duration.[32] This study was too small to draw any meaningful conclusions, and this trial will not be discussed further.

A second study was performed at the University of Rochester and randomized 114 patients with limb-threatening peripheral arterial occlusions of fewer than 7 days' duration to initial therapy with either surgery or intra-arterial urokinase.[33] The design of the study provided for the immediate correction of anatomical defects unmasked by thrombolysis with operation or balloon dilatation. The primary end points of the study were limb salvage and survival. A total of 57 patients were randomized to thrombolytic therapy and 57 patients to operative therapy. Thrombolytic therapy resulted in dissolution of the occluding thrombus in 40 (70%) of the patients. Although cumulative limb salvage was similar in the two treatment groups (82% at 12 months), cumulative survival was significantly improved in patients randomized to thrombolysis (84% vs. 58% at 12 months, $P = 0.01$). The mortality differences appeared primarily attributable to an increased frequency of in-hospital cardiopulmonary complications in the operative treatment group (49% vs. 16%, $P = 0.001$). The differences in the long-term mortality rate were clearly associated with the development of in-hospital, treatment-related cardiopulmonary complications such as myocardial infarction, pulmonary embolism, and pneumonia. When the two treatment groups were subdivided into four subgroups on the basis of the presence or absence of in-hospital cardiopulmonary complications, the primary determinant of long-term survival was the development of cardiopulmonary complications rather than the form of therapy. Thus, it appeared that the explanation for the improved survival in the thrombolytic group was the lowered frequency of in-hospital cardiac and pulmonary complications. The difference in the frequency of these complications may be related to a lower magnitude of intervention in the thrombolytic group, concurrent with a decreased fibrinogen concentration after thrombolytic infusion.

A third randomized trial was the Surgery versus Thrombolysis for Ischemia of the Lower Extremity (STILE) trial.[24] This multicenter, North American study randomized patients with acute and subacute lower-extremity ischemia to one of three treatment arms: surgery, intra-arterial urokinase, or intra-arterial rt-PA. The results of the two thrombolytic arms did not differ in any category and were subsequently grouped for a comparative analysis with surgery. The primary difference between the STILE trial and the Rochester trial was the inclusion of patients with symptoms of a longer duration in the former; the mean length of time between the onset of symptoms in the STILE trial averaged 50 days, vs. only 27 hours in the Rochester series. A second differentiating feature was the use of a composite measure of clinical outcome as the primary end point in the STILE trial. Whereas the primary outcome measure in the Rochester trial was amputation-free survival, the STILE trial used the development of any of a wide variety of untoward events to define the occurrence of the primary end point. Several of these components were objective and clinically relevant (death, major amputation, and hemorrhage); others were less well defined (ongoing ischemia, vascular complications, perioperative complications).

The broad spectrum of components defining the primary end point in the STILE trial accounted for a large percentage of patients attaining a negative outcome—36.1% in the surgical group vs. 61.7% in the thrombolytic group at 1 month. This difference was highly significant and forced the premature termination of the study at 393 patients, concluding that surgery was more efficacious than thrombolysis in the treatment of the ischemic extremity. The data did not, however, reveal any differences in mortality or amputation rates. Moreover, thrombolysis was associated with a significant reduction in the magnitude of the planned revascularization procedure; thrombolysis permitted a reduction in the magnitude of the planned procedure in 55.8% of the patients, compared with only 5.5% of surgical patients. The most interesting findings related to the outcome in the subgroups of patients seen with ischemia of fewer than or greater than 2 weeks' duration. When symptoms began within 14 days of treatment, thrombolytic intervention was associated with a significant reduction in the need for major amputation, 11.1% vs. 30.0% ($P = 0.01$). By contrast, patients seen beyond 14 days after the onset of symptoms were best served with surgery; the amputation rate was 3.0% in the surgical group vs. 12.1% in the thrombolytic group ($P = 0.01$). Mortality differences were not observed, irrespective of the duration of ischemia. The authors concluded that surgical revascularization was more effective and safer than thrombolytic intervention in patients with ischemia lasting 6 months or fewer. A secondary conclusion, equally compelling and derived on the basis of the subgroup analysis, recommended a treatment strategy of catheter-directed thrombolysis for patients seen within 14 days of symptom onset and surgical revascularization for all others.

The final and most recently reported randomized trial of thrombolysis vs. operative therapy for peripheral arterial occlusion was Thrombolysis or Peripheral Arterial Surgery (TOPAS).[34] The TOPAS trial was organized to evaluate recombinant urokinase vs. operation for the initial treatment of patients with limb-threatening lower-extremity peripheral arterial occlusion. The study was divided into two phases: phase I was a dose-ranging trial designed to evaluate three doses of recombinant urokinase (2,000, 4,000, 6,000 IU/min for 4 hours, followed by 2,000 IU/min) or surgery, and phase II was a direct comparison of the "best" dose and surgery. The phase I results were reported in 1996; the phase II results are unavailable at the time of this writing.

There were few significant differences in the three urokinase dose regimens of the TOPAS phase I trial. Recanalization was observed in approximately three fourths of the patients in each group at the time of the completion arteriogram. Complete clot lysis was achieved in two thirds of the patients in each group. When the data were stratified by type of occlusion, the 2,000-IU/min group appeared less effective for bypass graft occlusions, with complete clot lysis in only 13% of the grafts after 4 hours of administration. By contrast, complete clot lysis was observed at 4 hours in over 30% of grafts treated with 4,000 or 6,000 IU/min. No such dosage differences were observed in the native artery occlusions.

In-hospital survival rate was highest in the 4,000-IU/min urokinase group. Similarly, the 30-day survival was highest in the 4,000-IU/min group, but the differences did not persist beyond this follow-up point. Although TOPAS phase I was not designed to compare urokinase with

TABLE 2.
Comparison of Hospital Costs Associated With Thrombolytic Therapy[33]

Cost Category	Thrombolytic Group ($n = 57$)	Operative Group ($n = 57$)
Nonpharmaceutical costs	$17,176 ± $4,328	$16,365 ± $4,408
Medication, including urokinase	$4,995 ± $630	$3,410 ± $764
Medication—urokinase only	$2,653 ± 243	0
Total costs	$22,171 ± $4,959	$19,775 ± $5,253

surgery, mortality data were assessed to document the safety of the agent in comparison to that of initial surgical therapy in order to ethically begin phase II of the trial. In this regard, the 30-day survival and amputation-free survival rates were 100% and 90% for patients treated with 4,000 IU of urokinase per minute vs. 95% and 86% for patients treated surgically.

A close examination of the data from the thrombolytic trials suggests that different patient categories will benefit from one form of therapy over another. In a multivariate analysis of patients treated with intra-arterial thrombolysis, several variables were found to be predictive of successful arteriographic dissolution.[35] Technical factors appeared most important. Successful lysis was seldom achieved if the infusion catheter could not be threaded into the thrombus or if a guidewire could not be passed through the occlusive process. Several clinical factors also attained significance as independent predictors of arteriographic success. Vein grafts were less likely to undergo successful lysis than prosthetic grafts or native arteries. Lysis was more frequently achieved in nondiabetics than diabetics and in patients with fewer arterial segments involved.

The economics of thrombolysis have attained increased significance with the recent emphasis on the cost of health care. Thrombolysis appears to be associated with a similar length of hospital stay when compared with operative intervention.[33] The cost of hospitalization may be somewhat greater when thrombolytic therapy is used, principally as a result of the cost of the lytic agent (Table 2). When professional fees are considered, however, these differences vanish.[33]

THROMBOLYSIS FOR DEEP VENOUS THROMBOSIS

Deep venous thrombosis is responsible for patient discomfort in the form of pain and edema, as well as the potentially fatal sequelae of pulmonary embolism and the chronic debilitating symptom complex comprising the postphlebitic syndrome. Although the clinical entity of deep venous thrombosis has been recognized for centuries, anticoagulation with heparin did not become commonplace until 1960, when a controlled trial revealed a reduced incidence of pulmonary embolism with anticoagulant therapy.[36] Although anticoagulation is beneficial in decreasing the risk of pulmonary embolic events, dissolution of the original deep venous thrombus is uncommon (Table 3).[37] Moreover, when recanalization does occur, it is universally accompanied by destruction of functional venous valves.

TABLE 3.
Dissolution of Thrombi in Deep Venous Thrombosis

Author	Route/Agent	Cases	Clot Dissolution
Goldhaber[38]	Systemic heparin	91	16 (18%)
Meyerovitz[41]	Systemic rt-PA	74	17 (23%)
Goldhaber[53]	Systemic high dose UK	27	14 (52%)
Semba[48]	Catheter directed UK	25	23 (92%)

Abbreviation: UK, urokinase.

Thrombolytic therapy offers the opportunity to dissolve venous thrombi, potentially decreasing the magnitude of venous valvular dysfunction. This benefit, however, must be weighed against the increased risk of bleeding associated with thrombolytic administration. Technical difficulties in delivering adequate amounts of thrombolytic agent into the substance of the thrombus may limit efficacy and result in a higher risk-benefit ratio. Each of these issues must be addressed when considering the use of thrombolysis for acute deep venous thrombosis.

Whereas operation is the standard with which all new peripheral arterial interventions must be compared, heparin is the standard for comparison in the setting of deep venous thrombosis. To date, streptokinase is the only agent approved by the U.S. Food and Drug Administration. Thus, controlled trials have generally compared heparin and streptokinase, focusing on outcome measures such as phlebographic resolution of thrombus and the development of the postthrombotic syndrome.

Goldhaber and colleagues analyzed six well-defined, randomized trials of IV streptokinase and heparin for deep venous thrombosis.[38] The duration of the thrombotic process was fewer than 4 days in three of the studies and fewer than 14 days in all six studies. The streptokinase dose was generally 100,000 U/hr for a duration of 24 to 72 hours, and loading doses were used in each study. Phlebographically documented resolution of thrombus was rarely observed in patients treated with heparin, with frequencies ranging from zero to 38%. By contrast, streptokinase therapy resulted in clot dissolution in 53% to 88% of patients, accounting for a 3.7-fold increase in the frequency of dissolution with thrombolytic agents compared with heparin alone. Of the six randomized trials evaluated, three found statistically significant benefits in the frequency of phlebographic resolution of thrombus. The three studies without significant differences still found apparent benefits with thrombolytic agents, with P values ranging from 0.08 to 0.14. These results must be analyzed in the context of clinical benefit; the phlebographic resolution of a portion of deep venous thrombus is unlikely to translate into meaningful, clinically significant long-term benefit.

Francis and Marder reviewed the published studies comparing streptokinase with anticoagulation.[39] Substantial phlebographic improvement was documented in only 45% of the thrombolytic group, although only 5% of the anticoagulated patients achieved significant dissolution of thrombus. A subsequent review of 13 studies by Comerota[40] corroborated these findings, documenting significant or complete clot resolution in less than one half of the patients treated with thrombolytic agents.[40] Although some degree of clot lysis is to be expected with the systemic administration of thrombolytic agents, a study by Meyerovitz et al. documented greater than 80% lysis in only 17% of 110 venous segments in 50 patients treated with rt-PA.[41] These rather marginal results have been achieved at the cost of a significant incidence of bleeding complications, averaging approximately 20% in thrombolysed patients vs. less than 5% in patients receiving anticoagulation alone.[37] In the meta-analysis performed by Goldhaber et al., the risk of major bleeding was increased by a factor of 2.9 in patients receiving streptokinase vs. heparin ($P = 0.04$).[38]

Although the obvious short-term goal of thrombolysis is to achieve significant clot dissolution, the ultimate aims are to preserve valve function and provide long-term relief from the devastating complications of the postthrombotic syndrome. Major deep venous thrombosis is associated with the development of postthrombotic symptoms in 60% of patients vs. only 36% of patients treated with thrombolysis.[42, 43] These clinical findings are in concert with the physiologic data of Watz and Savidge.[44] These investigators performed descending phlebograms on patients treated with streptokinase or heparin. Normal proximal valve function was observed in 92% of the thrombolysed patients, vs. only 13% in patients treated with anticoagulation. The extent of thrombolytic dissolution is a predictor of subsequent postthrombotic symptoms, as clearly demonstrated in a study by Turpie and colleagues.[45, 46] In a randomized trial of rt-PA and heparin vs. heparin alone in the treatment of iliofemoral deep venous thrombosis, these authors observed a 25% incidence of postthrombotic symptoms in the patients who achieved greater than 50% clot lysis, compared with 56% in the patients in whom lysis was less than 50% ($P = 0.07$). Physiologic confirmation of the ability of thrombolysis to preserve valve function was provided by a study of Jeffery and associates.[47] Of 40 patients treated with thrombolysis, 12 (30%) achieved successful lysis. Doppler reflux was noted in only 9% of the patients with lysis, vs. 77% of those without ($P < 0.001$). Photoplethysmographic capillary refill to one-half baseline tracing, an index of venous valvular function, took 12 seconds in the patients with successful dissolution of thrombus, compared with only 5 seconds in patients without dissolution ($P < 0.001$).

A summary of the aforementioned data suggests that successful thrombolysis of venous clot is associated with a significant reduction in long-term venous sequelae. The most significant problem remaining, however, is the relatively low frequency of successful dissolution using standard, systemic protocols for thrombolytic administration. Experience with arterial thrombi has confirmed the importance of adequate contact of thrombolytic agent with the fibrin clot.[28] Corresponding data in the setting of venous thrombosis have been provided in the study by Meyerovitz and associates.[41] Data were analyzed from 139 thrombosed venous segments in patients randomized to rt-PA alone (34 patients), rt-PA plus heparin (16 patients), or heparin alone (12 patients). Initial and follow-up phlebography documented greater than 50% clot lysis in 25% of the patients treated with rt-PA; lysis was not observed in any of the segments treated with heparin alone. A prime correlate of successful lysis was the presence of a nonocclusive thrombus, where thrombolytic agent could reach the clot via the blood traversing the involved segment. Successful dissolution (greater than 50%) occurred in 59% of 29 nonocclusive thrombi, vs. only 14% of 81 obstructive thrombi.

The problem of thrombolytic access to a venous segment completely filled with occlusive thrombi has been addressed by Semba and Dake, using a catheter-directed technique of thrombolytic administration.[48] By embedding the catheter infusion ports into the substance of the clot, thrombolytic agent can be efficiently delivered into the occluding thrombus to achieve a high local concentration of plasminogen activator. The authors recommend a percutaneous approach to the right internal jugular vein, providing easy access to iliofemoral thrombi. Vena caval filters were not routinely used. Urokinase was infused into the thrombus, at doses of approximately 3,000 IU/min. Thrombolysis was followed by balloon angioplasty with or without a stent, performed to correct any underlying venous stenosis. Successful recanalization of the vein with less than a 30% residual stenosis was achieved in 85% of the 27 patients in the series, with an average duration of infusion of 30 hours. The age of the process did not appear to be a predictor of success; five of seven thrombi older than 4 weeks (mean duration, 1 year) were thrombolysed. Noninvasive and phlebographic follow-up was obtained at 3 months in 12 patients with initially successful lysis, and 11 (92%) maintained patency.

In summary, lower-extremity venous thrombi respond poorly to systemic thrombolytic therapy unless they are nonocclusive. The risks of bleeding may not justify the limited success and moderate long-term protection against postthrombotic sequelae. By contrast, large iliofemoral thrombi respond well to a catheter-directed approach. The risk of bleeding appears low and may be offset by a reduction in the frequency of postthrombotic symptoms. These observations form the basis of a rational protocol for the treatment of deep venous thromboses, using heparin and warfarin for infrainguinal, moderately symptomatic thrombi and catheter-directed thrombolysis for highly symptomatic iliofemoral venous thromboses.

REFERENCES

1. Tillett WS, Sherry S: The effect in patients of streptococcal fibrinolysin (streptokinase) and streptococcal desoxyribonuclease on fibrinous, purulent, and sanguineous pleural exudations. *J Clin Invest* 28:173, 1949.
2. Tillett WS, Sherry S, Christensen LR: Streptococcal desoxyribonuclease: Significance in lysis of purulent exudates and production by strains of hemolytic streptococci. *Proc Soc Exp Biol Med* 68:184, 1948.
3. Tillett WS, Johnson AJ, McCarty WR: The intravenous infusion of the streptococcal fibrinolytic principle (streptokinase) into patients. *J Clin Invest* 34:169–185, 1955.
4. Cliffton EE, Grossi CE: Investigations of intravenous plasmin (fibrinolysin) in humans; physiologic and clinical effects. *Circulation* 14:919, 1956.
5. Sherry S, Fletcher AP, Alkjaersig N: Developments in fibrinolytic therapy for thromboembolic disease. *Ann Intern Med* 50:560, 1959.

6. Cliffton EE: The use of plasmin in humans. *Ann N Y Acad Sci* 68:209–229, 1957.

7. Dotter CT, Rosch J, Seaman AJ: Selective clot lysis with low-dose streptokinase. *Radiology* 111:31–37, 1974.

8. Marder VJ: The use of thrombolytic agents: Choice of patient, drug administration, laboratory monitoring. *Ann Intern Med* 90:802–812, 1979.

9. Alkjaersig N, Fletcher AP, Sherry S: The mechanism of clot dissolution by plasmin. *J Clin Invest* 38:1086, 1959.

10. Marder VJ, Sherry S: Thrombolytic therapy: Current status-I. *N Engl J Med* 318:1512–1520, 1988.

11. Sherry S, Fletcher AP, Alkjaersig N: Fibrinolysis and fibrinolytic activity in man. *Physiol Rev* 39:343, 1959.

12. Sherry S, Lindemeyer RI, Fletcher AP: Studies on enhanced fibrinolytic activity in man. *J Clin Invest* 38:810, 1959.

13. Agnelli G, Buchanan MR, Fernandez F, et al: The thrombolytic and hemorrhagic effects of tissue type plasminogen activator: Influence of dosage regimens in rabbits. *Thromb Res* 40:769–777, 1985.

14. Goldhaber SZ, Heit J, Sharma GVRK, et al: Randomized controlled trial of recombinant tissue plasminogen activator versus urokinase in the treatment of acute pulmonary embolism. *Lancet* 2:293–298, 1988.

15. Kane KK: Fibrinolysis—a review. *Ann Clin Lab Sci* 14:443–449, 1984.

16. Kunlin J: Le traitement de l'arterite oblitérante par la greffe veineuse. *Arch Malad Coeur Vaiss* 42:371, 1949.

17. Dos Santos JC: Sur la desobstruction des thrombus arterielles anciennes. *Mem Acad Chir* 73:409, 1947.

18. Blaisdell FW, Steele M, Allen RE: Management of acute lower extremity arterial ischemia due to embolism and thrombosis. *Surgery* 84:822–834, 1978.

19. Jivegård L, Holm J, Schersten T: Acute limb ischemia due to arterial embolism or thrombosis: Influence of limb ischemia versus pre-existing cardiac disease on postoperative mortality rate. *J Cardiovasc Surg* 29:32–36, 1988.

20. Edwards JE, Taylor LM Jr, Porter JM: Treatment of failed lower extremity bypass grafts with new autogenous vein bypass grafting. *J Vasc Surg* 11:136–145, 1990.

21. McNamara TO, Bomberger RA, Merchant RF: Intra-arterial urokinase as the initial therapy for acutely ischemic lower limbs. *Circulation* 83:I-106S–I-119S, 1991.

22. Kandarpa K, Chopra PS, Aruny JE, et al: Prospective, randomized comparison of forced periodic infusion and conventional slow continuous infusion. *Radiology* 188:1–7, 1993.

23. Marder VJ, Sherry S: Thrombolytic therapy: Current status (II). *N Engl J Med* 318:1585–1595, 1988.

24. The STILE Investigators: Results of a prospective randomized trial evaluating surgery versus thrombolysis for ischemia of the lower extremity: The STILE trial. *Ann Surg* 220:251–268, 1994.

25. Graor RA, Risius B, Young JR, et al: Low-dose streptokinase for selective thrombolysis: Systemic effects and complications. *Radiology* 152:35–39, 1984.

26. Krings W, Roth FJ, Cappius G, et al: Catheter-lysis: Indications and primary results. *Int Angiology* 4:117–123, 1985.

27. Graor RA, Risius B, Lucas FV, et al: Thrombolysis with recombinant human tissue-type plasminogen activator in patients with peripheral artery and bypass graft occlusions. *Circulation* 74:15I–20I, 1986.

28. McNamara TO, Fischer JR: Thrombolysis of peripheral arterial and graft occlusions: Improved results using high-dose urokinase. *Am J Roentgenol* 144:769–775, 1985.

29. Sicard GA, Schier JJ, Totty WG, et al: Thrombolytic therapy for acute arterial occlusion. *J Vasc Surg* 2:65–78, 1985.

30. Ricotta J: Intra-arterial thrombolysis. A surgical view (comment). *Circulation* 83:1201–1211, 1991.

31. Lacombe M: Surgical versus medical treatment of renal artery embolism. *J Cardiovasc Surg* 18:281–290, 1977.

32. Nilsson L, Albrechtsson U, Jonung T, et al: Surgical treatment versus thrombolysis in acute arterial occlusion: A randomised controlled study. *Eur J Vasc Surg* 6:189–193, 1992.

33. Ouriel K, Shortell CK, DeWeese JA, et al: A comparison of thrombolytic therapy with operative revascularization in the treatment of acute peripheral arterial ischemia. *J Vasc Surg* 19:1021–1030, 1994.

34. Ouriel K, Veith FJ, Sasahara AA: Thrombolysis or peripheral arterial surgery: Phase I results. *J Vasc Surg* 23:64–75, 1996.

35. Ouriel K, Shortell CK, Azodo MVU, et al: Predictors of success in catheter-directed thrombolytic therapy of acute peripheral arterial occlusion. *Radiology* 193:561–566, 1994.

36. Barret D, Jordan S: Anticoagulant drugs in the treatment of pulmonary embolism: A controlled clinical trial. *Lancet* 1:1309, 1960.

37. Arnesen H: Heparin vs. streptokinase in the treatment of deep venous thrombosis: Short- and long-term results, in Comerota AJ (ed): *Thrombolytic Therapy*. Orlando, Fla, Grune & Stratton, 1988, pp 41–50.

38. Goldhaber SZ, Buring JE, Lipnick RJ, et al: Pooled analyses of randomized trials of streptokinase and heparin in phlebographically documented acute deep venous thrombosis. *Am J Med* 76:393–397, 1984.

39. Francis CW, Marder VJ: Fibrinolytic therapy for venous thrombosis. *Prog Cardiovasc Dis* 34:193–204, 1991.

40. Comerota AJ, Aldridge SC: Thrombolytic therapy for deep venous thrombosis: A clinical review. *Can J Surg* 36:359–364, 1993.

41. Meyerovitz MF, Polak JF, Goldhaber SZ: Short-term response to thrombolytic therapy in deep venous thrombosis: Predictive value of venographic appearance. *Radiology* 184:345–348, 1992.

42. Elliot MS, Immelman EJ, Jeffrey P, et al: A comparative randomized trial of heparin versus streptokinase in the treatment of acute proximal venous thrombosis: An interim report of a prospective trial. *Br J Surg* 66:838, 1979.

43. Comerota AJ: An overview of thrombolytic therapy for venous thromboembolism, in Comerota AJ (ed): *Thrombolytic Therapy*. Orlando, Fla, Grune & Stratton, 1988, pp 65–89.

44. Watz R, Savidge GF: Rapid thrombolysis and preservation of venous valvular function in high deep vein thrombosis. *Acta Med Scand* 205:293, 1979.

45. Turpie AGG, Jay RM, Carter CJ, et al: A randomized trial of recombinant tissue plasminogen activator for the treatment of proximal deep vein thrombosis. *Circulation* 72:III–193, 1985.

46. Turpie AG, Levine MN, Hirsh J, et al: Tissue plasminogen activator (rt-PA) vs heparin in deep vein thrombosis. Results of a randomized trial. *Chest* 97:172S–175S, 1990.

47. Jeffery P, Immelman E, Amoore J: Treatment of deep vein thrombosis with heparin or streptokinase: Long-term venous function assessment. *Proceedings of the Second International Vascular Symposium*, S20.3, 1986.

48. Semba CP, Dake MD: Iliofemoral deep venous thrombosis: Aggressive therapy with catheter-directed thrombolysis. *Radiology* 191:487–494, 1994.

49. Graor RA, Olin J, Bartholomew JR, et al: Efficacy and safety of intraarterial local infusion of streptokinase, urokinase, or tissue plasminogen activator for peripheral arterial occlusion: A retrospective review. *J Vasc Med Bio* 2:310–315, 1990.

50. Cragg AH, Smith TP, Corson JD, et al: Two urokinase dose regimens in native artery and graft occlusions. *Radiology* 178:681–686, 1991.
51. DeMaioribus CA, Mills JL, Fujitani RM: A reevaluation of intraarterial thrombolytic therapy for acute lower extremity ischemia. *J Vasc Surg* 17:888–895, 1993.
52. Faggioli GL, Peer RM, Pedrini L, et al: Failure of thrombolytic therapy to improve long-term vascular patency. *J Vasc Surg* 19:289–297, 1994.
53. Goldhaber SZ, Polak JF, Feldstein ML, et al: Efficacy and safety of repeated boluses of urokinase in the treatment of deep venous thrombosis. *Am J Cardiol* 73:75–79, 1994.

Rotary Atherectomy: A Downdate

Samuel S. Ahn, M.D.
Associate Clinical Professor of Surgery, UCLA Center for the Health Sciences, Section of Vascular Surgery, Los Angeles, California

Blessie Concepcion, B.S.
UCLA Center for the Health Sciences, Section of Vascular Surgery, Los Angeles, California

Atherectomy was conceived to address the limitations of the most commonly used procedure in treating peripheral arterial occlusive disease, percutaneous transluminal angioplasty (PTA). These limitations include its inability to treat lengthy diffuse or chronic occlusive disease,[1-3] inasmuch as acute occlusion occurs in 3% to 5% of cases[4-6] and restenosis in 30% to 40% within 6 months.[7-11] The concept of "debulking" or removing atheroma by using a mechanical, catheter-deliverable endarterectomy device was a very appealing alternative to PTA, which merely cracks, dissects, and stretches the vessel wall. Atherectomy applies remarkable technology designed to produce the aesthetic result of a smooth lumen without flaps, dissections, perforations, or other abnormalities and consequently reduce the likelihood of thromboembolization, restenosis, and reocclusion. Ablative "rotary" atherectomy uses a high-speed rotational device to micropulverize plaque into fragments small enough to be aspirated or removed harmlessly through the reticuloendothelial system. Rotary atherectomy devices include the Trac-Wright catheter and the Auth Rotablator.

The initial enthusiasm for these atherectomy devices was overwhelming, and clinical investigators reported promising early results. However, the optimism and euphoria quickly gave way to more somber, realistic expectations inasmuch as complications associated with atherectomy and clinical results beyond 6 months were reportedly dismal. This chapter will provide a critical review of the indications, results, complications, and limitations of the Trac-Wright catheter and the Auth Rotablator.

TRAC-WRIGHT CATHETER

DESCRIPTION OF THE DEVICE

First known as the Kensey atherectomy device and then as the Theratek catheter, the Trac-Wright catheter (Dow-Corning Wright, Arlington, Tenn) is composed of a rotating cam tip attached to a central driveshaft housed within a flexible polyurethane catheter. Powered by an electric motor, the

Advances in Vascular Surgery®, vol. 4

cam tip revolves at speeds up to 100,000 rpm. The rotating cam tip is designed to selectively micropulverize fibrous or firm atheromatous plaque without damaging the arterial wall (Fig 1). The polyurethane catheter contains a coaxial lumen through which contrast mixture is infused during the procedure to provide fluoroscopic guidance. A mixture of radiopaque contrast, dextran, urokinase, and heparin is infused at high rates and pressures to generate a radial jet from the rotating tip, that cools the rotating cam and also dilates the artery. The lateral pressure generated may approach 800 mm Hg at 100,000 rpm. Theoretically, the rotating cam follows the path of least resistance as it gently moves forward while remaining in the central channel. Thus there is no need for a leading guide wire.

The Trac-Wright catheter was available in 5, 8, and 10 French, which created a small lumen ranging from 1.7 to 3.3 mm and thus often required adjunctive PTA to create a satisfactory luminal wall that matched the normal portion of the artery. In these cases, the catheter generally acts as a pilot guide wire that debulks a hole to allow easier access for balloon angioplasty.

INDICATIONS

Clinical investigators have practically limited the application of the Trac-Wright catheter to the recanalization of long occlusive lesions (Table 1),[12–19] requiring adjunctive PTA in most of these lesions. Many of the patients treated with this device had claudication or limb-threatening ischemia. Their results show that the catheter should not be used to treat such complex lesions. The initial success rates are disappointingly low, and the patency rates are dismal because of high reocclusion rates (see Table 1). Furthermore, complications associated with the device in treat-

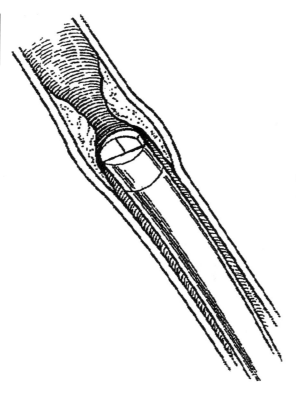

FIGURE 1.
The Trac-Wright catheter has a rotating cam tip that revolves at 100,000 rpm to pulverize atheromatous plaque.

TABLE 1.
Results of the Trac-Wright Catheter

Study	Lesions, N	Lesion Length, cm		Technical Success, %	Immediate Clinical Success, %	Clinical Patency %		
		Mean	Range			6 mo	12 mo	24 mo
Wholey[12]	12	—	15–40	100	67	—	—	—
Desbrosses[13]	46*	9.8	2–24	87	76	51	40	—
Cull[14]	46*	7.2	1–20	67	59	43	38	37.5
Snyder[15]	46	7.15	2–20	67	59	60	37.5	—
Lukes[16]	12*	—	6–20	58	33	25	25	—
Triller[17]	25*	8	5–15	80	76	59	38	—
Dyet[18]	22*	10.7	3–25	86	80	68	45	—
Meloni[19]	15*	6	—	87	—	51	51	51

*Adjunctive percutaneous transluminal angioplasty was performed on all treated lesions.

TABLE 2.

Complications of the Trac-Wright Catheter

Complications	Wholey[12]	Desbrosses[13]	Cull[14]	Snyder[15]	Lukes[16]	Triller[17]	Dyet[18]	Meloni[19]
Dissection	—	—	2/46 (4%)	—	—	5/25 (20%)	5/22 (23%)	1/15 (7%)
Embolization	1/12 (8%)	3/46 (7%)	—	—	—	5/25 (20%)	—	—
Hematoma	—	—	2/46 (4%)	3/46 (7%)	1/12 (8%)	—	—	—
Lymphocele	—	—	1/46 (2%)	—	—	—	—	—
Perforation	—	4/46 (9%)	11/46 (24%)	11/46 (24%)	4/12 (33%)	—	—	1/15 (7%)
Thrombosis	1/12 (8%)	—	—	—	—	—	—	—

ing long occlusive lesions are significant (Table 2). Nevertheless, the catheter has been successful in treating short (< 5 cm) stenotic or occlusive lesions (Table 3).

RESULTS

Although adjunctive PTA was performed in most of these clinical series, the reported initial technical and clinical success rates ranged widely from 58% to 100% and 33% to 80%, respectively (see Table 1).[12–19] These poor results may be attributed to the fact that most of the lesions treated in these clinical trials were long and occlusive. Desbrosses et al.[13] and Lukes et al.[16] reported early failures in treating calcified arteries. Intraoperative complications included dissection and vessel perforation, where extensive extravasation of contrast medium was observed fluoroscopically.[13–19] In these cases, atherectomy with the Trac-Wright catheter was aborted.

Overall, patency rates were most disappointing, with 25% to 68% reported at 6 months and 25% to 51% at 12 months (see Table 1).[12–19] Reocclusion of the treated arteries was a significant factor in these poor results.

COMPLICATIONS AND LIMITATIONS

As previously mentioned, the main complications associated with the Trac-Wright catheter are dissection and perforation (see Table 2). These complications reveal that the high-pressure fluid jet does not always keep the catheter safely in the central channel of the obstructed artery. Indeed, in an in vitro angioscopic study, Gehani et al.[20] noted that the catheter remained in the central coaxial position approximately 60% of the time and was causing critical intimal damage of the arterial wall. Furthermore, perforation induced by the rotating cam tip occurred mostly in heavily calcified lesions.[13–16, 19] The catheter follows the path of least resistance, which is often away from hard calcified plaque. The high risk of perforation and difficulty in recanalizing calcific lesions limit use of the catheter, particularly in the iliac and tibial arteries.

Theoretically, the Trac-Wright catheter micropulverizes atherosclerotic plaque into fine particles the size of red blood cells; the particles then pass harmlessly through the reticuloendothelial system. Several investigators have conducted in vitro studies to analyze the distribution and size of atheromatous debris after atherectomy with the Trac-Wright cath-

TABLE 3.
Indications for Use of the Trac-Wright Catheter

Amenable Lesions	Arterial Site	Complications/Limitations
Occlusion	Superficial femoral	Dissection
Short (< 5 cm)	Popliteal	Embolization
Stenosis		Perforation
Focal		Reocclusion

eter. Moellmann et al.[21] reported that nearly 80% of all particles ranged from 5 to 15 μm (approximately the size of red blood cells), over 20% of the particles were larger than 15 μm, and 2% were larger than 100 μm. Indeed, distal embolizations have been documented by some investigators[12, 13, 17] (see Table 2). Wholey et al.[12] reported one case of procedure-related embolization that subsequently led to amputation.

Reocclusion limits the applicability of this atherectomy device. Several investigators have reported the incidence of early reocclusions: Wholey et al.[12] reported reocclusion in 4 of 12 (33%), Desbrosses et al.[13] reported reocclusion in 5 of 46 (11%) within 48 hours, and Lukes et al.[16] reported reocclusion in 1 of 12 (8%) within 11 days. Furthermore, Moellmann et al.[21] reported a high 50% reocclusion and restenosis rate between 2 weeks and 10 months in treating 7 patients with occlusive and 3 with stenotic lesions. The Trac-Wright catheter has recently been removed from the market because it offers no true clinical benefit and has very limited application.

AUTH ROTABLATOR

DESCRIPTION OF THE DEVICE

The Auth Rotablator (Heart Technology, Inc., Bellevue, Wash) is a flexible, catheter-deliverable atherectomy device with a variable-sized, football-shaped metal bur on the distal tip. This high-speed rotary bur is studded with diamond chips ranging in size from 22 to 45 μm that function as multiple microknives. The rotating bur tracks along a central guide wire that prevents deflection of the bur away from the obstructive lesion (Fig 2). Burs are available in various sizes ranging from 1.25 to 6.0 mm. Progressively larger burs are used during the recanalization process until a satisfactory arterial lumen is obtained.

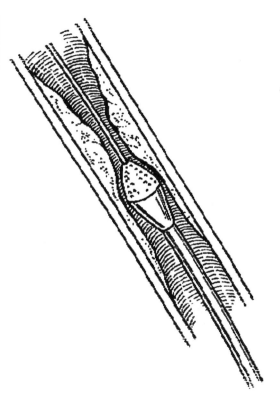

FIGURE 2.
The Auth Rotablator has a rotating bur that tracks along a central guide wire at 100,000 to 200,000 rpm to pulverize the atheromatous plaque.

The diamond-coated metal bur is welded to a flexible driveshaft that is encased within a protective plastic sheath to form a flexible catheter-deliverable system (Fig 3). The driveshaft is driven by a turbine housed within a plastic casing (Fig 4). Compressed air enters the turbine, which is capable of rotating the driveshaft in excess of 100,000 to 200,000 rpm. A strobe light built into the system measures and displays the revolutions per minute on a control panel. The revolutions per minute are controlled by air pressure, which is controlled by a dial on the control panel or by a separate foot pedal. The system also contains an irrigation port that leads to the plastic sheath around the rotating driveshaft. This irrigation solution thus lubricates and cools the rotating driveshaft and bur. A control knob on top of the plastic casing allows the surgeon to deliberately advance or retract the bur over the guide wire. The driveshaft has a built-in disengagement mechanism that stops the rotation at very low torque, thus preventing the artery from wrapping around the rotating bur or catheter. The guide wire comes separately and can be placed through the stenotic lesion entirely separate from the system and then integrated with the system by traversing the central part of the driveshaft and bur.

Atherectomy with the Rotablator assumes the concept of differential cutting in which the high rotating speed and the diamond microchips preferentially attack hard calcified atheroma and leave the surrounding viscoelastic tissue of normal arterial wall intact. Soft elastic tissue deflects

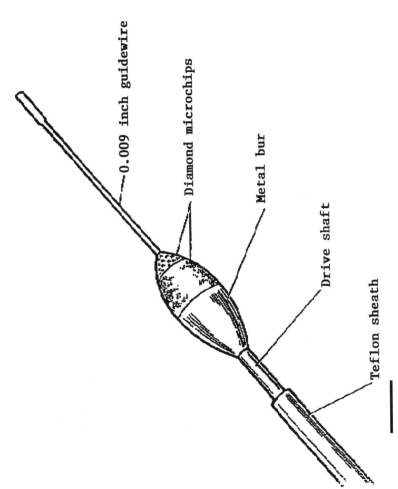

FIGURE 3.

The rotating metal bur is studded with diamond microchips and is welded onto a flexible driveshaft.

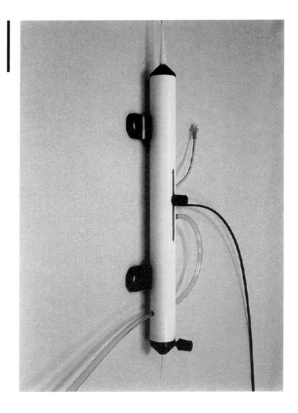

FIGURE 4.

The Auth Rotablator unit with the turbine housed within a plastic casing. The hard rigid tissue is cut off.

INDICATIONS

The Auth Rotablator is designed to treat hard calcified atheroma, especially in diabetic patients who have disabling claudication or limb-threatening ischemia. The device can be used in the superficial femoral, popliteal, and tibial arteries (Table 4). Experience with use in the iliac arteries is limited and generally not recommended.

Short stenotic lesions are ideally suited for treatment with the Auth Rotablator. Concentric and eccentric plaque also can be treated quite satisfactorily (see Table 4). Long, diffusely stenotic lesions appear uniquely suitable for this device because these lesions can readily be traversed by the guide wire and then followed with the atherectomy bur. Long total occlusions are difficult to traverse with the guide wire and are thus best suited for standard bypass procedures. Short total occlusions can be treated with the Rotablator only if the guide wire can readily traverse the occlusion.

TABLE 4.

Indications for Use of the Auth Rotablator

Amenable Lesions	Arterial Site	Complications/Limitations
Stenosis	Superficial femoral	Embolization
Long or short	Popliteal	Restenosis/reocclusion
Calcified atheroma	Tibial	Thrombosis
Concentric plaque		
Eccentric plaque		

TABLE 5.
Results of Use of the Auth Rotablator

Study	Patients, N	Lesions, N	Technical Success, %	Immediate Clinical Success, %	Clinical Patency, %		
					6 mo	12 mo	24 mo
Dorros[22]	43	82	95	88	—	—	—
Ahn[23]	20	42	93	72	66	47	12
White[24]	17	18	94	94	82	—	—
CRAG[25]	72	107	89	77	47	31	18.6
Henry[26]	150	212	97	85	58*	—	—
Myers[27]	34	36	94	92	68	60.7	—

*At 4 months, 163 lesions were evaluated for follow-up.
Abbreviation: CRAG, Collaborative Rotablator Atherectomy Group.

RESULTS

Several investigators reported promising technical but suboptimal immediate clinical success rates with the Auth Rotablator (Table 5).[22-27] Most of these series reported only a short follow-up of 6 months, and patencies at this time interval were poor, ranging from 47% to 82%. Furthermore, patencies at 1 year were worse: Ahn et al.[23] achieved a patency rate of 47% as a result of early thromboembolic complications; the Collaborative Rotablator Atherectomy Group (CRAG)[25] reported a disappointing 31% patency rate because of significant early failures and complications, and Myers et al.[27] achieved a rate of 61% from a small series of patients.

Ahn et al.[23] performed atherectomy with the Rotablator in patients with claudication, ulcer or gangrene, rest pain, and an asymptomatic failing graft. Twenty lesions ranged from 50% to 95% stenosis, and 5 lesions were occlusive. Although most of the residual lumen achieved was less than 20%, restenosis occurred in 9 of 20 (45%) and reocclusion in 4 of 20 (20%) within 18 months. Furthermore, intimal hyperplasia was clearly documented angioscopically or surgically in 4 of these cases and was suggestive in 9 cases arteriographically. The clinical patency rate at 2 years was a dismal 12%.

The CRAG[25] reported their experience with the Auth Rotablator from a multicenter trial. Angiographic success (residual lumen less than 25%) was achieved in 70 of 79 limbs (89%) and in 82 of 107 arteries (77%). The 9 limbs that demonstrated angiographic failure had a variety of technical problems, and in hospital thrombosis developed in 9 additional limbs, for an in-hospital success rate of 77% (61 of 79 limbs). Complications developed in approximately half of the patients, and half of these resulted in failure requiring an urgent or emergent surgical procedure within 30 days. Six of these patients underwent amputation, 2 of which were device related. Late failure was observed in 32 limbs within 15 to 41 months, 4 of which also resulted in an amputation. The clinical patency rate at 2 years was a most disappointing 18.6%. Interestingly, there was no statistically significant difference in the patency rates achieved between the limbs treated by atherectomy alone and those treated by atherectomy plus PTA or other vascular procedures.

COMPLICATIONS AND LIMITATIONS

In addition to the poor intermediate and long-term results just discussed, peripheral atherectomy with the Auth Rotablator currently has limited application because of its wide array of complications (Table 6). Significant early thromboses have been reported by Ahn et al.,[23] the CRAG,[25] and Henry et al.[26] Ahn et al.[23] reported 5 in-hospital cases of thromboses in 20 patients (25%), 4 of which were associated with hypercoagulable states and 1 subsequently necessitating a below-knee amputation. The CRAG[25] reported early thromboses in 9 of 79 patients (11%), 2 of which led to an amputation. Henry et al.[26] correlated the 12 thromboses in 150 patients (8%) in their series to a number of factors, including dissection, elastic recoil, intimal flaps, lengthy lesion, residual stenosis, or vasospasm.

TABLE 6. Complications Associated With Use of the Auth Rotablator

Complications	Dorros[22]	Ahn[23]	White[24]	CRAG[25]	Henry[26]	Myers[27]*
Bleeding	—	—	—	10/79 (13%)	—	1/34 (3%)
Cardiorespiratory	—	—	1/17 (6%)	—	—	—
Dissection	1/20 (5%)	—	—	5/79 (6%)	3/150 (2%)	—
Embolization	4/20 (20%)	—	—	8/79 (10%)	2/150 (1%)	—
Hematoma	10/43 (23%)	1/20 (5%)	1/17 (6%)	4/79 (5%)	—	—
Hemoglobinuria	27/43 (63%)	4/20 (20%)	—	10/79 (13%)	—	—
Infection	—	1/20 (5%)	—	1/79 (1%)	—	—
Limb loss (device related)	—	1/20 (5%)	—	2/79 (3%)	—	—
Perforation	2/43 (5%)	—	—	3/79 (4%)	1/150 (0.7%)	—
Pseudoaneurysm	—	—	—	1/79 (1%)	—	—
Spasm	10/43 (23%)	—	—	—	17/150 (11%)	—
Arterial tear	2/43 (5%)	—	—	—	—	—
Thrombosis	1/43 (2%)	5/20 (25%)	1/17 (6%)	9/79 (11%)	12/150 (8%)	—

*The number of patients in whom hemoglobinuria developed was not reported.

Abbreviation: CRAG, Collaborative Rotablator Atherectomy Group.

Arterial spasm has been encountered by Dorros et al.[22] in 23% and Henry et al.[26] in 11% of their cases (see Table 6). These spasms occurred mostly in small distal arteries and were attributed to the use of large burs, long rotational sequences, and/or the rotational speed.

Like all other atherectomy devices, the Auth Rotablator can cause dissection and perforation (see Table 6). The arterial wall did not always remain intact during the high-speed rotational ablation as previously reported.[28, 29] The CRAG[25] reported 9 initial technical failures, primarily as a result of dissection and perforation. Dissection can be avoided with greater care in use of the guide wire and introducer sheath. Perforations are often caused by bur entanglement and dislodgement, which can be avoided by not advancing the bur too rapidly.

Some investigators[22, 23, 25] reported cases of hemoglobinuria without any clinical sequelae (see Table 6). These cases were transient and developed in lesions that required larger burs and prolonged rotary sequences. This phenomenon may result from the high vortex forces created by the rapidly spinning bur. The larger bur has a faster circumferential speed and also has larger diamond bits, thus leading to the higher vortex forces. The prolonged atherectomy time can be minimized by using small burs initially and increasing the bur size incrementally. The smaller burs grind through the plaque easier and faster than the larger burs.

Previous studies[28] have indicated that embolic complications are not likely to occur with the Rotablator because the micropulverized particles are small enough to pass through the reticuloendothelial system. Contrary to this finding, some investigators[23, 25, 26] reported cases of embolic complications (see Table 6). The CRAG[25] reported eight embolic cases, three of which resulted in cutaneous necrosis and one in toe amputation.

Like PTA and all other atherectomy devices, restenosis and reocclusion are significant limiting factors of the Auth Rotablator. As previously mentioned, intimal hyperplasia may be the inciting factor. The CRAG[25] reported that such cases developed within 12 months. Recently, Henry et al.[26] reported a 24% restenosis rate, mostly in lesions 7 cm or larger in length, at a follow-up of 4 or more months.

DISCUSSION

Atherectomy was created to address restenosis, reocclusion, and other complications/limitations commonly associated with conventional PTA. A critical review of the literature reporting the experience with these high-speed rotary devices clearly establishes the feasibility of atherectomy in the treatment of peripheral arterial occlusive disease. However, in spite of the actual "debulking" of atheroma and leaving a smooth, polished intraluminal surface, the efficacy of rotary atherectomy devices still remains questionable. All the atherectomy devices, including the extirpative catheters, have failed to fulfill or uphold the aforementioned expectations. Although the initial technical and clinical results seem promising, patencies at intermediate and long-term follow-up are either similar or worse than those of conventional PTA.

Clearly, "debulking" or removing the atheroma to achieve less than 20% to 30% stenosis does not prevent restenosis or reocclusion. High-speed rotational ablation can cause considerable intimal damage, e.g., endothelial peeling and abrasion of smooth muscle cells, that subsequently leads to intimal hyperplasia and ultimately restenosis/reocclusion. Restenosis and reocclusion are inevitable in patients treated with conventional PTA or any of the atherectomy devices. However, these rates are significantly higher in patients treated with atherectomy.

With the significant early failure rates and complications as well as poor late patency results, rotary atherectomy is not generally recommended for the treatment of peripheral arterial occlusive disease. Further refinements in current devices and techniques need to be developed before rotary atherectomy becomes generally useful. For instance, a safety feature can be added to minimize dissection and perforation. Thromboembolic complications with the current rotary atherectomy devices can be minimized with the addition of a continuous extraction system for the atherectomized particles, similar to the situation with extirpative catheters. Most importantly, a plea for a more careful selection of patients is indicated before they undergo such a procedure. Obviously, rotary atherectomy, or any type of atherectomy for that matter, is not generally recommended for patients with multilevel disease and more advanced, complex lesions.

Of major concern regarding the use of these complex devices are who should perform the atherectomy and how can one obtain the proper training and credentialing. Unfortunately, no formal training is currently available in endovascular surgery techniques such as atherectomy. Vascular practitioners currently rely on postgraduate courses offered by various institutions and books on endovascular techniques. With endovascular surgery gaining more recognition and acceptance within the medical community, efforts by many medical societies are currently under way to provide endovascular training programs in which participants can actually perform the techniques themselves on various training models. Recently, the Society for Vascular Surgery and the International Society for Cardiovascular Surgery organized the First Endovascular Surgery Workshop with an emphasis on intensive, hands-on instruction by experienced faculty using a special life-sized training model. However, a consensus of the proper training and credentialing requirements has still not been established. Ultimately, hospital administrators with their policies presently determine the proper training and credentialing requirements for their physicians before granting them the privilege to perform such procedures in their facilities. Thus both hospital administrators and vascular surgeons must keep themselves abreast of all pertinent issues and discuss them rationally before such policies are made.

REFERENCES

1. Ellis SG, Rubin GS, King SB, et al: Angiographic and clinical predictor of acute closure after native vessel coronary angioplasty. *Circulation* 77:372–379, 1988.
2. Johnston KW, Rae M, Hogg-Johnston SA, et al: Five year results of a prospective study of percutaneous transluminal angioplasty. *Ann Surg* 206:403–413, 1987.

3. Jeans WD, Armstrong S, Cole SEA, et al: Fate of patients undergoing transluminal angioplasty for lower limb ischemia. *Radiology* 177:559–564, 1990.

4. Gardiner GA, Meyerovitz MF, Harrington DP, et al: Dissection complicating angioplasty. *Am J Radiol* 145:627–631, 1985.

5. Bredlau CE, Roubin GS, Leimgruber PP, et al: Inhospital morbidity and mortality in patients undergoing elective coronary angioplasty. *Circulation* 62:1044–1052, 1985.

6. Cowley MJ, Dorros G, Kelsey SF, et al: Acute coronary events associated with percutaneous transluminal coronary angioplasty. *Am J Cardiol* 53:12C–16C, 1984.

7. Mosley JG, Gulati SM, Raphael M, et al: The role of percutaneous transluminal angioplasty for atherosclerotic disease of the lower extremities. *Ann Coll R Surg Engl* 67:83, 1985.

8. Johnston KW, Rae M, Hogg-Johnston SA, et al: Five year results of a prospective study of percutaneous transluminal angioplasty. *Ann Surg* 206:403–413, 1987.

9. Hewes RC, White RI, Murray RR, et al: Long term results of superficial femoral artery angioplasty. *Am J Radiol* 146:1025–1029, 1986.

10. Blackshear JL, O Callaghan WG, Califf RM: Medical approaches to prevention of restenosis after coronary angioplasty. *J Am Coll Cardiol* 9:834–848, 1987.

11. Leimgruber PP, Roubin GS, Hollman J, et al: Restenosis after successful coronary angioplasty in patients with single-vessel disease. *Circulation* 73:710–717, 1986.

12. Wholey MH, Smith JAM, Godlewski P, et al: Recanalization of total arterial occlusions with the Kensey dynamic angioplasty catheter. *Radiology* 172:95–98, 1989.

13. Desbrosses D, Petit H, Torres E, et al: Percutaneous atherectomy with the Kensey catheter: Early and midterm results in femoropopliteal occlusions unsuitable for conventional angioplasty. *Ann Vasc Surg* 4:550–552, 1990.

14. Cull DL, Feinberg RL, Wheeler JR, et al: Experience with laser-assisted balloon angioplasty and a rotary angioplasty instrument: Lessons learned. *J Vasc Surg* 14:332–339, 1991.

15. Snyder SO, Wheeler JR, Gregory RT, et al: The Trac-Wright atherectomy device, in Ahn SS, Moore WS (eds): *Endovascular Surgery.* Philadelphia, WB Saunders, 1992, pp 287–294.

16. Lukes P, Wihed A, Tidebrant G, et al: Combined angioplasty with the Kensey catheter and balloon angioplasty in occlusive arterial disease. *Acta Radiol* 33:230–233, 1992.

17. Triller J, Do DD, Maddern G, et al: Femoropopliteal artery occlusion: Clinical experience with the Kensey catheter. *Radiology* 182:257–261, 1992.

18. Dyet JF: High speed rotational angioplasty in occluded peripheral arteries. *J Intervent Radiol* 7:1–5, 1992.

19. Meloni T, Carbonnato P, Mistretta L, et al: Arterial recanalization with the Kensey catheter. *Radiol Med* 86:509–512, 1993.

20. Gehani AA, Davies A, Stoodley K, et al: Does the Kensey catheter keep a coaxial position inside the lumen? An in vitro angioscopic study. *Cardiovasc Intervent Radiol* 14:222–229, 1991.

21. Moellmann D, Kuhn FP, Bomer D: Distribution and size of particles after dynamic angioplasty in cadaveric arteries with the Kensey catheter system: A comparison with clinical experience. *Cardiovasc Intervent Radiol* 15:201–204, 1992.

22. Dorros G, Iyer S, Zaitoun R, et al: Acute angiographic and clinical outcome of high speed percutaneous rotational atherectomy (Rotablator). *Cathet Cardiovasc Diagn* 22:157–166, 1991.

23. Ahn SS, Yeatman LR, Deutsch LS, et al: Intraoperative peripheral rotary atherectomy: Early and late clinical results. *Ann Vasc Surg* 6:272–280, 1992.

24. White CJ, Ramee SR, Escobar A, et al: High speed rotational ablation (Rotablator) for unfavorable lesions in peripheral arteries. *Cathet Cardiovasc Diagn* 30:115–119, 1993.

25. The Collaborative Rotablator Atherectomy Group: Peripheral atherectomy with the Rotablator: A multicenter report. *J Vasc Surg* 19:509–515, 1994.

26. Henry M, Amor M, Ethevenot G, et al: Percutaneous peripheral atherectomy using the Rotablator: A single center experience. *J Endovasc Surg* 2:51–66, 1995.

27. Myers KA, Denton MJ: Infrainguinal atherectomy using the Auth Rotablator: Patency rates and clinical success for 36 procedures. *J Endovasc Surg* 2:67–73, 1995.

28. Ahn SS, Auth D, Marcus D, et al: Removal of focal atheromatous lesions by angioscopically guided high speed rotary atherectomy: Preliminary experimental observations. *J Vasc Surg* 7:292–300, 1988.

29. Ahn SS, Arca M, Marcus D, et al: Histologic and morphologic effects of rotary atherectomy on human cadaver arteries. *Ann Vasc Surg* 4:563–569, 1990.

Superficial Femoral Vein—An Alternate Vascular Conduit

A.R. Downs, M.D., F.R.C.S.C., F.A.C.S.

Professor of Surgery, Department of Surgery, Health Sciences Centre, University of Manitoba, Winnipeg, Manitoba

R.P. Guzman, M.D., F.R.C.S.C., F.A.C.S., R.V.T.

Assistant Professor of Surgery, Department of Surgery, Health Sciences Centre, University of Manitoba, Winnipeg, Manitoba

M ost vascular surgeons remain skeptical about use of the superficial femoral vein as a conduit for arterial and venous reconstruction because of the fear of consequences of venous obstruction when the superficial femoral vein is removed. Historically, the superficial femoral vein has been ligated for the treatment of venous thromboembolic disease,[1] and documented evidence of chronic venous insufficiency as a result of superficial femoral vein obstruction is lacking.[2]

Schulman et al.[3–5] deserve credit for demonstrating the safety of superficial femoral vein removal for femoral popliteal arterial grafting in several publications. Sladen et al.[6,7] have also had considerable experience with use of the superficial femoral vein and has advocated its use for infrainguinal arterial reconstruction in limb salvage operations when the saphenous vein has not been available in secondary operations.

PERSONAL EXPERIENCE

We first used the superficial femoral vein for replacement of an internal jugular vein.[8] A 15-cm segment of vein was removed and no leg swelling occurred. Since 1989, we have used the superficial femoral vein on 19 occasions for arterial and venous reconstruction (Table 1). All infrainguinal reconstructions have been done in the absence of the saphenous vein or when the saphenous vein was inadequate in length. Of the 12 infrainguinal reconstructions, 8 have been secondary procedures after failed grafts (Table 2).

Seven patients received composite grafts with the saphenous, basilic, or cephalic veins (Table 2, Figs 1 to 3). The length of superficial femoral vein used has varied from 5 to 40 cm. Almost all of the patients have had end-stage ischemia with pain at rest and tissue necrosis (see Table 2).

Two early postoperative occlusions have occurred and resulted in amputation. A 79-year-old female with severe cardiac disease suffered a postoperative graft rupture with hemorrhage and shock. Graft occlusion oc-

Advances in Vascular Surgery®, vol. 4

TABLE 1.
Superficial Femoral Vein Conduit Sites

Infrainguinal	12
Iliofemoral	2
Aortofemoral	1
Trauma	1
Vein replacement	3
Total	19

TABLE 2.
Superficial Femoral Vein Conduit

Patient	Site	Length of SFV (cm)	Indication	Patient (mo)	Swelling Early	Late
A.P. (R)	SF-BKP	38	Rest pain	78	1	0
(L)	CF-BKP	39	Rest pain	72	3	0
L.E. (L)	CF-BKP	40 (48)* S	Rest pain, ulcers	51	4	0
H.E. (L)	CF-BKP	21 (48) S	Rest pain	57	1	0
(R)	CF-BKP	26 (61) S	Claudication	36	2	0
A.G. (L)	PF-PT	37 (51) S	Rest pain	36	1	0
A.R. (L)	SF-PER	30 (60) B	Rest pain, necrosis	0	Died 6/12	2 Amp.
E.M. (L)	SF-BKP	23	Rest pain, gangrene	20	2	1
A.G. (R)	CF-BKP	16 (45) B	Rest pain, gangrene	20	4	1
B.J. (R)	PF-BKP	19 (44) C	Rest pain	0	2	Amp.
L.T. (R)	XCF-BKP	27 (63) S	Rest pain	11+	2	1
D.M. (R)	SF-SF	5	Trauma	22	0	0
W.B. (L)	SF-BKP	23	Popliteal aneurysm	Recent	0	0
R.T.	CI-F	25	Claudication	60	1	0
G.O.	EI-F	9.5	Claudication	42	1	0
D.L.	A-F	34	Rest pain, necrosis	36	3	1
G.C.	IJV	5	Bilateral radical neck	3	0	Died
M.F.	SMV	5	Cancer of the duodenum	3	0	Died
P.G.	SR Shunt	8	Portal hypertension	0	0	0

*Values in parentheses are the total lengths of composite grafts.

†Thrombectomy at 8 and 14 weeks.

Abbreviations: SVF, superficial femoral vein; *SF,* superficial femoral artery; *BKP,* below-knee popliteal artery; *CF,* common femoral artery; *S,* saphenous composite vein; *PT,* posterior tibial artery; *PF,* profunda femoris artery; *PER,* peroneal artery; *B,* basilic composite vein; *Amp.,* amputation; *C,* cephalic composite vein; *XCF,* cross common femoral artery; *CI,* common iliac artery; *F,* femoral artery; *EI,* external iliac artery; *A,* aorta; *IJV,* internal jugular vein; *SMV,* superior mesenteric vein; *SR,* splenorenal vein.

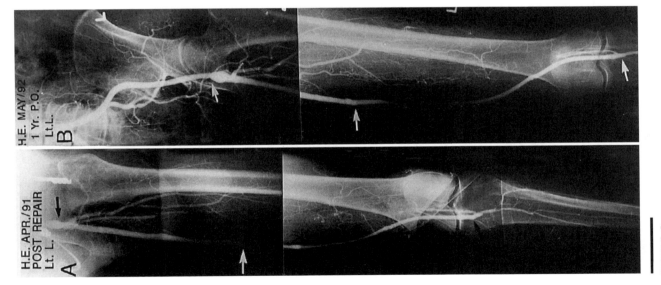

FIGURE 1.

Patient H.E. with a composite common femoral artery–below-knee popliteal artery bypass. **A**, reversed saphenous vein (distal), 27 cm, plus a reversed superficial femoral vein (proximal), 21 cm—after repair. **B**, 1 year postoperatively. *Arrows indicate anastomoses.*

curred and was followed by an above-knee amputation. She died 6 months later of cardiac failure, but no other patients have died. The second graft occlusion occurred in a 62-year-old female with a composite graft. Revision was unsuccessful, and a below-knee amputation was required. Venous obstruction did not appear to be the cause of graft failure

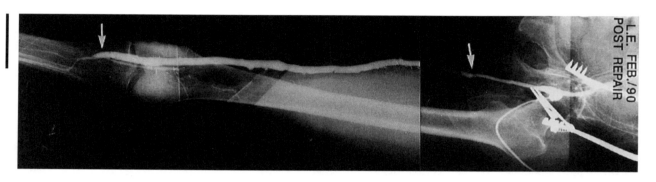

FIGURE 2.

Patient L.E. with a composite common femoral artery–below-knee popliteal artery bypass with reversed saphenous vein (proximal), 8 cm, and reversed superficial femoral vein (distal), 40 cm—after repair. *Arrows* indicate anastomoses.

because edema was not severe. All other grafts in the arterial system have remained open, with the longest graft patency being 78 months. The preoperative and postoperative ankle indices in 11 infrainguinal reconstructions are listed in Table 3. There has been only one late graft occlusion, which was treated successfully with thrombolysis and thrombectomy (see Fig 3).

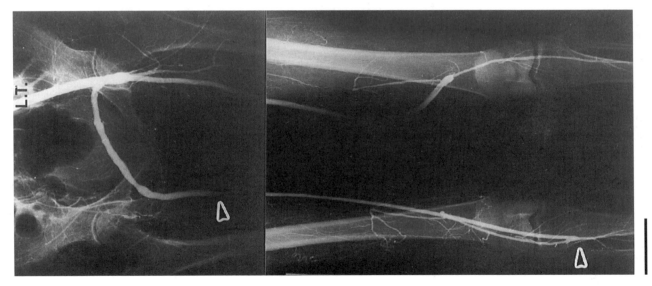

FIGURE 3.
Patient L.T. with a composite cross common femoral artery–below-knee popliteal artery bypass: reversed superficial femoral vein 27 cm, and reversed saphenous vein 36 cm—after repair. *Arrows* indicate anastomoses.

POSTOPERATIVE EDEMA AND VENOUS STASIS

Three patients had marked postoperative swelling with cyanosis and skin blistering (Fig 4). High leg elevation and postoperative heparin have been used to successfully resolve the swelling. Distal tibial vein thrombosis has been demonstrated in two patients by venography (Fig 5). The edema resolved in all of these patients, who have now had no leg swelling for

TABLE 3.
Superficial Femoral Vein Conduit; Ankle-Brachial Indices

Patient	Site	Preoperative	Postoperative	Runoff
A.P. (R)	SF-BKP	0.54	0.72	2
(L)	CF-BKP	0.5	0.9	2
L.E. (L)	CF-BKP	0.23	0.92	1 AT
H.E. (L)	CF-BKP	0.46	1.15	1 PT
(R)	CF-PT	0.51	1.2	1 PT
L.G. (L)	PF-PT	0.34	1.25	1 PER
A.R. (L)	SF-PER	0.3	Occluded	1 PER, AKA
E.M. (L)	SF-BKP	0.49	0.98	1 PT
A.G. (R)	CF-BKP	0.34	0.9	1 AT
B.J. (R)	PF-BKP	0.33	Occluded	1 AT, BKA
L.T. (R)	XCF-BKP	0.2	0.95	2 AT, PER

Abbreviations: SF, superficial femoral artery; *BKP,* below-knee popliteal artery; *CF,* common femoral artery; *AT,* anterior tibial artery; *PT,* posterior tibial artery; *PF,* profunda femoris artery; *PER,* peroneal artery; *AKA,* above-knee amputation; *BKA,* below-knee amputation; *XCF,* cross common femoral artery.

20, 51, and 72 months postoperatively (see Fig 5). The usual degree of postoperative edema in a patient who has undergone a repeat iliofemoral graft with the superficial femoral vein is seen in Fig 6, A and B. Late changes in the superficial femoral vein graft, such as elongation and kinking, have been demonstrated angiographically (Fig 7, A and B). This graft remains patent at 78 months.

OTHER COMPLICATIONS

Two patients suffered postoperative hemorrhage from blowout of a ligated tributary. Large tributaries should be suture-ligated to avoid this complication.

TECHNIQUE OF SUPERFICIAL FEMORAL VEIN REMOVAL

The technique of removal has been well described by Schulman et al.[4] and Sladen and colleagues.[6] The superficial femoral vein is identified adjacent to the superficial femoral artery in the groin and is dissected distally for an adequate length of vein. The vein can be dissected down to the tibial veins including the popliteal vein, to provide a length up to 40 cm. When the popliteal vein is bifid, the medial segment is used. The thigh has a few large, short, thin-walled tributaries that must be handled carefully and suture-ligated with 6-0 Prolene to avoid injury to the vein and blood loss. The appropriate length of vein is removed and dilated with heparin saline to overcome dissection-induced spasm. If the vein is greater than 1 cm in diameter, it is reduced in size with an indwelling catheter to a 7-mm diameter if it is to be used for distal reconstruction. Although Schulman and Sladen and their associates[4,6] have used the nonreversed vein, we continue to use the reversed technique in the arterial system to avoid any intimal injury.

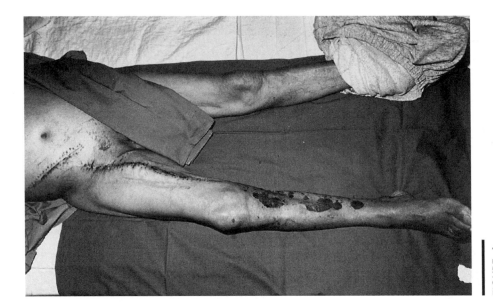

FIGURE 4.

Patient A.G. has postoperative swelling with blisters, an iliofemoral prosthetic graft, and a femoral popliteal reversed superficial femoral vein graft—10 days postoperatively.

It is absolutely essential to identify the deep femoral vein before dividing the superficial femoral vein. The deep femoral vein, with continuity to the common femoral vein and its collateral flow from the tibial veins, is the key to avoiding severe venous congestion early postoperatively and late venous and nerve dysfunction related to prolonged ischemia because of distal arterial thrombosis and required reoperation. The late function is good, although sensory impairment is still present in the foot.

DISCUSSION

The concern about early and late venous obstruction has not been borne out in our small experience. Severe edema in 4 of 7 patients reported by Coburn et al.[9] serves as a warning that these complications can occur. They have advised against using the popliteal vein below the knee, although in four patients we have done so without an adverse outcome. It is absolutely essential to maintain patency of the deep femoral vein and its continuity with the common femoral vein. The report of Schanzer et

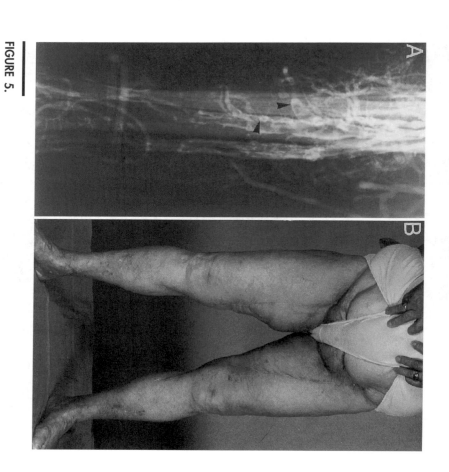

FIGURE 5.

Patient A.P. **A,** postoperative venogram showing calf vein thrombosis (*arrows*). **B,** 6 years after bilateral femoral-popliteal grafts with a reversed superficial femoral vein.

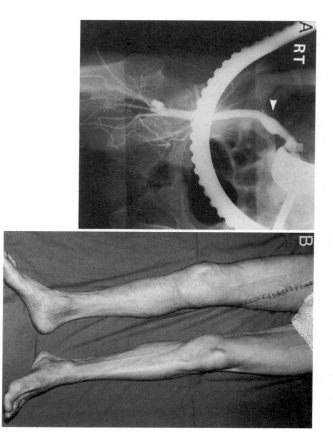

FIGURE 6.

Patient R.T. **A,** iliofemoral graft using a reversed superficial femoral vein (*arrow* indicates anastomosis). **B,** postoperative mild leg swelling.

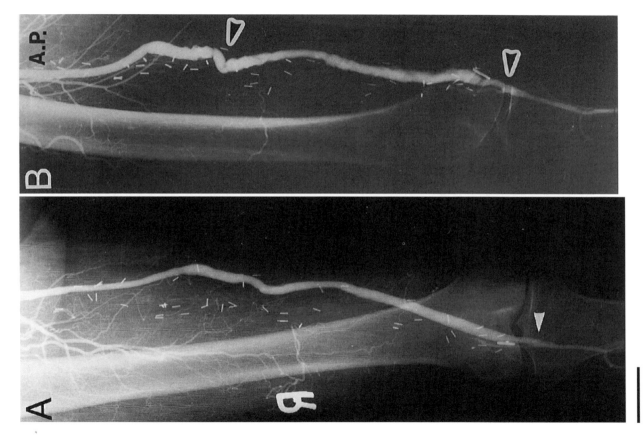

FIGURE 7.

Patient A.P. **A,** reversed superficial femoral vein 6 months postoperatively. **B,** reversed superficial femoral vein 66 months postoperatively—elongation of the graft is seen. *Arrows* indicate anastomoses.

al.[10] on the functional status of the venous system after superficial femoral vein removal lends strong support to the safety of this procedure. We strongly recommend high elevation of the limb for the first 4–6 days postoperatively and compression wrapping from the toes to the thigh. Heparin is not used routinely postoperatively unless severe swelling is present or hypercoagulability is a concern. External support should be used with ambulation, and a fitted stocking as suggested by Sladen[6] would probably be appropriate.

OTHER SITES OF USE

We have used the superficial femoral vein in secondary reconstruction for aortoiliac occlusion in three patients in whom prosthetic grafts repeatedly occluded. These grafts are probably preferable to the saphenous vein simply because of their size, which is more appropriate for iliac replacement. Their function up to 5 years has been very satisfactory. Aneurysms have not occurred, although long-term performance is not available. Clagett et al.[11] have used the superficial femoral vein for aortic replacement, and Sladen and colleagues[6,7] have used it for cross femoral grafts in the presence of infection. We have recently used it for popliteal aneurysm repair, and it is suited for this because it is a large conduit and a shorter graft can be used.

The superficial femoral vein is extremely well suited for venous reconstruction, and I believe it should replace the spiral vein concept.

CONCLUSION

We believe that sufficient evidence is now available to confirm Schulman's pioneering work[3–5] on the use of the superficial femoral vein as a conduit for arterial and venous reconstruction.

REFERENCES

1. Szilagyi DE, Alsop JF: Early and late sequelae of therapeutic vein ligation for thrombosis of veins of lower limbs. *Arch Surg* 59:663–666, 1949.
2. Masuda E, Kistner R, Ferris E: Long term effects of superficial femoral vein ligation: Thirteen-year followup. *J Vasc Surg* 16:741–749, 1992.
3. Schulman ML, Badhey MR: Deep veins of the leg as femoro-popliteal bypass grafts. *Arch Surg* 116:1141–1145, 1981.
4. Schulman ML, Badhey MR, Yatco R, et al: An 11-year experience with deep leg veins as femoropopliteal bypass grafts. *Arch Surg* 121:1010–1015, 1986.
5. Schulman ML, Badhey MR, Yatco R: Superficial femoro-popliteal veins and reversed saphenous veins as primary femoropopliteal bypass grafts: A randomized comparative study. *J Vasc Surg* 6:1–10, 1987.
6. Sladen JG, Reid JDS, Maxwell TM, et al: Superficial femoral vein: A useful autogenous harvest site. *J Vasc Surg* 20:947–952, 1994.
7. Sladen JG, Downs AR: Superficial femoral vein. *Semin Vasc Surg* 8:209–215, 1995.
8. Al-Ghamdi SA, Beecroft WA, Downs AR: Internal jugular vein reconstruction using a superficial femoral vein graft. *Can J Surg* 34:621–624, 1991.
9. Coburn M, Ashworth C, Francis W, et al: Venous stasis complications of the use of the superficial femoral and popliteal veins for lower extremity bypass. *J Vasc Surg* 17:1005–1009, 1993.
10. Schanzer H, Chiang K, Mabrouk M, et al: Use of lower extremity deep veins as arterial substitutes: Functional status of the donor leg. *J Vasc Surg* 14:624–627, 1991.
11. Clagett GP, Bowers BL, Lopex-Viego M, et al: Creation of a neo-aorto-iliac system from lower extremity deep and superficial femoral veins. *Ann Surg* 218:239–249, 1993.

Femorotibial Reconstruction for Claudication

Michael S. Conte, M.D.
Assistant Professor of Surgery, Yale University School of Medicine, New Haven, Connecticut

Michael Belkin, M.D.
Assistant Professor of Surgery, Harvard Medical School, Brigham and Women's Hospital, Boston, Massachusetts

The modern era of vascular surgery is marked by an expanding array of interdisciplinary therapies, improved medical and anesthetic management, and the expectation of consistent, durable results for the full range of interventions performed. These accomplishments have resulted simultaneously in both improved patient outcomes and a progressive broadening of indications as risk-benefit ratios have improved. Surgical therapy for asymptomatic carotid stenosis, now firmly based on the clear demonstration of benefit and low morbidity when performed by competent surgeons, is one such example. Perhaps more than any other area within vascular surgery, infrainguinal arterial reconstruction has been a benchmark for the sustained technical progress over the last quarter century. As vascular surgeons were demonstrating the ability to reconstruct progressively more distal vessels in the lower extremity, advances in the identification and treatment of cardiovascular risk factors have been enabling patients with atherosclerosis to live longer, fuller lives. The promise of our specialty is to continue to extend survival and improve quality of life for all patients with disabling circulatory disorders.

Whereas risk-benefit analysis of arterial reconstruction for limb-threatening ischemia clearly justifies intervention for most patients, the role of surgery for intermittent claudication remains controversial. In large part, this is based on an understanding of the benign course of this symptom in most patients, as documented in a number of historical reports. Nonetheless, aortofemoral reconstruction for claudication is commonly justified both by the excellent long-term results and a perception among some that aortoiliac occlusive disease is associated with a greater risk of progression to critical ischemia. Similarly, as modern results of femoropopliteal bypass have begun to approach those obtained with aortofemoral surgery, disabling claudication has increasingly become accepted as an appropriate indication for many patients. Current series from a number of institutions demonstrate that tibial reconstruction can be performed with morbidity, mortality, and long-term patency equivalent to

Advances in Vascular Surgery®, vol. 4

those observed for more proximal bypasses. Increasingly, it has become appreciated that infrainguinal bypass patency is most clearly linked to operative indication, conduit quality, and aggressive graft surveillance, and far less strongly to the level of the distal anastomosis per se. These observations suggest that a select subgroup of patients with severe claudication and anatomy warranting bypass to the tibial level might be well served by an aggressive approach.

This chapter will critically examine the role of femorotibial reconstruction for claudication and attempt to place it in an appropriate context with the other available treatment options. The natural history of claudication will first be reviewed, with emphasis on the contrast of modern and historical series, clinical-anatomical correlates, and the identification of subgroups at increased risk for progression. Conservative treatment approaches will be briefly considered. Patient selection considerations and results of arterial reconstruction will be reviewed and contrasted by anatomical level: aortoiliac, femoropopliteal, and femorotibial. An attempt will be made to develop a balanced approach to the management of patients with disabling claudication by consideration of surgical risk, anticipated quality-of-life improvement, risk of progression to critical ischemia, arteriographic and technical factors, and expected results.

CLAUDICATION: NATURAL HISTORY AND BASIC CONSIDERATIONS

With the increasing age of the American population, cardiovascular disease and its various manifestations can be expected to continue to increase in prevalence. The Framingham Study documented the high prevalence of claudication associated with increased age, male sex, diabetes mellitus, and smoking.[1] Mortality rates from cardiovascular causes are declining, likely a result of improved recognition and treatment of risk factors as well as better therapies for specific disease entities.[2] Thus, patients with atherosclerosis may live longer and be more functional at advanced age. This trend may have important implications for the demand for durable interventions for patients with disabling claudication.

Early studies documenting the generally benign natural history of claudication relied predominantly on clinical evaluation and physical examination to identify patient cohorts.[3–5] These studies made important observations of increased cardiovascular mortality and low risk of limb loss associated with claudication. The lack of objective (i.e., noninvasive laboratory) assessment of the severity of lower-extremity occlusive disease is a significant limitation of these reports, resulting in a tendency to underestimate the expected morbidity for claudicants encountered in a clinical vascular surgery practice. More recent reports have employed noninvasive studies and multivariate analysis in an attempt to more accurately define the natural history of arterial claudication for specific subgroups of patients.[6–9] Despite the difficulty in comparing these data because of referral patterns, demographics, and prevalence of co-morbidities, some generalizations can safely be made. The annual risks of mortality and limb loss can be reasonably approximated at 5% and 1%, respectively. Roughly 20% to 30% of patients will come to operation within 5 years for severe clinical deterioration, of whom about half will have progressed to rest pain, ulceration, or gangrene. More than half of these patients will remain stable or even improve in symptoms with time and conservative treatment; the remainder can be expected to experience increasing disability.

These general observations are of limited usefulness in practice, however, because claudicants are a markedly heterogeneous group with regard to survival as well as risk of progression in the affected limb. Numerous studies have attempted to define clinical or laboratory variables that are predictive of outcome for claudicants.[6-8, 10-13] Although the literature does not reveal uniform agreement on their relative importance, several risk factors for progression to critical ischemia have been clearly identified: diabetes mellitus, continued smoking, hemodynamic indices (low at baseline and/or temporally declining), and presence of multilevel occlusive disease. These factors appear to act synergistically when in combination, which is often how they are encountered in clinical practice. Hemodynamic assessment in the noninvasive laboratory assumes primary importance in the initial evaluation and subsequent follow-up, providing objective evidence of the levels and severity of arterial occlusion over time. Although useful for characterizing groups of patients at high risk, these tools remain quite limited in their ability to predict the rate of progression of lower-extremity atherosclerosis in the individual patient. Unfortunately, atherosclerosis often clinically progresses in discrete periods of rapid deterioration, and not along a definable curve of slow decline that can be measured in the laboratory and predictably intercepted in a timely fashion.

An unresolved question remains that of the relationship of the level of occlusive disease to long-term outcomes. The literature is divided on this point, with several studies indicating a poorer natural history for aortoiliac disease[3, 4] and others indicating that the degree of distal involvement is more predictive of clinical progression.[5, 14] In the absence of firm evidence on this point, other factors must be considered in formulating an approach based on level of disease. For one, long-term survival may be linked to the level of lower-extremity atherosclerosis, with several studies suggesting increased mortality for patients with more distal occlusive disease.[15] In addition, patients with isolated aortoiliac disease tend to be younger and have fewer co-morbidities than do those with tibial occlusions and, thus, may be more likely to experience full functional benefit from intervention.

Diabetic claudicants are a subgroup at particularly high risk for critical ischemia and limb loss. Studies have documented a 5-10-fold higher risk of progression to these end points for diabetic as opposed to nondiabetic claudicants.[11, 13] It is quite sobering to note that the ravages of atherosclerosis are also responsible for a twofold higher annual mortality rate in diabetic vs. nondiabetic claudicants (50% vs. 75% survival at 6 years),[13] adding to the complexity of therapeutic decision-making. Diabetic claudicants who smoke are in an extremely precarious group, underscoring the paramount importance of tobacco cessation.

The mechanisms underlying the profound negative influence of diabetes remain somewhat unclear, although several important factors are likely to be operative. Vascular disease in diabetics affects the arterial tree at all levels: large vessels develop atherosclerotic plaque, muscular arteries are subject to medial calcinosis, and the microcirculation develops basement membrane thickening and intimal proliferation. Of particular significance is the pattern of macrovascular involvement in the lower extremities, which is commonly multisegmental and diffuse, with a predilection for the popliteal trifurcation and tibial vessels. Diabetic claudicants are less likely to have isolated superficial femoral artery disease and more often harbor coexistent tibial disease as well. In contrast to the focal lesions often seen in nondiabetics, tibial disease in diabetic patients more often affects longer segments of at least two of the three tibial arteries.[16] Occlusive disease of the plantar arch is threefold more common.[17] The net result of this pattern in the diabetic claudicant is often a more tenuous collateral network with limited reserve, which is prone to sudden deterioration to critical ischemia. Peripheral neuropathy may further complicate the clinical picture by masking early symptoms of worsening ischemia and producing mechanical foot deformities that predispose to ulceration. Diabetics thus represent an important and challenging group for determining the appropriate timing of intervention to avoid tissue necrosis and maximize functional benefit in carefully selected patients who seem likely to have long-term survival potential.

CLAUDICATION: CONSERVATIVE THERAPY

The cornerstones of conservative management of claudication are smoking cessation, exercise, and appropriate management of associated cardiovascular risk factors (e.g., hypertension, hyperlipidemias). The critical importance of smoking cessation can hardly be overstated. Some 80% of claudicants smoke, and those who continue to use tobacco are at several-fold higher risk for mortality, amputation, or deterioration to critical ischemia.[10, 18] These inauspicious statistics are equalled by the disappointing failure to achieve sustained tobacco abstinence in most patients, even when supervised behavior-modification programs are used.[19] The promise of nicotine analogues in this regard remains incompletely fulfilled to date.

The benefits of programmed regular exercise training for claudicants are generally agreed on, although the underlying mechanism for improved walking capacity remains subject to debate. Potential mechanisms include improved muscle metabolism and hemorrheologic effects; it appears unlikely that collateral vessel formation is increased to a significant degree. Several studies have documented symptomatic improvement in patients undergoing supervised physical training programs.[20] In general the maximal benefit attained is apparent within the first several months and is likely to be less for patients with more long-standing claudication and poorer hemodynamic indices. Obviously, compliance with any long-term regimen is an important issue, and highly motivated study patients may not be representative of the spectrum of claudicants encountered in clinical practice. The benefits of exercise, although less dramatic than with arterial reconstruction, may be additive in combination with surgery[21] and have a broad range of positive effects on cardiovascular health.

Of the various classes of pharmacologic agents that have been studied, the hemorrheologic drugs, and pentoxifylline in particular, have been the most extensively evaluated. Despite a large number (more than 10) of randomized trials, most of which were placebo-controlled, the benefits of pentoxifylline remain somewhat unclear. Factors limiting the applicability of these study results include wide variability in the estimates of treatment effects, disparate outcome measurements, significant placebo effects, and inability to correlate effect with clinical variables.[20] In general, the improvement in walking distance that is attributed to pentoxifylline appears unpredictable and of modest degree compared with the effects of placebo. These limitations may not justify the cost of the drug to the individual, particularly if it were to be used for the duration of active life. Patients who are already taking pentoxifylline when first encountered and are convinced of its benefits should arguably be continued with the drug unless direct reconstruction is undertaken or cost becomes an issue. Patients who continue to experience severe symptoms despite adherence to conservative treatment, and who are not judged as good candidates for reconstruction, may derive some benefit from pentoxifylline, and a therapeutic trial seems justifiable.

ARTERIAL RECONSTRUCTION FOR CLAUDICATION

GENERAL CONSIDERATIONS FOR PATIENT SELECTION

It should be clear from this discussion that patients with claudication form an extremely heterogeneous group with respect to important comorbidites, anticipated survival, risk to the affected limb, degree of disability, and potential functional benefit to be achieved by reconstruction. Careful assessment of each of these factors, in combination with a risk-benefit estimate for the proposed intervention, is required to determine the best approach for the individual patient.

The important clinical variables associated with a poorer prognosis for the affected limb have already been mentioned. Noninvasive hemodynamic testing (segmental limb pressures, pulse-volume recordings, treadmill exercise testing) is critical to provide objective assessment of disease severity. Patients being monitored under conservative therapy who clearly deteriorate to severe disability or incipient limb threat warrant an aggressive approach. Two other important factors—the presence of diabetes and the level of arterial occlusion—may have simultaneous effects on anticipated patient mortality and disease progression that tend to offset each other in the decision analysis. Patients with long-standing diabetes with multiple end-organ manifestations and predominantly distal lower-extremity arterial disease are at higher risk to both life and limb, often mandating a careful surveillance strategy with intervention reserved for deterioration. The critical determination often becomes that of estimating the anticipated survival of patient vs. limb, with chronologic age being far less paramount than the extent of organ-system dysfunction present. Clinical experience, judicious assessment of co-morbidities, and input from other physician caretakers are the essential components of this difficult decision process.

The functional assessment is the next most critical component of the management decision. Certainly the degree of disability present, particularly when it limits the activities of daily living or the patient's ability to carry out his occupation, may mitigate for an aggressive approach. Although this aspect may be relatively straightforward to ascertain, a more difficult issue is that of predicting functional outcome after intervention. As most claudicants will not progress to critical ischemia, functional quality-of-life improvement becomes the primary benefit to be sought from reconstruction. A careful consideration of the limitations imposed by other co-morbid factors—particularly cardiac disease, chronic pulmonary conditions, and musculoskeletal conditions, all of which are common in the atherosclerotic population—is required. This assessment is often made difficult by the degree of impairment imposed by severe claudication, leading to disappointing outcomes for both patient and surgeon after successful revascularization has only unmasked another equally limiting medical condition. Detailed consultation with each of the other involved medical specialists should be sought, and functional tests of cardiac and pulmonary reserve may be useful.

The anticipated quality-of-life improvement for specific interventions, along with the durability of these effects, is only recently becoming defined as outcome measures become an important and standard feature of reported series. Two recently reported series suggest that patients with lower-extremity vascular disease have low baseline perceptions of quality of life and functional well-being as compared with age-matched controls. Schneider et al., reporting on a series of 60 patients who underwent successful aortofemoral bypass at least 6 months prior, found persistently impaired physical function, role function, and health perception, and greater bodily pain in these patients compared with controls without peripheral vascular disease.[22] Gibbons et al. reported their assessment of quality-of-life measures after infrainguinal reconstruction.[23] They found that the baseline perception of health status was an important predictor of postoperative functional status, with only 45% of patients feeling "back to normal" by 6 months. Although leg pain improved and ulcers healed, complaints of persistent leg swelling were common and viewed as a significant problem by many. Clearly, much more information on quality-of-life outcomes for patients with lower-extremity vascular disease is needed to accurately predict the functional results of conservative and interventional treatments.

The decision to proceed to arteriography is predominantly based on the above considerations. The final factor in any decision for intervention, the anticipated risk-benefit for the proposed procedure, plays a role both before and after the angiogram. Given the significantly greater long-term patency of percutaneous interventions above the inguinal ligament, coupled with the low morbidity of these approaches, patients with aortoiliac disease may be considered for arteriography somewhat more readily than similarly disabled patients with infrainguinal disease. In general, however, arteriography is reserved for patients deemed suitable for a surgical approach if required. In the final analysis, the surgeon must recommend an approach based on the anatomy defined and the anticipated risks and benefits of the options available. It will be argued here that anatomical criteria are increasingly becoming a less significant component of this complex decision, as technical improvements have resulted in operative morbidities and patency rates approaching similar values for proximal and distal reconstructions.

RESULTS

Aortoiliac Disease

Both percutaneous and surgical treatment options for aortoiliac disease enjoy excellent long-term success. Percutaneous transluminal angioplasty (PTA) is an excellent option for patients with discrete iliac stenoses (5-year patency averaging 70%), and the addition of stents may improve long-term results by 10% or more.[24] Short, focal common iliac stenoses seem to respond best, whereas long-segment external iliac stenoses or occlusions have markedly inferior long-term outcomes.

The gold standard for aortoiliac reconstruction remains aortofemoral bypass grafting. Numerous large series reported from a variety of institutions (Table 1) have documented the outstanding long-term performance of these operations.[15, 25–28] Secondary patency rates at 5 and 10 years may be anticipated to be 85% and 75%, respectively. Long-term limb loss rates are under 10% and often are linked to progression of infrainguinal disease. Nonetheless, in carefully considering aortofemoral bypass within the spectrum of approaches for patients with claudication, some additional factors are germane. For one, although operative mortality rates are commendably low in all modern series (2% to 5%), few would argue that

TABLE 1.
Comparative Results of Vascular Reconstructions in Claudicants

	n	Claudicants (%)	Survival		2° Patency		Limb Loss > 5 yrs. (%)
			5 Yr. (%)	10 Yr. (%)	5 Yr. (%)	10 Yr. (%)	
Aortofemoral							
Szilagyi et al.[25]	1,647	65	59	33	85	80	6.5
Brewster et al.[26]	582	56	—	—	88	75	—
Martinez et al.[15]	376	72	79	48	88	78	4
Nevelsteen et al.[27]	352	42	65	37	80	62	8
Crawford et al.[28]	719	100	76	56	87	81	3
Femoropopliteal							
Kent et al.[30]	167	100	88	—	78 (*)	—	2.4
Taylor et al.[31]	88	100	67	—	83 (†)	—	—
Donaldson et al.[32]	240	32	70	—	86 (‡)	—	2.2
Sladen et al[33]	100	100	79	—	84	79	5
Femorotibial							
Conte et al.[37]	57	100	54	—	86	—	0

*Reported as primary patency only.
†Patency results not analyzed separately for claudicants (31% of total series).
‡Patency results not analyzed separately for claudicants (32% of total series).
(Courtesy of Conte MS, Belkin M, Donaldson MC, et al: J Vasc Surg 21:873–881, 1995.)

direct aortic reconstruction often incurs greater perioperative stresses than do infrainguinal procedures. In addition, the frequency with which secondary procedures are required for pseudoaneurysm (as high as 10%, not indicated in patency calculations) should not be ignored and is additive to revisions required to maintain patency.

Femoropopliteal Disease

Patients with occlusive disease limited to the superficial femoral artery (SFA) and/or proximal popliteal artery may be considered for percutaneous or surgical approaches. Percutaneous transluminal angioplasty of short-segment SFA stenoses is associated with reasonably good patency rates (averaging 50% at 5 years), although early restenosis remains a significant problem in 20% to 30% of patients within the first year.[29] In patients with favorable anatomy and disabling symptoms, PTA offers a low-risk option for an initial approach. Results for angioplasty are far inferior when applied to long-segment (greater than 10 cm) stenoses, multiple stenoses, distal popliteal lesions, or complete occlusions of the SFA, in which circumstances it is not recommended.

Surgical options include bypass grafting and endarterectomy. Despite continued interest in endarterectomy in other countries, with several centers reporting truly outstanding results comparable to those obtained with bypass, this operation is rarely performed in the United States for SFA/popliteal disease. This dissatisfaction is based on a history of significantly inferior results using a variety of instruments and techniques, with high rates of restenosis secondary to intimal hyperplasia noted.

Modern results of femoropopliteal bypass grafting are illustrated in Table 1, which compares data from several selected series with reference to claudication.[30–33] Presently, 5-year cumulative patency rates greater than 80% can be anticipated for autogenous vein bypasses to the popliteal level, with operative mortality around 2%. In general, patency rates are not demonstrably different for diabetics or for above- vs. below-knee vein grafts. By way of contrast, prosthetic bypasses are significantly inferior when placed to the below-knee popliteal artery, arguing strongly against their use for claudication in that circumstance. In the presence of adequate autogenous vein, the choice of above- vs. below-knee popliteal for the distal anastomosis should be based solely on the angiographic appearance of the recipient artery and runoff. Given the propensity for disease progression in the popliteal per se, the below-knee artery will be chosen more frequently by these criteria.

Femorotibial Disease

The dramatically improved results for femorotibial reconstruction with autogenous vein witnessed over the last 10–15 years mark a significant achievement for vascular surgery. Excellent results have been reported using both reversed and in situ vein techniques.[34,35] We recently reported on the long-term experience with in situ vein grafting at Brigham and Women's Hospital (BWH), in which secondary patency rates for femorotibial bypasses were 77% and 67% at 5 and 9 years, respectively.[36] Similar results have been achieved with this technique in a number of institutions.

Recently, we reviewed the BWH experience with femorotibial bypass performed for the indication of disabling claudication, in an attempt to define a role for this aggressive approach.[37] Fifty-three patients underwent 57 reconstructions within the 16-year period from 1977 to 1993, comprising 5% of all infrainguinal vein reconstructions during this period. For comparison, two other concurrent series of vein grafts were identified: 261 femoropopliteal grafts performed for claudication (FP/CLAUD) and 369 femorotibial grafts performed for limb salvage (FT/LS). Demographics and distribution of risk factors for the three patient groups are summarized in Table 2. Of the 57 grafts in the current series, 40 were performed using the greater saphenous vein in situ and 12 were reversed; the remainder used ectopic vein. Distal anastomoses were distributed to the tibioperoneal trunk in 7 (12%), anterior tibial in 10 (18%), posterior tibial in 27 (47%), and peroneal artery in 13 (23%) of cases.

There were no perioperative deaths in the series, and major morbidity occurred in five patients (myocardial infarction, 1; renal failure, 1; pulmonary embolism, 1; cerebrovascular event, 2). Hemodynamic indices improved significantly from a mean of 0.56 ± 0.15 at baseline to 0.97 ± 0.23 postoperatively ($P < 0.0001$). Follow-up information was complete for 45 of the grafts for a mean of 30 months and range up to 4,170 days.

Survival rates were similar for patients undergoing femorotibial bypass for either claudication or limb salvage (54% vs. 61% at 5 years, respectively) and were notably inferior to survival in the FP/CLAUD group (78% at 5 years, $P < 0.055$; Fig 1), suggesting again that patient survival may be linked to the level of lower-extremity arterial occlusion. Primary and secondary graft patencies for the three groups were calculated by the life-table method and are demonstrated graphically on Figures 2 and 3.

TABLE 2.
Patient Demographics and Distribution of Risk Factors

	Present Series (n = 53)	FP/Claud (n = 261)	FT/LS (n = 369)
Male-female ratio	44:9	172:89	241:128
Age: mean (range)	66(44–85)	63(32–82)	68(26–97)
Risk Factors (n [%])			
Smoking*	33(58)	198(76)	186(50)
Diabetes mellitus	14(25)	49(19)	180(49)
Hypertension	40(70)	146(56)	206(56)
Coronary artery disease	25(44)	129(49)	174(47)
Prior CABG	4(7)	18(7)	40(11)
COPD	7(12)	34(13)	45(12)
Renal failure	3(5)	9(3)	25(7)
Baseline ABI, mean	0.56	0.58	0.54
Median	0.57	0.56	0.44

*Defined as positive if patient reported smoking within one year prior to procedure

Abbreviations: *CABG*, coronary artery bypass graft; *COPD*, chronic obstructive pulmonary disease; *ABI*, ankle-brachial index; *FP/Claud*, femoropopliteal grafts performed for claudication; *FT/LS*, femorotibial grafts performed for limb salvage. (Courtesy of Conte MS, Belkin M, Donaldson MC, et al: *J Vasc Surg* 21:873–881, 1995.)

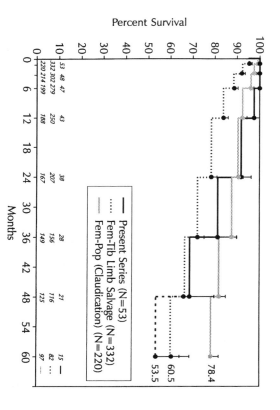

FIGURE 1.

Patient survival for three concurrent groups of infrainguinal vein bypasses performed at Brigham and Women's Hospital, 1976–1993. (Courtesy of Conte MS, Belkin M, Donaldson MC, et al: *J Vasc Surg* 21:873–881, 1995.)

Primary and secondary patency rates at 5 years were 81% and 86% for the present series, similar to those achieved in the FP/CLAUD group (74% and 81%) and markedly superior to those observed in the FT/LS group (51%, 61%, *P* < 0.001). Thus, graft performance was closely linked to the indication for bypass and not significantly associated with the level of the distal anastomosis in this series.

Cumulative palliation, defined as successful by the presence of a patent graft in a surviving patient at each time point, is another useful

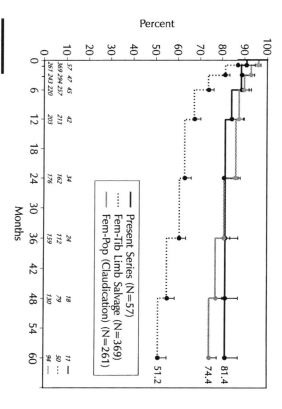

FIGURE 2.

Cumulative primary graft patency for three concurrent groups of infrainguinal bypasses. (Courtesy of Conte MS, Belkin M, Donaldson MC, et al: *J Vasc Surg* 21:873–881, 1995.)

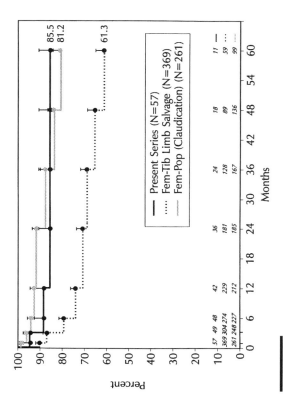

FIGURE 3.

Cumulative secondary graft patency for three concurrent groups of infrainguinal bypasses. (Courtesy of Conte MS, Belkin M, Donaldson MC, et al: *J Vasc Surg* 21:873–881, 1995.)

measure by which to analyze interventions for claudication when limb "salvage" statistics lack meaning. In the present series of tibial bypasses performed for claudication, cumulative successful palliation was achieved for 71% of patients at 3 years, comparing favorably with the 78% observed in the FP/CLAUD group as well as other data reported in the literature for femoropopliteal grafts.[34] These data are illustrated on Figure 4.

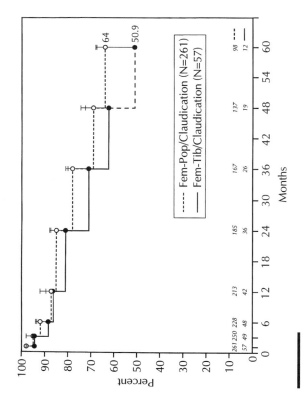

FIGURE 4.

Cumulative palliation achieved for two concurrent groups of infrainguinal by-passes.

In an attempt to garner some subjective assessment of functional outcomes in these patients, follow-up interviews were obtained in 21 of 24 surviving patients. Although admittedly prone to a number of important sources of bias (telephone survey, retrospective, time interval from procedure as long as 3 years), the striking uniformity of the responses adds some insight to the standard graft patency analysis. Of the 21 respondents, 15 reported increased maximal walking distance, 4 were unchanged in this measure, and 2 had deteriorated (1 due to worsening arthritis, the other to claudication in the contralateral limb). Role functioning and independence were improved in 12 patients and unchanged in 9; a full 86% (18 of 21) expressed overall satisfaction with their operation and would choose to do it again under similar circumstances. Overall health status and degree of impairment caused by other co-morbid conditions did not change appreciably for the interviewed patients (Table 3).

Incomplete availability of the preoperative angiograms in this retrospective study precludes precise characterization of the runoff in these patients. Nonetheless, we would consider the presence of a continuous tibial vessel to the ankle as minimal angiographic criteria for considering bypass to the tibial level for claudication. An example of the preoperative arteriographic findings in this select patient group is shown in Figure 5: SFA occlusion, an isolated popliteal segment, and reconstitution of the proximal posterior tibial artery that is continuous to the ankle. Patients with a patent but diffusely diseased popliteal segment, another common pattern in this series, are likely better served by choosing a proximal tibial site for the distal anastomosis, regardless of indication.

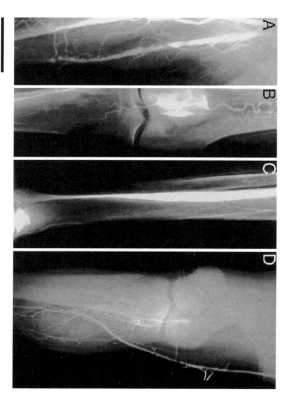

FIGURE 5.

Preoperative (A–C) and intraoperative (D) arteriograms of a patient in the femorotibial reconstruction series described. Vein bypass to the proximal posterior tibial artery was performed with a good technical result.

TABLE 3. Changes in Health Perception Preoperatively and Postoperatively

	Improved - 1 Level	Improved - 2 Levels	Improved - 3 Levels	Worse - 1 Level	Worse - 2 Levels	Worse - 3 Levels	Unchanged
Overall health status	3	1	1	3	1	0	12
Maximal walking distance	2	7	6	2	0	0	4
Impairment of walking:							
Claudication	1	4	10	1	0	0	6
Joint pain/stiffness	0	0	0	1	2	1	17
Chest pain/shortness of breath	0	0	0	0	0	0	21
Weakness in legs	0	0	0	1	0	0	20
Role functioning/independence	7	4	1	0	0	0	9

	YES	NO
Would recommend surgery to others?	18	3

KEY TO RESPONSE SCALES IN OUTCOME SURVEY:

ITEM	LEVELS	DESCRIPTION
Overall health	1–5	Excellent–poor
Maximal walking distance	1–6	# Blocks: ≥ 5, 2–5, 1–2, 1/2–1, < 1/2, rest pain
Causes of walking impairment:		
Claudication	1–5	Very much–none
Joint pain/stiffness	1–5	Very much–none
Chest pain/shortness of breath	1–5	Very much–none
Weakness in legs	1–5	Very much–none
Role functioning/independence	1–5	Excellent–poor
Recommend this surgery to others?		Yes/No

(Courtesy of Conte MS, Belkin M, Donaldson MC, et al: *J Vasc Surg* 21:873–881, 1995.)

SUMMARY: ROLE OF FEMOROTIBIAL BYPASS IN THE TREATMENT OF DISABLING CLAUDICATION

An aggressive approach to claudication is warranted in the younger, good-risk patient with disabling symptoms and minimal co-morbidities that might detract from the expected functional benefits of reconstruction. Elevated risk for progression to critical ischemia, such as low hemodynamic indices (e.g., ankle-brachial index less than 0.6) and the presence of diabetes, is an important factor favoring intervention before deterioration and tissue necrosis. Most claudicants are best served by initial conservative management to effect smoking cessation, institution of daily exercise, and treatment of associated cardiovascular risk factors. The key variables to be considered in selecting patients for intervention are anticipated survival, risk for progression in the affected limb, degree of disability, anticipated functional outcome, and risk-benefit potential for the particular approach.

Cost-effectiveness is an additional parameter that must be considered, particularly in the current health care environment. Limited resources, capitated contracts, and disincentives for specialist referral are increasingly prevalent market forces that may ultimately determine the availability and use of many types of elective interventions. At the societal level, a cost-benefit analysis may be argued to support a steadfast conservative approach to claudicants who are no longer in the workforce and for whom claudication is an individual quality-of-life issue. The difficulty with such an analysis is the inability to quantify the potential negative effects of increasing debility, inactivity, and progressive loss of independence. In terms of cost, percutaneous options may not offer any significant advantage over surgical approaches for patients with infrainguinal occlusions.[38] It seems clear that economic factors will exert a net negative influence on the use of all types of intervention for claudicants. More detailed functional outcomes information is needed on large populations of patients to enable accurate subgroup analysis of the benefits obtained vs. the health care costs incurred.

Presently, percutaneous endovascular options (e.g., PTA) offer far superior results and are more frequently appropriate for patients with inflow as opposed to outflow disease. The possibility of an endovascular approach for the patient with aortoiliac disease may be estimated to some extent by noninvasive testing (i.e., tracings consistent with iliac stenosis vs. occlusion) and may be a factor favoring earlier intervention. By and large, however, patients are referred for arteriography assuming a surgical approach may be required. For those whose disease is predominantly infrainguinal in nature, the technical considerations that most heavily influence the anticipated outcome are the availability and quality of autogenous vein conduit and the arterial anatomy. Patients lacking greater saphenous vein by virtue of prior coronary bypass or lower-extremity revascularizations should only be considered for intervention for incapacitating symptoms or deterioration to impending limb threat. Duplex ultrasound mapping is useful for assessment of the quality of ectopic venous conduits in this circumstance. Infrageniculate bypass for claudication is contemplated only when the availability of an adequate length of good-quality autogenous vein is considered highly likely.

Our reported experience with tibial bypass for claudication confirms the notion that the anatomical level of the distal anastomosis is less critical to graft performance than the presenting indication (and presumably runoff) and quality of conduit used. Based on the aforementioned criteria, claudicants selected for arteriography who demonstrate severe popliteal disease and suitable tibial outflow should be considered for femorotibial grafting if adequate saphenous vein can be reasonably expected. Conversely, in the presence of adequate vein, we would *favor* performing the distal anastomosis to a nondiseased tibial artery rather than a significantly diseased popliteal. Our results indicate that, in carefully selected patients, composing a small percentage of claudicants in our practice, autogenous vein bypass to the tibial level has excellent and durable results that compare favorably with those of more proximal reconstructions for claudication.

REFERENCES

1. Dawber TR: *Framingham Study.* London, Harvard University Press, 1980.
2. US Bureau of the Census: Statistical Abstract of the United States: 1993, 113th ed. Washington, DC, US Government Printing Office, 1993:91.
3. Boyd AM: The natural course of arteriosclerosis of the lower extremities. *Proc R Soc Med* 55:591–593, 1962.
4. Singer A, Rob C: The fate of the claudicator. *BMJ* 2:633–636, 1960.
5. Imparato AM, Kim GE, Davidson T, et al: Intermittent claudication: Its natural course. *Surgery* 78:795–799, 1975.
6. Cronenwett JL, Warner KG, Zelenock GB, et al: Intermittent claudication: Current results of nonoperative management. *Arch Surg* 119:430–436, 1984.
7. Rosenbloom MS, Flanigan P, Schuler JJ, et al: Risk factors affecting the natural history of intermittent claudication. *Arch Surg* 123:867–870, 1988.
8. Jonason T, Ringqvist I: Factors of prognostic importance for subsequent rest pain in patients with intermittent claudication. *Acta Med Scand* 218:27–33, 1985.
9. McDaniel MD, Cronenwett JL: Basic data related to the natural history of intermittent claudication. *Ann Vasc Surg* 3:273–277, 1989.
10. Juergens JL, Barker NW, Hines EA Jr: Arteriosclerosis obliterans: Review of 520 cases with special reference to pathogenic and prognostic factors. *Circulation* 21:188–195, 1960.
11. Schadt DC, Hines EA Jr, Juergens JL, et al: Chronic atherosclerotic occlusion of the femoral artery. *JAMA* 175:937–940, 1961.
12. McAllister FF: The fate of patients with intermittent claudication managed nonoperatively. *Am J Surg* 132:593–595, 1976.
13. Jonason T, Ringqvist I: Diabetes mellitus and intermittent claudication. *Acta Med Scand* 218:217–221, 1985.
14. Humphries AW, deWolfe VG, Young JR: Evaluation of the natural history and the results of treatment in occlusive arteriosclerosis involving the lower extremities in 1850 patients, in Weslowski D (ed): *Fundamentals of Vascular Grafting.* New York, McGraw-Hill, 1963, pp 423–440.
15. Martinez BD, Hertzer NR, Beven EG: Influence of distal arterial occlusive disease on prognosis following aortobifemoral bypass. *Surgery* 88:795–805, 1980.

16. Haimovici H: Patterns of arteriosclerotic lesions of the lower extremity. *Arch Surg* 95:918–933, 1967.

17. Ferrier TM: Comparative study of arterial disease in amputated limbs from diabetics and non-diabetics (with special reference to feet arteries). *Med J Aust* 1:5–11, 1967.

18. Jonason T, Bergstrom R: Cessation of smoking in patients with intermittent claudication: Effects on the risk of peripheral vascular complications, myocardial infarction and mortality. *Acta Med Scand* 221:253–260, 1987.

19. Radack K, Wyderski RJ. Conservative management of intermittent claudication. *Ann Intern Med* 113:135–146, 1990.

20. Radack K, Wyderski RJ: Conservative management of intermittent claudication. *Ann Intern Med* 113:135–146, 1990.

21. Lundgren F, Dahllof AG, Lundholm K, et al: Intermittent claudication: Surgical reconstruction or physical training? *Ann Surg* 209:346–355, 1989.

22. Schneider JR, McHorney CA, Malenka DJ, et al: Functional health and well-being in patients with severe atherosclerotic peripheral vascular occlusive disease. *Ann Vasc Surg* 7:419–428, 1993.

23. Gibbons GW, Burgess AM, Guadagnoli E, et al: Return to well-being and function after infrainguinal revascularization. *J Vasc Surg* 21:35–45, 1995.

24. Rutherford RB, Durham JD, Kumpe DA: Endovascular interventions for lower extremity ischemia, in Rutherford RB (ed): *Vascular Surgery.* Philadelphia, WB Saunders, 1992, pp 858–874.

25. Szilagyi DE, Elliot JP, Smith RF, et al: A thirty-year survey of the reconstructive surgical treatment of aortoiliac occlusive disease. *J Vasc Surg* 3:421–436, 1986.

26. Brewster DC, Darling RC: Optimal methods of aortoiliac reconstruction. *Surgery* 88:642–653, 1980.

27. Nevelsteen A, Suy R, Daenen W, et al: Aortofemoral grafting: Factors influencing late results. *Surgery* 88:642–653, 1980.

28. Crawford ES, Bomberger RA, Glaeser DH, et al: Aortoiliac occlusive disease: Factors influencing survival and function following operation over a twenty-five year period. *Surgery* 90:1055–1067, 1981.

29. Hunink MGM, Meyerovitz MF: Infrainguinal percutaneous transluminal balloon angioplasty, in Whittemore AD (ed): *Advances in Vascular Surgery.* St Louis, Mo, Mosby–Year Book, 1994, Vol 2, pp 135–159.

30. Kent KC, Donaldson MC, Attinger CE, et al: Femoropopliteal reconstruction for claudication: The risk to life and limb. *Arch Surg* 123:1196–1198, 1988.

31. Taylor LM, Porter JM: Clinical and anatomic considerations for surgery in femoroopopliteal disease and the results of surgery. *Circulation* 83:63I–69I, 1991.

32. Donaldson MC, Mannick JA, Whittemore AD: Femorodistal bypass with in-situ greater saphenous vein: Long term results using the Mills valvulotome. *Ann Surg* 213:457–465, 1991.

33. Sladen JG, Gilmour JL: Fate of claudicants after femoropopliteal vein bypass: Prospective, long-term follow-up of 100 patients. *Can J Surg* 28:401–404, 1985.

34. Taylor LM, Edwards JM, Porter JM: Present status of reversed vein bypass grafting: Five-year results of a modern series. *J Vasc Surg* 11:193–206, 1990.

35. Shah DM, Darling RC III, Chang BB, et al: Long-term results of in situ saphenous vein bypass: analysis of 2058 cases. *Ann Surg* 222:438–448, 1995.

36. Belkin M, Conte MS, Donaldson MC, et al: The impact of gender on the results of arterial bypass with in-situ greater saphenous vein. *Am J Surg* 170:97–102, 1995.

37. Conte MS, Belkin M, Donaldson MC, et al: Femorotibial bypass for claudication: Do results justify an aggressive approach? *J Vasc Surg* 21:873–881, 1995.
38. Hunink MG, Wong JB, Donaldson MC, et al: Revascularization for femoropopliteal disease. A decision and cost-effectiveness analysis. *JAMA* 274:165–171, 1995.

The Impact of Duplex Surveillance on Infrainguinal Vein Bypass Surgery

Joseph L. Mills, M.D.

Associate Professor of Surgery, Chief, Section of Vascular Surgery, University of Arizona Health Sciences Center, Tucson

I ntermediate and late failures after infrainguinal arterial bypass surgery with autogenous venous conduits are often preceded by the development of intrinsic graft lesions. Some of these lesions are prone to progression and, undetected, may become hemodynamically significant and reduce graft flow velocity with resultant graft thrombosis. Szilagyi et al. first described the occurrence and progression of such intrinsic structural defects in a serial arteriographic study of 377 arterialized vein conduits implanted for lower extremity revascularization.[1] Breslau and DeWeese in 1965 were the first to report successful, direct surgical repair of a "failing" vein graft caused by an intrinsic graft stenosis.[2] These two fundamental observations, that vein graft failure was often heralded by the development and progression of intrinsic graft lesions and that such lesions could be successfully repaired, were generally underappreciated because of the lack of an accurate, reproducible screening tool to identify grafts at risk. Repetitive clinical evaluations, including the measurement of Doppler-derived ankle pressures, were insufficiently sensitive, and serial arteriographic studies were too expensive and invasive. The application of duplex scanning, a powerful noninvasive method of performing serial postoperative evaluations of infrainguinal vein grafts, has evolved over the last decade into the gold standard for postoperative graft surveillance.

Convincing data now exist to support careful postoperative duplex surveillance of both in situ and reversed vein conduits after infrainguinal revascularization.[3] Diligent postoperative surveillance in concert with timely intervention when significant, progressive lesions are identified appears to have significantly improved assisted-primary patency rates after infrainguinal vein grafting. Nevertheless, many vascular surgeons hesitate to recommend intensive graft surveillance for their patients. This reluctance may stem from the logistics involved in instituting such a protocol in a busy vascular practice, concerns over the additional costs to the patient and the health care system, or doubts about the efficacy of graft revision in asymptomatic patients. The purpose of this chapter is to provide the rationale and justification for a duplex graft surveillance protocol, describe the currently recommended technique and methods of graft surveillance, delineate the evolution of threshold noninvasive crite-

Advances in Vascular Surgery®, vol. 4
© 1996, Mosby–Year Book, Inc.

ria for intervention, and summarize the overall impact that duplex surveillance has had not only on assisted-primary patency rates but also on our broader understanding of vein graft function and the mechanisms of graft failure.

RATIONALE AND JUSTIFICATION FOR DUPLEX SURVEILLANCE

Duplex surveillance is based on several underlying premises that deserve critical re-examination before concluding that intensive postoperative graft monitoring is justified. The major premises include the following: (1) vein graft failure most often results from the development of intrinsic graft stenosis; (2) high-grade vein graft stenoses will lead to graft thrombosis if not revised; (3) vein graft stenosis is frequently clinically silent and not reliably detectable before graft occlusion by history, physical examination, and simple noninvasive measurements; (4) vein graft stenoses and low-flow states can be accurately identified, graded, and monitored for progression by duplex surveillance; (5) prophylactic revision of patent but "failing" vein grafts yields results superior to those obtained after thrombectomy or thrombolysis and revision of occluded vein grafts; and (6) vein graft patency and limb salvage rates are significantly improved by a postoperative duplex surveillance protocol. If these premises are sound, then not only is duplex surveillance of infrainguinal vein grafts justifiable, it is also mandatory.

Postoperative studies using serial arteriography and duplex scanning convincingly demonstrate that intrinsic vein graft strictures are the most common cause of vein graft failure; these strictures account for 60% of the failures in the first 5 postoperative years.[4] Of particular importance is the observation that nearly 75% of these lesions develop within the first postoperative year.[4–6] The incidence of postimplantation lesions is surprisingly high, ranging from 12% to 37%, depending on which threshold criteria are used to define graft stenosis.[5–7] The data linking unrepaired vein graft stenosis with subsequent graft thrombosis are especially persuasive. Mattos et al. recently reported a 4-year patency rate of 83% in infrainguinal vein grafts with normal postoperative duplex scans as compared with 57% in those grafts with stenoses detected by color duplex scanning.[8] Both Taylor et al.[6] and Moody et al.[9] reported a short-term graft thrombosis rate exceeding 20% in bypasses with unrepaired stenoses detected by duplex surveillance. Idu, Buth, and associates observed that all vein grafts with stenosis of over 70% of the vessel's diameter that were identified by duplex scanning eventually occluded if the lesion was not repaired.[10,11]

Vein graft strictures are frequently progressive in nature. In their classic study using serial postoperative arteriography, Szilagyi et al. noted that certain specific intrinsic graft lesions, which they termed fibrotic stenosis and valvular fibrosis, were particularly threatening to long-term graft patency, and resulted in graft occlusion 75% of the time.[1] Indirect and direct evidence support the premise that progressive vein graft stricture most often remains clinically silent until graft thrombosis and recurrent limb ischemia ensue. Veith et al. reported a series of 191 patients with recurrent limb ischemia after lower extremity revascularization.

Prompt arteriography identified patent, but failing grafts in 38 (20%) cases.[12] Therefore, in 80% of the patients, thrombosis of the graft had already occurred when recurrent limb ischemia developed. Reliance on clinical symptoms alone is therefore not sufficiently sensitive to detect vein grafts harboring intrinsic lesions or low-flow states with a predisposition to sudden graft thrombosis. Graft surveillance protocols using pulse palpation, pulse volume recording (PVR), and Doppler-derived ankle-brachial index (ABI) determinations have been used to successfully identify failing vein grafts before graft occlusion. Multiple studies, however, have shown these techniques to be less sensitive than either duplex scanning alone or duplex surveillance in combination with ABI and PVR measurements. Bandyk et al. reported that 30% of the lesions detected by their duplex surveillance protocol that led to graft revision were not associated with a decreased ABI.[7] Mills et al., in an analysis of 48 failing grafts in a series of 379 reversed vein bypasses monitored with duplex surveillance, noted that only 29% of these failing grafts were associated with a decrease in resting ABI of greater than 0.15.[13] Barnes and associates monitored 232 infrainguinal bypass grafts with serial postoperative ABI measurements and determined that an ABI diminution greater than 0.2 did not correlate well with graft occlusion.[14] It appears unequivocal, then, that serial postoperative duplex surveillance is currently the most sensitive method of detecting vein graft stenosis.

DETECTION AND GRADING OF VEIN GRAFT STENOSIS

Graft surveillance should consist of measurement of Doppler-derived ABIs and color duplex interrogation of the adjacent inflow and outflow arteries, both anastomoses, as well as the venous conduit in its entirety. Such surveillance allows one to obtain morphologic and hemodynamic information of considerable prognostic significance. These examinations should be performed with sufficient frequency and completeness to detect the presence and monitor the progression of lesions before the advent of graft occlusion. Because the period of greatest risk is during the initial 12 to 18 months after graft implantation, most surveillance protocols call for more frequent evaluations (every 3 months) during this interval, with less frequent examination of grafts with normal scans (every 6 months) thereafter. Although changes in ABI are by themselves relatively insensitive, they are of prognostic importance in patients with compressible arteries in conjunction with information derived from duplex scanning.

Depending on the depth of the graft, longitudinal color Doppler imaging of the complete reconstruction (including adjacent proximal and distal arteries) should be performed with either a 5.0- or 7.5-MHz linear-array probe. Representative center-stream velocity spectra should be recorded at multiple graft segments, with careful examination of the anastomotic regions of the vein graft. Velocity spectra measurements should be made at a Doppler angle of 60 degrees or less. In addition, if a focal color-flow disturbance (mosaic color pattern) or "flow jet" is noted at any site, careful interrogation with measurement of peak systolic velocity (V_p) and velocity ratio (V_r) should be performed. A V_p that exceeds 150 cm/

sec and a V_r greater than 1.5 are abnormal. Such sites of flow disturbance can thus be identified, graded, and monitored for progression with the use of these simple duplex-derived measurements (Fig 1). In addition, the detection of an end-diastolic velocity greater than 20 cm/sec has been shown to correlate closely with the presence of angiographic stenosis with

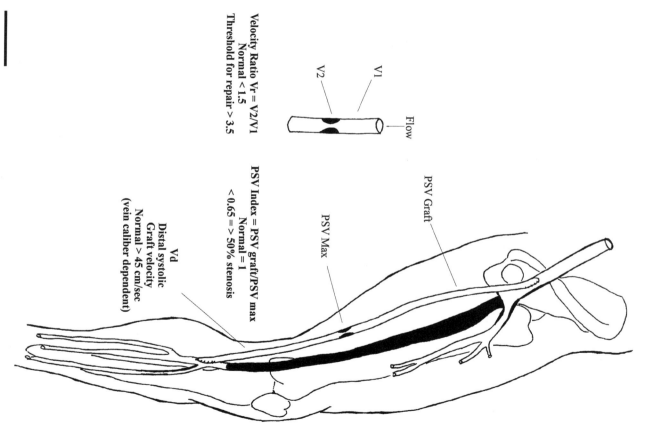

Velocity Ratio Vr = V2/V1
Normal < 1.5
Threshold for repair > 3.5

PSV Index = PSV graft/PSV max
Normal = 1
< 0.65 = > 50% stenosis

Vd
Distal systolic
Graft velocity
Normal > 45 cm/sec
(vein caliber dependent)

FIGURE 1.

Sites of flow disturbance can be graded for hemodynamic significance by simple duplex-derived measurements, including peak systolic velocity (PSV), velocity ratio (V_r), PSV index, and distal graft velocity (V_d).

greater than 70% diameter reduction.[11] Once a stenosis is identified, the patient should return to the vascular laboratory for repeat surveillance at 6-week intervals until either regression or stabilization of the lesion is documented or progression to threshold criteria for intervention occurs.

After infrainguinal vein bypass surgery, a spectrum of clinically unsuspected abnormalities can be present in the venous conduit (retained valve, fibrotic valve, stenotic vein segment), in the adjacent arteries (clamp injury or endarterectomy end point), or at anastomotic sites (suture stenosis or intimal defect). These lesions may reduce graft flow and precipitate graft thrombosis or may act as a nidus for the development of progressive, myointimal hyperplasia.[3,5] Serial postoperative duplex surveillance allows one to detect and monitor such early-appearing defects for progression, as well as identify de novo lesions that arise in the vein graft at sites without preexisting abnormalities or flow defects. Although precise threshold criteria warranting prophylactic intervention to prevent graft thrombosis are currently evolving, published criteria are in significant agreement, as outlined in Table 1.[15–18]

I generally recommend repair of all lesions with a V_p greater than 300 cm/sec and V_r over 3.5, especially if distal graft velocity is low (less than 45 cm/sec) and/or the ABI has fallen more than 0.2. Surveillance allows one to stratify vein grafts into broad categories of risk based on hemodynamic information. Asymptomatic patients with normal ABIs and normal duplex scans are at minimal risk of sudden graft occlusion. In contrast, patients with grafts harboring a high-grade stenosis, a low-flow state in the distal end of the graft, and a fall in ABI of greater than 0.2 are at highest risk for failure. In fact, abundant evidence suggests that lesions with duplex-derived velocity spectra of a high-grade stenosis and greater than 70% diameter reduction by angiography uniformly result in graft occlusion if left unrepaired.

Thus patients at either end of the spectrum are relatively simple to

TABLE 1.
Published Duplex Criteria for High-Grade Infrainguinal Vein Graft Stenosis

Criteria	References
Primary	
$V_p > 300$ cm/sec, $V_r > 3.0$	18
$V_p > 300$ cm/sec, $V_r > 3.5$	16
$V_p > 250$ cm/sec, $V_r > 3.4$	17
EDV > 20 cm/sec at the site of stenosis	11
PSVI < 0.65	10,11
Secondary	
Reduction in distal graft $V_d < 45$ cm/sec	16–18
Reduction in ABI ≥ 0.2	16–18

Abbreviations: V_p, peak systolic velocity; V_r, velocity ratio; *EDV*, end-diastolic velocity; *PSVI*, peak systolic velocity index = PSV graft/PSV max; V_d, distal graft flow velocity; *ABI*, ankle-brachial index.

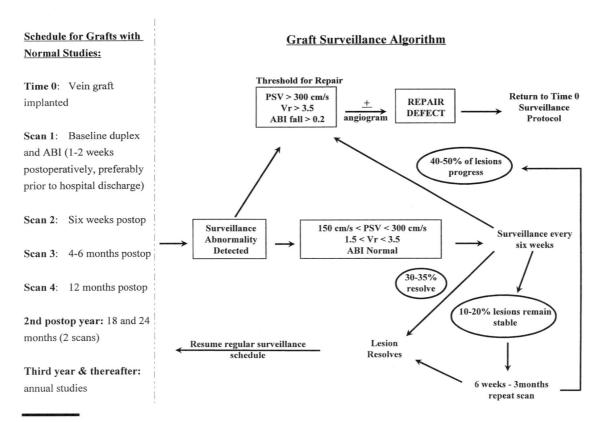

Schedule for Grafts with Normal Studies:

Time 0: Vein graft implanted

Scan 1: Baseline duplex and ABI (1-2 weeks postoperatively, preferably prior to hospital discharge)

Scan 2: Six weeks postop

Scan 3: 4-6 months postop

Scan 4: 12 months postop

2nd postop year: 18 and 24 months (2 scans)

Third year & thereafter: annual studies

Graft Surveillance Algorithm

Threshold for Repair

PSV > 300 cm/s
Vr > 3.5
ABI fall > 0.2

$\pm$ angiogram

REPAIR DEFECT

Return to Time 0 Surveillance Protocol

40-50% of lesions progress

Surveillance Abnormality Detected

150 cm/s < PSV < 300 cm/s
1.5 < Vr < 3.5
ABI Normal

Surveillance every six weeks

30-35% resolve

10-20% lesions remain stable

Resume regular surveillance schedule

Lesion Resolves

6 weeks - 3months repeat scan

FIGURE 2.

Algorithm for infrainguinal vein graft surveillance. *Abbreviations: PSV,* peak systolic velocity; V_r, velocity ratio; *ABI,* ankle-brachial index.

manage. The greatest dilemma occurs with patients in the intermediate-risk groups. We currently examine patients with lesions having a V_p of 150 to 300 cm/sec and a V_r less than 3 at 4- to 6-week intervals to detect rapid progression. The hemodynamic course of lesion regression or progression to threshold levels generally occurs within 3 or 4 months, a time period that allows appropriate intervention. Approximately 15% to 20% of grafts will require revision, and the rate of sudden graft occlusion in a series of patients monitored and treated in this manner will be extremely low. The principles just outlined have led to the development of an algorithm that is useful in the management of patients monitored in an infrainguinal vein graft surveillance protocol (Fig 2). Grafts found to have residual stenosis with V_p greater than 300 cm/sec and V_r greater than 3.5 should usually be revised, especially if the overall graft flow velocity is low or the postoperative ABI is less than expected.

VEIN GRAFT REVISION

The success of graft revision after graft occlusion has been poor. Even after a responsible lesion is uncovered following successful thrombectomy or thrombolysis and appropriately repaired, intermediate and long-term "secondary" patency rates are less than 25% to 40%.[19] In contrast, the "assisted-primary" patency rates of stenotic, hemodynamically failing vein grafts repaired before graft thrombosis are 80% to 85% at 5 years, which approximates the patency of vein grafts that never required revision.[20] Surgical revision appears to be clearly superior to balloon angioplasty.[21]

Focal, fibrotic circumferential lesions require excision and interposition vein graft placement. Selected midgraft lesions can be handled with excision of the fibrotic valve leaflet and vein patch angioplasty. Focal, juxta-anastomotic lesions, which usually occur on the venous side of either the distal or the proximal anastomosis, usually require resection and replacement with either vein graft interposition or reimplantation of the graft into an alternative site. In the case of a proximal juxta-anastomotic stenosis, the anastomosis can sometimes be moved more distally onto the common femoral, superficial femoral, or deep femoral arteries, depending on local anatomic considerations. It is extremely important to document that the repair has restored normal graft hemodynamics, either with intraoperative duplex scanning or with a complete arteriogram of the repair as well as evaluation of the rest of the conduit to make sure that no additional lesions are present. Although selected lesions can be repaired with duplex scanning alone, it is frequently helpful to perform arteriography before vein graft revision to make sure that no inflow and outflow lesions are present. Also, a high-grade stenosis can sometimes mask other lesions in the conduit. When the high-graft lesion is repaired, if the entire conduit has not been investigated, on occasion another lesion may be "unmasked." Successful repair restores normal graft flow velocities and normal hemodynamics and improves the ABI if this was abnormal preoperatively. Revision operations that restore hemodynamics result in excellent 5-year patency, with multiple groups reporting assisted-primary rates of at least 80% at 5 years. This is clearly superior to the approximately 40% to 50% 1- to 2-year patency rates reported after balloon angioplasty. Balloon angioplasty may have a role in selected patients with focal fibrotic midgraft lesions, particularly when they occur at a later time interval after placement of the graft. Most lesions that appear early after bypass are best treated operatively. It is also my impression that early-appearing stenoses are more malignant and should be monitored very closely. When the repair threshold is reached, prompt repair should be carried out to prevent graft thrombosis.

Only one randomized prospective trial of duplex vein graft surveillance has been performed.[22] Numerous other clinical studies attest to the efficacy of duplex surveillance in maintaining long-term graft patency.[5, 6, 9, 13, 20] Abundant natural history data dating back to the initial report of Szilagyi et al. document the graft-threatening potential of high-grade fibrotic graft strictures.[1] In addition, recent work by Idu, Buth, and associates has documented that nearly all grafts with greater than 70% stenosis ultimately occluded if not repaired.[10, 11] It would be inappropriate to perform a graft surveillance trial in which high-grade lesions were not repaired. In addition, in a vascular unit that performs careful graft surveillance, it is uncommon for patients to require surgery for graft occlusion. In my own practice, nearly all graft revisions of infrainguinal vein grafts are performed after detection of a high-grade stenosis. In a unit performing approximately 100 reconstructions per year, fewer than 10% of the revisions are required for occluded grafts. Although some of these may represent missed lesions, in other cases, lesions were detected but not repaired. If a graft with a known defect occludes and the occlusion is of short duration, it is not unreasonable to perform catheter-directed thrombolysis and then revision of the previously identified graft defect. These patients should then be maintained on a regimen of sodium warfarin because the thrombotic episode damages the endothelium and use of oral anticoagulation may improve late patency. Nevertheless, the focus of a surveillance protocol should be to identify high-grade lesions and to repair them before graft thrombosis and thus avoid this management difficulty.

Current recommendations for vein graft surveillance are based on our own studies as well as those of others and are outlined in the algorithm in Figure 2. I believe that obtaining early duplex scans is critically important to document the hemodynamic status of a newly placed vein bypass graft.[5, 23] Although early graft occlusion is rare with meticulous intraoperative technique and monitoring, it is still worthwhile to obtain duplex study before hospital discharge or at least at the time of the patient's first postoperative clinic visit. It is our experience and that of others that approximately 30% of grafts harbor intrinsic defects that are present early after implantation.[5, 6, 10] It is these defects that are very likely to progress to a more severe stenosis. For this reason it is important to expeditiously identify these high-risk grafts. Thus the surveillance protocol as outlined places primary importance on the early identification of high-risk grafts with close follow-up for detected abnormalities. In my experience, if the graft scan is normal for the first 6 to 9 months, it is very uncommon for lesions to subsequently develop during the following 1 to 2 years. For this reason, after the first 1- to 2-year follow-up period, graft surveillance can be decreased in frequency to once or twice per year.

It is also my impression that certain types of grafts are at higher risk for early failure and should be monitored more closely. First-time femoropopliteal bypasses with excellent-quality ipsilateral greater saphenous vein appear to exhibit a much lower incidence of graft stenosis. If the early scans are normal, the graft surveillance protocol can probably be relaxed for such grafts. The highest-risk grafts include alternate conduits such as arm vein or spliced lesser and greater saphenous veins, as well as redo or reoperative distal bypasses. As many as 60% to 75% of arm vein conduits may harbor valve or short-segment sclerotic defects, which if not identified will result in intermediate graft occlusion. For this reason, reoperative bypass grafts and arm vein grafts are frequently tunneled subcutaneously so that they can be easily monitored. Should repair be necessary, it is relatively simple to accomplish because of the graft's subcutaneous location.

SUMMARY

The preceding analysis has established the six major premises that were outlined in the initial rationale and justification for duplex surveillance for infrainguinal bypass grafts. Because all these premises are sound and supported by strong natural history and clinical data, it would appear that duplex surveillance of infrainguinal grafts is not only justifiable but mandatory. I believe the current approach to graft surveillance has been best summarized by P.L. Harris in the *British Journal of Surgery*:

> If the purchaser of a new motor can expect guaranteed after-sales service targeted against possible early mechanical breakdown, surely the recipient of a vein graft has the right to expect after-care, which is at least as attentive and effective in averting disaster. Until the problem of fibrous stenoses has been eliminated all together, vein graft surveillance should be an integral component of every vascular surgical service.[24]

REFERENCES

1. Szilagyi DE, Elliott JP, Hageman JH, et al: Biologic fate of autogenous vein implants as arterial substitutes: Clinical, angiographic, and histo-pathologic observations in femoro-popliteal operations for atherosclerosis. *Ann Surg* 178:232–246, 1973.
2. Breslau RC, DeWeese JA: Successful endophlebectomy of autogenous venous bypass graft. *Ann Surg* 162:251–254, 1965.
3. Bandyk DF: Essentials of graft surveillance. *Semin Vasc Surg* 6:92–102, 1993.
4. Mills JL, Fujitani RM, Taylor SM: The characteristics and anatomic distribution of lesions that cause reversed vein graft failure: A five-year prospective study. *J Vasc Surg* 17:195–206, 1993.
5. Mills JL, Bandyk DF, Gahtan V, et al: The origin of infrainguinal vein graft stenosis: A prospective study based on duplex surveillance. *J Vasc Surg* 21:16–25, 1995.
6. Taylor PR, Wolfe JHN, Tyrrell MR, et al: Graft stenosis—justification for 1-year surveillance. *Br J Surg* 77:1125–1128, 1990.
7. Bandyk DF, Schmitt DD, Seabrook GR, et al: Monitoring functional patency of in-situ saphenous vein bypasses: The impact of a surveillance protocol and elective revision. *J Vasc Surg* 9:286–296, 1989.

8. Mattos MA, van Bemmelen PS, Hodgson KJ, et al: Does correction of stenoses identified with color duplex scanning improve infrainguinal graft patency? *J Vasc Surg* 17:54–66, 1993.

9. Moody P, Gould DA, Harris PL: Vein graft surveillance improves patency in femoro-popliteal bypass. *Eur J Vasc Surg* 4:117–121, 1990.

10. Idu MM, Blankenstein JD, de Gier P, et al: Impact of a color-flow duplex surveillance program on infrainguinal vein graft patency: A five-year experience. *J Vasc Surg* 17:42–53, 1993.

11. Buth J, Disselhoff B, Sommeling C, et al: Color-flow duplex criteria for grading stenosis in infrainguinal vein grafts. *J Vasc Surg* 14:716–728, 1991.

12. Veith FJ, Weiser RK, Gupta SK, et al: Diagnosis and management of failing lower extremity arterial reconstruction prior to graft occlusion. *J Cardiovasc Surg* 25:381–384, 1984.

13. Mills JL, Harris EJ, Taylor LM Jr, et al: The importance of routine surveillance of distal bypass grafts with duplex scanning: A study of 379 reverse vein grafts. *J Vasc Surg* 12:379–389, 1990.

14. Barnes RW, Thompson BW, MacDonald CM, et al: Serial noninvasive studies do not herald postoperative failure of femoropopliteal or femorotibial bypass grafts. *Ann Surg* 210:486–494, 1989.

15. Grigg MJ, Nicolaides AN, Wolfe JHN: Detection and grading of femorodistal vein graft stenoses: Duplex velocity measurements compared with angiography. *J Vasc Surg* 8:661–666, 1988.

16. Gahtan V, Payne LP, Roper LD, et al: Duplex criteria for predicting progression of vein graft lesions: Which stenoses can be followed? *J Vasc Technol* 19:211–215, 1995.

17. Papanicolaou G, Zierler RE, Beach KW, et al: Hemodynamic parameters of failing infrainguinal bypass grafts. *Am J Surg* 169:238–244, 1995.

18. Sladen JG, Reid JDS, Cooperberg PL, et al: Color flow duplex screening of infrainguinal grafts combining low- and high-velocity criteria. *Am J Surg* 158:107–112, 1989.

19. Whittemore AD, Clowes AW, Couch NP, et al: Secondary femoropopliteal reconstruction. *Ann Surg* 193:35–42, 1981.

20. Bergamini TM, George SM, Massey HT, et al: Intensive surveillance of femoropopliteal-tibial autogenous vein bypasses improves long-term graft patency and limb salvage. *Ann Surg* 221:507–518, 1995.

21. Perler BA, Osterman FA, Mitchell SE, et al: Balloon dilatation versus surgical revision of infrainguinal autogenous vein graft stenosis: Long-term follow-up. *J Cardiovasc Surg* 31:656–661, 1990.

22. Lundell A, Lindblad B, Berquist D, et al: Femoropopliteal-crural graft patency is improved by ABI intensive surveillance program: A prospective randomized study. *J Vasc Surg* 21:26–34, 1995.

23. Wilson WG, Davies AH, Carrie IC, et al: The value of pre-discharge duplex scanning in infrainguinal graft surveillance. *Eur J Endovasc Surg* 10:237–242, 1995.

24. Harris PL: Vein graft surveillance—all part of the service. *Br J Surg* 79:97–98, 1992.

The Septic Diabetic Foot: "Foot-Sparing Surgery"

Gary W. Gibbons, M.D.

Clinical Chief, Division of Vascular Surgery, Chairman, Quality Assurance, Department of Surgery, New England Deaconess Hospital; Associate Clinical Professor of Surgery, Harvard Medical School, Boston, Massachusetts

Geoffrey M. Habershaw, D.P.M.

Chief, Division of Podiatry, New England Deaconess Hospital; Clinical Instructor in Surgery, Harvard Medical School, Boston, Massachusetts

Many of the estimated 16 million individuals in the United States with diagnosed and undiagnosed diabetes will have pathologic changes of their lower extremities, making them more vulnerable to the development of serious foot problems. The human and financial costs of lower extremity problems, especially amputation, are staggering. Diabetic foot ulcers are common and are estimated to affect about 15% of all diabetic individuals during their lifetime.[1] Clinical epidemiologic studies suggest that foot ulcers precede about 85% of nontraumatic lower extremity amputations in diabetics.[2] The average length of hospitalization for diabetic patients with ulcer conditions was 59% longer than for diabetics without them. Toe, foot, and ankle amputations are more common in individuals with diabetes than without diabetes. More than half of the major lower leg amputations occur in diabetics, with amputation rates increasing with age, in males compared with females, and among members of racial and ethnic minorities compared with whites. Within 12 months after amputation, 9% to 20% of diabetic individuals had a new ipsilateral or contralateral leg amputation, requiring a separate hospitalization. At 5 years, 28% to 51% of diabetic amputees required a second leg amputation. Five-year mortality after amputation was 39% to 68%. The problem is so significant that the American Diabetes Association and the U.S. Department of Health and Human Services propose a 40% reduction in major amputations in the diabetic population by the year 2000.[3] Methods to achieve this goal are available and are best achieved by a multidisciplinary approach.[4]

HOST CONSIDERATIONS

The triad of neuropathy, vascular insufficiency, and an altered response to infection either singularly or, more often, collectively makes the diabetic uniquely susceptible to foot problems.[5] It is important to note that diabetic patients can effectively live with these pathogenic conditions (stressing the importance of prevention). Minor trauma is the single most important contributor to cutaneous ulceration, especially when associated with other pathophysiologic, behavioral, and educational risk factors.[6]

NEUROPATHY

Peripheral neuropathy is present in more than 80% of diabetic patients with foot lesions. Sensory, motor, and autonomic neuropathy represent the greatest risk for ulcer development. Not only are pain and pressure sensations lost, but proprioception, the position sense of the foot, is lost. The result is that diabetics seemingly disown their feet, delaying early awareness and treatment of a problem.

Motor neuropathy affects all the muscles of the foot, resulting in characteristic deformities such as hammering of the toes and hallux rigidous. This motor neuropathy results in abnormal bony prominences and loss of normal foot architecture. Autonomic neuropathy (mainly autosympathectomy) is characterized by dry skin, absence of sweating, and increased capillary filling secondary to cutaneous arteriovenous shunting.

PERIPHERAL VASCULAR DISEASE

Peripheral vascular disease is 20 times more common in diabetic patients. Pecoraro and colleagues noted that critical ischemia was associated with 62% of cases with nonhealing ulceration and was a causal factor in 46% of amputations.[7] The relationship between the major arterial circulation and the relative adequacy of the cutaneous circulation of the foot requires understanding, because adequate cutaneous perfusion not only depends on the underlying arterial circulation but may be significantly influenced by other factors, including skin integrity, pressure necrosis from repetitive mechanical pressure, tissue edema, and uncontrolled infection. Vascular surgeons must consider the distinction between the relative adequacy of the cutaneous circulation and its relationship with the major arterial circulation. Unrecognized and untreated ischemia increases the risk of major amputation.

INFECTIONS

Ulceration is rarely caused by infection, but open ulcers serve as a portal of entry for pathogenic bacteria. Defects in leukocyte function and wound repair have been identified in diabetic patients.[8] Uncontrolled diabetes adversely affects infection, and infection adversely affects diabetic control (an important clinical marker). Most importantly is the need to understand that systemic signs and symptoms of a septic process in the diabetic patient develop late or may be absent, making unexplained hyperglycemia the only reliable sign of a potentially limb- and life-threatening infection.[9] In our series of diabetic patients with documented pedal osteomyelitis, less than one third had an elevated white blood cell count and only 8% had a significant temperature elevation (greater than 100°F). The lack of systemic signs or symptoms of infection does not warrant early discharge, especially when the patient's blood sugar levels have not been well controlled.

PREVENTION

Patient and physician education and understanding correlate directly with the successful management of foot problems.[10] The simple technique for testing for sensory neuropathy with a monofilament can be used to identify patients at risk for ulceration and therefore most in need of preventive intervention.[5] It also underscores the beneficial results of a multidisciplinary team approach. This approach includes diabetes management, control of other associated risk factors, periodic vascular examinations, and proper foot care. As an integral member of the team, vascular surgeons should educate their diabetic patients as to the importance of proper hygiene, daily shoe and foot inspection, wearing of appropriate shoes, and rotation of shoes at least twice a day to vary the stress and pressure points.

MEDICAL AND SURGICAL TREATMENT OF INFECTED DIABETIC FOOT ULCERS

The diagnosis and initial course of treatment of an infected diabetic foot ulcer are determined by its extent, severity, and the adequacy of the circulation.[11] Previous classifications of foot ulcers, such as Wagner's, are complex and exclude ischemia, treatment initiatives, or outcomes. We created two simplified algorithms to encompass today's practice. We divide foot ulcers into two categories: non–limb-threatening, for which the patient is initially treated as an outpatient (Table 1); and limb-threatening, which requires immediate hospitalization (Table 2).

TABLE 1.
Management of Non–limb-threatening Diabetic Foot Ulcers

Clinical Characteristics	Patient Characteristics
Superficial	Reliable
Minimal or no cellulitis	Conforms to treatment
No bone or joint involvement	Vigilant support system
No significant ischemia	
No systemic toxicity	

Therapy

Rest of injured part (non–weight-bearing)
Culture and sensitivities
Empirical broad-spectrum oral antibiotics: specific antibiotic selected based on results of cultures and response of wounds
Careful débridement
Local wound dressings
Intensive follow-up
Podiatric appliances and modified footwear

TABLE 2.

Management of Severe Limb-threatening Diabetic Foot
Ulcers

Clinical Characteristics	Patient Characteristics
Deep ulcer	Unreliable
>2-cm cellulitis/lymphangitis	Immunocompromised
Bone or joint involvement	Poor support system
Significant ischemia/gangrene	
Systemic toxicity±	

Therapy

Immediate admission and complete bedrest
Control blood glucose levels and stabilize medically
Appropriate cultures and sensitivities
Empiric broad-spectrum IV antibiotics; specific
  antibiotic based on sensitivities and response
Plain radiographs
Early surgical débridement, dependent drainage, and/or
  open amputation
Meticulous wound care
Early evaluation for ischemia
Selected revascularization and foot-sparing
surgery/conservative amputations/revisions
Intensive follow-up
Podiatric appliances and modified footwear

INSPECTION

Because of neuropathy and the frequent lack of systemic signs and symptoms of infection, thorough inspection of the wound is mandatory to determine its severity. The extent of tissue destruction and infection may not be fully appreciated merely from just observing the ulcer or affected callous. The lack of systemic signs and symptoms does not automatically place the ulcer in the non–limb-threatening category.

Sensory neuropathy allows most inspections to be done locally, at the bedside, with little or no anesthesia. Good light, sterile forceps, probe, and scissors are required. All encrusted areas should be unroofed and the wound inspected with a probe to determine the extent of deep tissue destruction and possible bone, joint, or tendon involvement. The importance of inspection and its findings must be communicated with the patient and family to eliminate any misconceptions on the part of the patient that the practitioner caused the ulcer underneath a hard callous during the débridement.

NON–LIMB-THREATENING INFECTIONS

Superficial ulcers with minimal cellulitis (less than 2 cm) may be initially treated in the outpatient setting, provided there is no significant ischemia and the patient has no systemic toxicity from infection. The patient must be compliant and reliable and have an appropriate support system. Complete rest of the injured part is mandatory, and all treatment efforts will fail unless weight-dependent ulcers are allowed to rest completely. The loss of sensation and propioception preclude partial weight-bearing. This requires crutches, a walker, or a wheelchair, and not a cane. For some patients, a prolonged period with no weight put on the affected foot is unrealistic, and specialized dressings such as contact casting or felted foam allow continued ambulation while effectively relieving pressure at the site of the ulcer.[5]

The wound is cultured with the initial débridement, and an oral antibiotic is administered. Our culture data as well as others demonstrate that *Staphylococcus aureus* and *Streptococcus* species are the most common pathogens cultured from these wounds. Antibiotic selection must be appropriate, and the most expensive antibiotic doesn't mean that it is the best.

Antibiotics are only an adjunct to proper wound care. For cracks and fissures, we prefer antibiotic ointments or lanolinized creams. Open ulcers are treated with plain gauze wetted with saline or diluted isotonic antiseptic solutions changed once or twice a day. We avoid full-strength solutions or other occlusive dressings that stay on for days and preclude examination of the wound. The efficacy of topically applied growth factors has not been conclusively proven. Heat, soaks, or whirlpools in any form are contraindicated because they can burn or macerate tissue and lead to the spread of bacteria.

For patients with no significant improvement within 24–48 hours, hospitalization must be considered. If there is improvement, regular follow-up must be maintained. Further vascular evaluation and follow-up are recommended for any patient with questionable peripheral vascular compromise, especially if the healing is slow or fails. Obviously proper nutrition, control of edema, as well as physical therapy and conditioning, are essential elements of healing.

If healing is achieved, weight-bearing should be initiated slowly to prevent recurrent breakdown or an acute Charcot foot (neuropathic joint disease of the diabetic). Podiatric or orthotic consultation for modification of footwear is recommended to protect high-risk sensitive areas. Some member of the health care team must follow these patients at regular intervals, examining both feet, because the uninvolved extremity is always at risk.

LIMB-THREATENING ULCERS

Immediate hospitalization is recommended when inspection reveals a potential limb-threatening ulceration. These ulcers are characterized by larger, deeper wounds, with spreading cellulitis (greater than 2 cm). The presence of lymphangitis or ulcers that allow a probe to penetrate the bone, joint, or tendon sheaths are also limb-threatening. Gangrene, substantial ischemia, or immunocompromise are included in this category, as well as an unreliable patient or the lack of a support system. An early, aggressive, inhospital treatment algorithm for these patients is justified because it reduces the risk of major amputation.

Inpatient management requires complete bed rest and medical stabilization. Immediate blood sugar control most often requires insulin and not oral agents. Although medical stabilization is important, it must not delay emergent surgical débridement and drainage of infection. The return of the blood sugar levels toward normal is an excellent indicator that infection has been controlled. Deep aerobic and anaerobic culture specimens are obtained during the initial débridement, and this includes sending deep tissue or bone whenever possible. We obtain blood cultures in patients manifesting systemic signs and symptoms.

Most diabetic patients with limb-threatening foot sepsis have polymicrobial infections (greater than three isolates per ulcer). More than 90% of these patients have gram-positive bacteria on culture, of which the most common are *S. aureus* and *Streptococcus* species. Gram-negative enteric bacteria are found in about 50% of these wounds, and anaerobic bacteria in 50% to 70%. We prefer the use of broad-spectrum IV antibiotics or combinations to ensure maximum delivery to the infected site.[12] This is especially important for patients demonstrating diabetic gastroenteropathy. We recommend the most effective antibiotic or combinations with the fewest side effects.[13] Changes are made based on sensitivity reports and the response of the wound. We tend not to use aminoglycocides because of their potential renal toxicity, especially in patients needing arteriography. Antibiotic costs cannot be ignored. Antibiotics are only adjunctive to early and effective surgical débridement and management.

SURGICAL MANAGEMENT

Diabetic patients do not tolerate undrained infection. Deeply infected ulcers with extensive cellulitis, lymphangitis, tissue necrosis, and pus constitute a surgical emergency. Aggressive surgical débridement and drainage of the infected area should be performed, preferably in the operating room, as expeditiously as possible. Surgical intervention should not be delayed because of a misguided pursuit of radiologic imaging tests or medical stabilization. Fortunately little or no anesthesia is needed, and this débridement must be done before any vascular evaluation. Systemic toxicity will not improve until there is adequate surgical débridement and drainage, and an excellent parameter to follow is the stabilization of blood sugar levels.

Incisions must be carefully placed to ensure adequate débridement and yet conserve as much healthy tissue as possible. The location of the ulcer, the extent of the infection and its control, as well as the adequacy of the circulation, determine the final result.[14] A neuropathic foot with excellent circulation is managed differently from the same infection in an ischemic foot, but again, initial control of infection has the highest priority regardless of the circulatory status. We have abandoned previous surgical teaching that anatomical surgical landmarks be used for débridement, foot reconstruction, and amputations in favor of carefully placed incisions to ensure adequate débridement while conserving as much healthy tissue as possible.[15] Even small skin flaps are saved that may later be used in foot reconstruction. A deep, necrotic diabetic wound cannot be adequately débrided through small stab wounds and the use of drains. Any viable area should be left untouched and protected, even if this means multiple operative procedures to control the infection. In the end, most patients will accept a deformed, "funny-looking" foot in preference to amputation.

Patients whose infection has destroyed much of the foot architecture should be emotionally prepared for an open guillotine amputation. The presence of gas by plain radiographic examination, physical examination, or during débridement, or a foul, fetid odor confirms anaerobic or facultative growth but does not necessarily indicate that guillotine amputation be performed. It is imperative that the débridement and drainage extend proximally to the fullest extent of infection and gas.

OSTEOMYELITIS

Most health care professionals would agree that inadequately diagnosed and treated osteomyelitis complicating a diabetic foot ulcer increases the risk for local as well as major amputation. Early diagnosis is critical. Reports documenting the success of any one of a number of radiologic imaging tests in diagnosing osteomyelitis have not correlated bone histopathology and/or microbiology as part of the diagnostic evaluation. We have demonstrated that probing to bone or joint has the same positive and negative predictive values as any of the currently used radiologic imaging studies and is more cost-effective.[16] The current radiologic imaging techniques should be reserved for situations in which the diagnosis is uncertain, such as in the case of Charcot's disease.

Treating diabetic osteomyelitis has also engendered controversy. Previous reports supporting long-term antibiotic therapy to cure osteomyelitis lack definitive diagnosis by histopathology and/or microbiology. These reports also accept almost a 30% major amputation failure rate and a 20% minor amputation rate after treatment.[17, 18] Failure was predictable in patients with bacteremia, open wounds after treatment, gangrene, and ischemia. Relying on antibiotics alone to cure osteomyelitis is also costly, with a 6-week course of outpatient IV antibiotic therapy costing a minimum of $12,000.

Our multidisciplinary team believes that all devitalized bone, including the bony cortex of any protruding metatarsal or phalanx, be débrided carefully during the operative procedure. If the vascular integrity is adequate, granulation tissue will cover the bone and the wound will respond. Removal of the infected bony prominence is not considered a failure because it probably was responsible for initiating the pressure that resulted in the ulceration.[19] Its removal will prevent local recurrence. In our experience, early aggressive surgical débridement reduces the duration of adjunctive IV antibiotic therapy to a median of 2 weeks.

Dressings are used to provide a moist wound environment conducive to healing. We use the same protocol as noted for outpatient non–limb-threatening ulcers. Dressings do not replace débridement, and it is important to continually inspect the wound. Hyperbaric oxygen is costly and its use unsupported by randomized trials for the routine treatment of infected diabetic foot ulcers. Nutritional replenishment, control of edema, as well as physical therapy and conditioning, are all adjuncts to successful wound healing. One should also remember that the other foot and leg are at risk during all phases of treatment.

VASCULAR EVALUATION AND TREATMENT

The incidence of lower extremity arterial disease (LEAD) in diabetic patients is at least 10 times that of nondiabetic patients.[2] The incidence increases with older age, longer duration of diabetes, and presence of other atherogenic risk factors such as hypertension, cigarette smoking, and dyslipidemia. In population-based studies, absent foot pulses were found in about 20% to 30% of diabetic patients.[2] Also, in patients with LEAD, the mortality rate is two to three times greater than that in the general population.

The association of LEAD and diabetes reinforces the importance of prevention. Periodic vascular examination, including noninvasive testing when appropriate, identifies patients at risk so they can be observed more carefully or referred to a vascular surgeon. The clinical presentation of patients with major artery occlusions or hemodynamically significant stenoses varies depending on their activity level and the adequacy of collateral pathways. Establishing the diagnosis of ischemia in the diabetic is made more difficult by the presence of peripheral and autonomic neuropathy. We believe that clinical evaluation, judgment, and experience remain the most important means for assessing vascular insufficiency in the diabetic lower extremity. Noninvasive evaluation by whatever means is complementary to one's clinical evaluation. A general rule of thumb is that vascular consultation and arteriography are indicated when there is a question of ischemia complicating a diabetic foot problem.

Unrecognized and untreated ischemia increases the risk for major amputation. Pecoraro and colleagues noted that ischemia was the only causal factor that could be singularly responsible for amputation in their study.[7] We noted that ischemia complicated more than 50% of cases of documented pedal osteomyelitis.[16] Again it must be remembered that adequate cutaneous perfusion depends not only on the underlying arterial circulation but may be critically influenced by the effects of neuropathy and an altered response to infection.

Although the pathology of atherosclerosis is similar in both diabetic and nondiabetic patients, several distinguishing features characterize diabetic lower extremity macrovascular disease. In the diabetic patient, there is a predilection for occlusive disease to involve primarily the tibial and peroneal arteries between the knee and the foot. This is evidenced by the finding that 40% of diabetic patients with gangrene have a palpable popliteal pulse. The dorsalis pedis artery and foot vessels are usually spared. No occlusive microvascular disease of the diabetic foot exists that precludes revascularization. This misconception from the early 1950s has been refuted by many observers and was carefully reviewed by LoGerfo and Coffman in 1984.[20] Tooke has noted that there is a hemodynamic effect of macrovascular disease on microvascular function.[21] He believes that microvascular dysfunction begins early in diabetic life, with increased microvascular pressure and flow leading to endothelial injury with sclerosis (basement-membrane thickening) and limited capillary capacity with loss of autoregulatory function, including the abolition of a vasoconstrictor response. This microvascular dysfunction is not an occlusive lesion and does not preclude revascularization but rather supports an aggressive approach. Simply put, tissue perfusion in the ischemic diabetic foot can be restored with appropriate modern vascular reconstructive techniques.

Diabetic LEAD is also associated with a diminished ability for collateral circulation to develop, especially around the distal profunda femoris artery and the infrageniculate arteries. Calcification involving the intimal plaque and media (medial calcinosis or Mönckeberg's sclerosis), although probably neuropathic in origin, frequently involves diabetic arteries at all levels but often spares the foot vessels. Medial calcinosis often results in erroneous noninvasive testing results, especially elevating segmental systolic pressures and the ankle-brachial ratio. It also complicates surgical bypass techniques and laser or balloon angioplasty treatment.

Diabetic patients without severe claudication or rest pain can live with peripheral vascular disease until a traumatic event initiates an ulcer or a fissure. Vascular consultation and evaluation should be strongly considered in patients whose ulcers are thought to have an ischemic component or that fail to heal within a specific period (assuming that appropriate treatment has been rendered). This includes incisions from local procedures that fail to heal and areas that recurrently break down. There are a small number of diabetic patients who, despite palpable foot pulses at rest because of collateral circulation, have severe enough ischemia so as not to heal when there is any increased demand.[22] Precision arteriography, visualizing the foot vessels, remains the most effective means for definitive evaluation of lower extremity ischemia. With current arteriographic techniques, more than 90% of diabetic patients with ischemic foot lesions are shown to have surgically correctable occlusive disease.[23] A diabetic patient with threatened limb loss and only an audible dorsalis pedis Doppler signal without arteriographic visualization still has a 59% chance of a successful bypass.[24]

Aortoiliac (inflow) disease in diabetic patients is managed in the same manner as in nondiabetic patients.[25,26] Adjunctive profundaplasty can be of benefit for the relief of ischemic rest pain but contributes little to the resolution of tissue ulceration and necrosis. Sophisticated and aggressive distal revascularization techniques have demonstrated excellent graft patency and limb salvage in the diabetic leg.[27-29] Our own approach is to seek inflow from the most distal nondiseased portion of the femoral or popliteal artery, both of which are frequently spared in diabetics, as previously mentioned.[30] We extend the bypass graft to the most proximal tibial outflow vessel in direct continuity with the pedal circulation. Rather than bypassing to a blind popliteal segment or peroneal vessel, we prefer to proceed to direct pedal artery grafting in situations where pulsatile pedal flow is essential to promote the healing of ulcerations, minor amputations, or to facilitate reconstructive foot surgery. Since its inception in 1985, the pedal artery bypass now constitutes 25% of our revascularization procedures. Initial 3-year results for this procedure show an 87% graft patency and 92% limb salvage. Using life-table analysis, our most recent tabulation of 384 dorsalis pedis artery bypass grafts, with a mean follow-up of 22 months, yielded 5-year primary and secondary patency rates of 68% and 81%, respectively. Limb salvage in this group has remained at 92% at 3 years and exceeds 87% at 5 years.[31] Regional as well as general anesthesia are equally safe, and with routine invasive monitoring in this high-risk group, the operative mortality has been 1.8% with a cardiac morbidity of 5.4%. These complication rates are at least similar to those of diabetic patients undergoing major amputation alone, and support an aggressive approach to limb salvage.

Diabetic patients are rarely candidates for distal balloon or laser angioplasty for limb salvage, because of their vulnerability for diffuse infrapopliteal disease and medial calcification, both of which limit the success of these procedures.

In summary, the importance of ischemia complicating primary or recurring diabetic foot ulceration and/or the healing of local procedures cannot be understated. Early recognition and aggressive surgical drainage of pedal sepsis are critical to achieving maximum limb salvage in this high-risk population. Débridement of devitalized tissue in the face of ischemia may result in a larger soft tissue defect, so prompt and thorough evaluation and treatment of ischemia follow. Fitting and wearing shoes are easier when the foot remains intact. If as much of the anatomy of the foot can be preserved, it is not necessary to use custom-molded shoes. Most important, foot-sparing surgery is better accepted by patients who fear any type of amputation.

FOOT-SPARING SURGERY IN THE DIABETIC

Since 1984, our multidisciplinary team approach to the diabetic foot has demonstrated a significant reduction in every category of amputation at the New England Deaconess Hospital and Joslin Diabetes Center.[4] There are advantages to preserving as much of the foot as possible. The forces that traverse the foot during walking are dissipated over a maximal surface area when the distal tissue is preserved. Débridement of devitalized tissue in the face of ischemia, to facilitate forefoot reconstructions, and to heal minor amputations if needed.[32]

BASIC FOOT MECHANICS

The foot is a dynamic vaulted arch that functions to allow the body to traverse over irregular terrain and remain upright. This function is accomplished by the motions of pronation and supination. While the skin of the forefoot is fixed to the ground during gait, the musculoskeletal elements are constantly in motion. This leads to the production of sheer forces against the skin, which may lead to ulceration in the diabetic patient with neuropathy. Structural deformities such as long metatarsals, short metatarsals, plantar-flexed metatarsals, bunions, hammer toes, and rigid joints contribute to the increased forces against the skin. Also, intrinsic muscle wasting occurs, which attenuates pressure points by allowing the development of hammer toes and prominent metatarsal heads. All of these factors combine to cause the skin to be exposed to repetitive moderate stress and callous formation. The lack of sensation makes the diabetic unable to feel the pain of the callous, which leads to blister formation and eventual ulceration and infection. Repetitive moderate stress on the skin is the most common cause of ulceration in the neuropathic patient who has lost protective sensation.

SURGICAL CONSIDERATIONS

Prophylactic surgery on the neuropathic foot to reduce musculoskeletal deformities in the presence of sensory neuropathy without current skin breakdown or history of chronic ulceration is not recommended. Preventive measures as mentioned previously are the first line of defense. In addition, all neuropathic ulcerations deserve appropriate conservative management (see Table 1) as initial therapy. Forefoot-sparing surgery includes toe arthroplasty replacing toe amputation; metatarsal osteotomy or, when necessary, metatarsal phalangeal joint resection replacing ray amputation; and panmetatarsal head resection replacing the transmetatarsal amputation. When nonsurgical intervention fails to allow chronic ulceration or chronically recurrent ulceration to heal, these procedures should be considered before acute cellulitis or deep space infection occurs. These are elective procedures in the neuropathic patient with normal circulation, as well as for the previous ischemic patient who has undergone vascular reconstruction.

TOE ULCERATION

Ulceration of the lesser digits occurs dorsally, distally, or interdigitally. Dorsal ulceration is most likely caused by shoe gear rubbing at the apex of a hammered toe. The ulcer may be excised if it is less than 1 cm in diameter, and an arthroplasty performed by removal of the proximal phalangeal head. It may be closed when no deep abscess or necrotic tissue is encountered. This may also be done for ulceration at the distal aspect of the toe, provided there is no bony exposure. Arthroplasty may also be done for ulceration at the tip or at the interphalangeal joint of the great toe.

THE HALLUX

Loss of the great toe in the neuropathic diabetic, especially when combined with the metatarsophalangeal joint, has in our experience been associated with potential long-term morbidity and disability. It may predispose to alterations in gait that can lead to biomechanical imbalances elsewhere, such as neuropathic fractures, Charcot changes in the midfoot, or ulcerations to adjacent areas of increased pressure, either on the adjacent digits or beneath the lateral metatarsal heads. We resort to any foot-sparing surgery, including sesamoidectomy with or without metatarsophalangeal joint resection, that will save the great toe and especially prevent a ray amputation.[33]

METATARSAL SURGERY

The forefoot functions as a three-column structure, each of which has an independent range of motion. The medial column includes the great toe, first metatarsal, and medial cuneiform. The central column includes the second, third, and fourth toes, the metatarsals, and the middle and lateral cuneiforms. The lateral column includes the fifth toe and fifth metatarsal. Surgery on any one metatarsal affects the others. This results from alterations in the distribution of forces of the remaining metatarsals during gait. Therefore, anticipation of potential problems because of transfer ulcerations should always be part of the overall treatment plan.

Lesser ulceration of metatarsal two through five is best treated with isolated metatarsal osteotomy.[34] Osteotomy of the fifth metatarsal is least likely to allow for transfer lesions to the fourth metatarsal because it has an independent range of motion. Osteotomy of the second, third, or fourth metatarsals creates a much greater chance for development of transfer lesions because the central column is rigidly fixed in the tarsus.

Osteotomy is most easily performed from the dorsum with a double-action bone-cutting forceps placed around the surgical neck of the metatarsal. Osteotomy performed too proximal to the shaft of the metatarsal most certainly leads to transfer ulceration of the adjacent metatarsal head. Multiple osteotomies are not done as an initial procedure. This procedure may be considered if a transfer ulcer has developed below the third metatarsal head after a second metatarsal osteotomy. Osteotomy of the third and fourth metatarsal should then be considered.

If the ulceration probes into the bone or the joint, in which case osteomyelitis is highly probable, metatarsal head resection should be performed. Transfer ulceration is very common after metatarsal head resection, with the possible exception of the fifth metatarsal head. In most cases, the ulceration is excised with an elliptical incision, and the head of the metatarsal and the base of the proximal phalanx removed. If the wound is clean and infection controlled, it is closed using a proximal drain as necessary. Weight-bearing is not allowed for 3–4 weeks to ensure healing.

PANMETATARSAL HEAD RESECTION

This salvage procedure is recommended only when lesser procedures such as single or multiple osteotomies have failed to allow the forefoot to remain ulcer-free. The procedure is designed to remove all pressure points across the forefoot by excision of all the metatarsal heads. There are three advantages of this procedure compared with transmetatarsal amputation (TMA): preservation of the toes and the distal soft tissue, which contributes to dissipation of forces during gait; greater ease of fitting a shoe; and avoidance of an amputation.[35] The procedure is performed usually from the dorsum with three or four linear incisions over the distal metatarsal shafts. If chronic osteomyelitis is present in an isolated or in multiple metatarsals, a combination of dorsal and plantar incisions is used.

TRANSMETATARSAL AMPUTATION REVISION

In diabetic patients, the indications for TMA, a forefoot amputation originally developed at the Deaconess Hospital, have changed. It is still an excellent solution when there is nonreconstructible ischemic forefoot necrosis; when there is extensive tissue loss in the forefoot prohibiting more direct foot salvage; and to control acute sepsis so as to save limb and life. It should not be performed for chronic neuropathic ulcers. A complication of TMA is ulceration at bony prominences or spicules at the cut surfaces of the metatarsal shafts, and revision of these areas often becomes necessary. This is best done as an exostectomy of the involved metatarsal or metatarsals. The ulcers are left alone when no deep sepsis or osteomyelitis exists but are excised and partially closed when these conditions exist.

Transmetatarsal amputation is prone to reulceration because of the lesser surface area on the plantar surface of the foot. The forces are therefore increased over a smaller surface area. Achilles tendon lengthening has been a valuable adjunct to TMA revision. This procedure functions by shortening the stride length of the patient and thereby diminishing the driving force of the gastroc-soleus complex at the distal aspect of the TMA. All patients who have had this procedure are able to continue to walk and function as before, but with a shorter step. A padded ankle-foot orthosis is used in recalcitrant cases.

CHARCOT FOOT SURGERY

Reconstructive surgery for the Charcot foot is recommended when it is clear that amputation is otherwise inevitable. Chronic ulcers on the Charcot foot occur most commonly at the proximal medial column or first metatarsocuneiform joint or the proximal lateral column below the cuboid. If the ulcers are superficial, exostectomy may be done through an adjacent incision. First metatarsocuneiform exostectomy is done from a medial approach. A generous portion of the plantar medial aspect of this joint is removed.

Ulceration below the cuboid is treated by removal of the plantar peroneal ridge just proximal to the course of the peroneus longus tendon. Exostectomy should also be generous. Excision of the ulcer is based on its size and depth. Closure may be difficult if the excised ulcer is greater than 2 cm in diameter. All exposed bone must be excised, and closure depends on the findings at the time of surgery. Working with plastic surgeons allows for the use of various reconstructive flap procedures to allow closure. Non–weight-bearing is maintained until the plantar ulceration is closed, which is usually 3–4 weeks. Other procedures for Charcot foot reconstruction include midfoot osteotomies, triple arthrodesis, or pantalar arthrodesis, which are all performed with rigid internal or external fixation. Strict non–weight-bearing is required for at least 4 months postoperatively. Therefore, although Charcot foot deformities can cause some of the most deformed and unstable feet, they should no longer be thought of as a therapeutic nightmare because durable foot salvage is obtainable.

REAR FOOT

Ulcerations of the heel result from a variety of mechanisms, including iatrogenic. The heel is very susceptible to dry fissures and cracking secondary to autonomic neuropathy and ischemia. Pressure ulcers can easily develop in patients confined to bed, and both heels warrant protection at all times. Because the heel is mainly fat, ulcerations progress rapidly, leading to significant soft-tissue defects and often to associated osteomyelitis of the calcaneus. Initial conservative management is the same as for other ulcers (see Figs 1 and 2), including suspension of the heel from the mattress. When osteomyelitis is present, partial calcanectomy with or without primary closure of the ulceration is the most effective way of managing recalcitrant ulcers. By working with plastic surgeons, rotational, advancement, or now free flaps may be used to cover and heal large soft-tissue defects, especially those associated with extensive bone loss.

SHOEING

Once ulcerations or surgical incisions are closed and weight-bearing can begin, a postoperative shoe with a molded plastazoate insert is made. Partial weight-bearing is begun using a walker or crutches, but this shoe is not meant to be used for normal activity. Progression to full weight-bearing usually takes about 2 weeks, and it is vital for neuropathic and ischemic patients to then change their shoes and socks every 3–4 hours. Pressure points are changed by rotating different pairs of shoes. Friction is minimized because all shoes begin to fatigue at 3–4 hours, allowing the foot to slide and causing increased friction and shear. During shoe rotation, the patient or someone can check the feet, especially sensitive high-risk areas, to be sure that all is okay. These simple maneuvers allow patients and their families to participate maximally in the management of their insensate feet and further lessen the incidence of reulceration. More frequent shoe rotation also allows patients to wear more conventional shoes, especially when they combine shoe rotation with a walking or running shoe. No shoe can guarantee prevention of reulceration in the neuropathic foot.

Molded shoes are used for the neuropathic patient who no longer has a conventionally shaped foot. This is usually the case for patients in whom a Charcot fracture has developed, who need shoes designed with soft materials with removable molded soft inserts to accommodate bony prominences, which invariably occur on the plantar midfoot.

THE FUTURE

The multidisciplinary team approach to the diabetic foot presented in this chapter has demonstrated appropriateness, efficiency, and effectiveness.[36, 37] Our algorithm includes immediate aggressive débridement and drainage of infection, combined with appropriate antibiotics, proper wound care, early evaluation of ischemia, and modern surgical revascularization techniques to restore pulsatile arterial flow to the foot. Foot-sparing surgery achieves healing; preserves length, appearance, and function; and avoids amputation. The emotional and physical well-being of the diabetic patient is best preserved by a health care system that champions quality care to reduce the cost of care.

REFERENCES

1. Palumbo PJ, Melton LJ: Peripheral vascular disease and diabetes, in Harris M, Hamman RF (eds): *Diabetes in America*. Washington, DC, 1985, US Government Printing Office, NIH Publication No 85-1468, pp XV, 1–21.
2. Reiber GE, Boyko EJ, Smith DG: Lower extremity foot ulcers and amputations, in Diabetes, in Harris M, Hamman RF (eds): *Diabetes in America*. Washington, DC, 1995, US Government Printing Office, NIH Publication No 95-1468, pp XVIII, 1–19.
3. Department of Health and Human Services: *Healthy People, 2000. National*

Health Promotion and Disease Prevention Objectives. DHHS Publication No (PHS) 91-50212, 1991.

4. LoGerfo F, Gibbons G, Pomposelli F, et al: Trends in the care of the diabetic foot: Expanded role of arterial reconstruction. *Arch Surg* 127:617–621, 1992.

5. Caputo GM, Cavanagh PR, Ulbrecht JS, et al: Assessment and management of foot disease in patients with diabetes. *N Engl J Med* 331:854–860, 1994.

6. Bolton AJM: The diabetic foot. *Med Clin North Am* 72:1513–1530, 1988.

7. Pecoraro RE, Reiber GE, Burgess EM: Pathways to diabetic limb amputation: Basis for prevention. *Diabetes Care* 13:513–521, 1990.

8. Fylling CP (guest ed): Wound healing: An update. *Diabetes Spectrum* 5:328–359, 1992.

9. Gibbons GW: Diabetic foot sepsis. *Semin Vasc Surg* 5:244–248, 1992.

10. Reiber GE: Diabetic foot care: Financial implications and practice guidelines. *Diabetes Care* 15:295–315, 1992.

11. Karchmer AW, Gibbons GW: Foot infections in diabetics: Evaluation and management, in Remington JS, Swartz MH (eds): *Current Clinical Topics in Infectious Diseases*, ed 14. Boston, Blackwell Scientific, 1994, pp 1–22.

12. Grayson ML, Gibbons GW, Habershaw GM, et al: Use of ampicillin/sulbactam vs. imipenem/cilastatin in the treatment of limb-threatening foot infections in diabetic patients. *Clin Infect Dis* 18:683–693, 1994.

13. Grayson ML: Diabetic foot infections: Antimicrobial therapy, in Eliopoulos GM, (ed): *Infectious Disease Clinics of North America. Infections in Diabetes Mellitus.* Philadelphia, WB Saunders, 1995, pp 143–162.

14. Gibbons GW: The diabetic foot: Amputation and drainage of infection. *J Vasc Surg* 5:791–793, 1987.

15. Gibbons GW, Marcaccio EJ, Habershaw GM: Management of the diabetic foot, in Callow AD, Ernst CB (eds): *Vascular Surgery Theory and Practice.* Stanford, Conn, Appelton and Lange, 12:167–179, 1995.

16. Grayson ML, Gibbons GW, Balogh K, et al: Probing to bone in infected pedal ulcers: A clinical sign of underlying osteomyelitis in diabetic patients. *JAMA* 273:721–723, 1995.

17. Bamberger DM, Daus GP, Gerding DN: Osteomyelitis in the feet of diabetic patients. Long-term results, prognostic factors and the role of antimicrobial and surgical therapy. *Am J Med* 83:653–660, 1987.

18. Peterson LR, Lissack LM, Canter K, et al: Therapy of lower extremity infections with ciprofloxacin in patients with diabetes mellitus, peripheral vascular disease or both. *N Engl J Med* 311:1615–1619, 1984.

19. Gibbons GW, Habershaw GM: Diabetic foot infections: Anatomy and surgery, in Eliopoulos GM (ed): *Infectious Disease Clinics of North America. Infections in Diabetes Mellitus.* Philadelphia, WB Saunders, 1995, pp 131–142.

20. LoGerfo F, Coffman J: Vascular and microvascular disease of the diabetic foot: Implications for foot care. *N Engl J Med* 311:1615–1619, 1984.

21. Tooke JE: European consensus document on critical limb ischemia: Implications for diabetes. *Diabetic Med* 7:544–546, 1990.

22. Andros G, Harris RW, Dulawa LB, et al: The need for arteriography in diabetic patients with gangrene and palpable foot pulses. *Arch Surg* 119:1260–1263, 1984.

23. Taylor L, Porter J: Results of lower extremity bypass in the diabetic patient. *Semin Vasc Surg* 5:226–233, 1992.

24. Pomposelli FB, Jepson SJ, Gibbons GW, et al: Efficacy of the dorsal pedal bypass for limb salvage in diabetic patients. *J Vasc Surg* 11:745–752, 1990.

25. Mannick J, Whittemore AD, Donaldson MC: Aortofemoral bypass for atherosclerotic aorto iliac disease, in Ernst CB, Stanley JC (eds): *Current Therapy of Vascular Surgery*, ed 2. Philadelphia, BC Decker, 1991, pp 391–394.

26. Gibbons GW: Vascular surgery of the diabetic lower extremity, in Frykberg R (ed): *The High Risk Foot in Diabetes Mellitus.* New York, Churchill-Livingstone, 1990, pp 273–297.

27. Leather RP, Karmody AM: In situ saphenous vein arterial bypass for the treatment of limb ischemia, in Mannick JA, et al (eds): *Advances in Surgery.* Year Book, Chicago, 1986, pp 175–219.

28. Veith VJ, Gupta SK, Wengerter KR, et al: Femoral-popliteal-tibial occlusive disease, in Moore WS (ed): *Vascular Surgery.* Philadelphia, WB Saunders, 1991, pp 364–390.

29. Taylor LM Jr, Edwards JM, Porter JM: Present status of reversed vein bypass grafting: Five-year results of a modern series. *J Vasc Surg* 11:193–206, 1990.

30. Pomposelli F, Jepsen S, Gibbons G, et al: A flexible approach to infrapopliteal vein grafts in patients with diabetes mellitus. *Arch Surg* 126:724–729, 1991.

31. Pomposelli FB, Marcaccio EJ, Gibbons GW, et al: Dorsalis pedis arterial bypass: Durable limb salvage for foot ischemia in patients with diabetes mellitus. *J Vasc Surg* 21:375–384, 1995.

32. Rosenblum BI, Pomposelli FB, Giurini JM, et al: Maximizing foot salvage by a combined approach to foot ischemia and neuropathic ulceration in patients with diabetes mellitus: A five year experience. *Diabetes Care* 17:983–987, 1994.

33. Rosenblum BI, Giurini JM, Chrzan JS, et al: Preventing loss of the great toe with the hallux interphalangeal joint arthroplasty. *J Foot Ankle Surg* 33:557–560, 1994.

34. Tillo TH, Giurini JM, Habershaw GM, et al: Review of metatarsal osteotomies for the treatment of neuropathic ulcerations. *J Am Podiatr Med Assoc* 80:211–217, 1990.

35. Giurini JM, Basile P, Chrzan JS, et al: Panmetatarsal head resection: A viable alternative to the transmetatarsal amputation. *J Am Podiatr Med Assoc* 83:101–107, 1993.

36. Gibbons GW, Marcaccio EJ, Burgess AM, et al: Improved quality of diabetic foot care, 1984 vs 1990: Reduced length of stay and costs, insufficient reimbursement. *Arch Surg* 128:576–581, 1993.

37. Gibbons GW, Burgess AM, Guadagnoli E, et al: Return to well-being and function after infrainguinal revascularization. *J Vasc Surg* 21:35–45, 1995.

PART VI

Complications of Deep Vein Thrombosis

Current Management of Phlegmasia Cerulea Dolens

Anthony J. Comerota, M.D., F.A.C.S.

Professor of Surgery, Chief, Section Vascular Surgery, Director, Center for Vascular Diseases, Temple University Hospital, Philadelphia, Pennsylvania

P hlegmasia cerulea dolens is the clinical syndrome of a cyanotic, painful, swollen leg in a patient with occlusive venous thrombosis, usually involving the common femoral vein and more proximal veins. The iliofemoral venous segment is frequently obliterated, with associated extensive infrainguinal venous thrombosis. There is often semantic argument about the term phlegmasia cerulea dolens,[1] because it refers to a combination of clinical signs and symptoms rather than defined pathology. To avoid semantic disagreement, this chapter discusses the treatment of patients with acute iliofemoral deep venous thrombosis (DVT), most of whom have the clinical presentation of phlegmasia cerulea dolens.

Acute iliofemoral DVT, which often presents as phlegmasia alba dolens or phlegmasia cerulea dolens, is associated with the most severe acute symptoms of DVT as well as the most troublesome postthrombotic sequelae.[2,3] When one understands the natural history of acute DVT as related to postthrombotic sequelae, this observation is not surprising.

The underlying pathophysiology of the postthrombotic syndrome is ambulatory venous hypertension.[4] The pathologic components contributing to ambulatory venous hypertension are obstruction of the deep venous system and incompetence of the venous valves.[4,5]

The presence of both obstruction and incompetence produces the most severe postthrombotic sequelae.[4,5] In prospective natural history studies, it has been observed that if clot in the deep venous system lyses within a reasonably short period (2–3 months), it is possible to preserve valvular function in the deep system.[6,7]

Traditional teaching indicates that bed rest, leg elevation, and anticoagulation is adequate for recovery of patients with iliofemoral venous thrombosis. This is based on the opinion that little can be done to clear the deep venous system, and many physicians treating acute DVT do not manage the serious postthrombotic sequelae. Our personal observations however, indicate that when treated with anticoagulation alone, many patients have persistent acute symptoms, have significant postthrombotic symptoms after hospital discharge, and those who are physically active have varying degrees of venous claudication. It has been our opinion that in patients initially seen with acute iliofemoral DVT, the clot should be eliminated.[8]

Figure 1 illustrates the deep venous system of a 32-year-old woman

Advances in Vascular Surgery®, vol. 4
© 1996, Mosby–Year Book, Inc.

A.J. Comerota

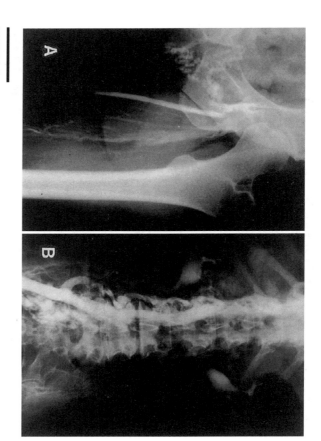

FIGURE 1.

Postthrombotic ascending phlebogram on a 32-year-old woman who had iliofemoral-femoral popliteal deep venous thrombosis 11 months earlier. **A,** occlusion of entire femoral popliteal deep venous system with patent saphenous vein that is occluded at the saphenofemoral junction. Small cross-pubic collaterals are noted. **B,** Occlusion of entire left iliac venous system with failure of recanalization.

who had acute iliofemoral DVT 11 months earlier. The DVT was treated with bed rest, leg elevation, and standard anticoagulation. This young woman had such severe postthrombotic symptoms that she left her job and had difficulty caring for her two young children. The patient was referred for evaluation for a venous bypass to relieve her venous claudication. Unfortunately, options for venous reconstruction are limited; therefore, the appropriate time to intervene is when acute thrombosis occurs, rather than attempt to manage the subsequent post-thrombotic sequelae.

It seems intuitive that the thrombus in the iliofemoral venous system of these patients should be removed. Surgeons have attempted to achieve this objective by performing venous thrombectomy to restore patency and reduce acute and long-term sequelae.[9, 10] Although initial reports were favorable, venous thrombectomy fell into disfavor in the United States because of unacceptable operative morbidity and frequent rethrombosis associated with progressive venous insufficiency.[11, 12]

Systemic thrombolysis was then used in an effort to pharmacologically clear the deep venous system. This too was met with disappointing results.[13] Our observations were similar, in that systemic thrombolysis often failed to achieve its goal. Anticoagulation with IV heparin followed by long-term oral anticoagulation with warfarin compounds became the standard for these patients.

As thrombolytic therapy developed and drug delivery systems improved, it became evident that direct intrathrombus delivery of plasminogen activators significantly increased success compared with systemic delivery. Likewise, with the refinement of vascular surgical technique, improved intraoperative imaging capability, correction of residual iliac venous stenoses, and a better understanding of postoperative anticoagulation, the results of venous thrombectomy are improved and associated with reduced operative morbidity.

The goals of treatment for iliofemoral DVT are (1) to prevent pulmonary embolism, (2) to relieve acute symptoms of venous obstruction, and (3) to prevent postthrombotic sequelae. These goals can be achieved if (1) the thrombus is removed, (2) unobstructed venous drainage is provided (importantly, from the profunda femoris vein to the vena cava), (3) stenotic iliac vein lesions are corrected, and (4) recurrent thrombosis is avoided. Available treatment options that can achieve early clearing of thrombus with restoration of unobstructed venous drainage are catheter-directed thrombolysis or venous thrombectomy. The problem of recurrent thrombosis is avoided by aggressive anticoagulation, correction of an un-

ALGORITHYM FOR Rx OF ILIOFEMORAL DVT

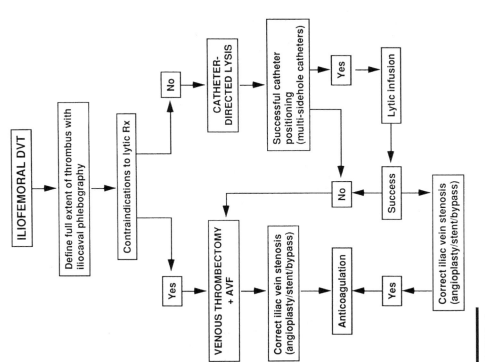

FIGURE 2.

Algorithm for treatment of patients with iliofemoral deep venous thrombosis. *Abbreviation: AVF*, arteriovenous fistula.

derlying iliac vein stenosis, judicious use of arteriovenous fistulae, and the application of external pneumatic compression devices. Our algorithm for the treatment of patients with iliofemoral venous thrombosis is demonstrated in Figure 2.

Before initiating anticoagulation, blood samples should be obtained for a complete hypercoagulable evaluation. Objective diagnosis of acute DVT is generally accomplished with venous duplex imaging; however, all patients should have the contralateral iliofemoral venous segment and vena cava examined phlebographically. This gives important information about the status of the contralateral iliac vein and vena cava and demonstrates the proximal extent of the thrombus. An introducer sheath is left in the contralateral femoral vein for access for infusion catheters.

CATHETER-DIRECTED THROMBOLYSIS

TECHNIQUE

Thrombolytic techniques have evolved over the years, and catheter delivery of plasminogen activators into the clot has demonstrated significantly improved results compared with systemic thrombolysis in virtually every vascular bed where thrombolytic therapy has been used. Catheter-directed thrombolysis for acute DVT conceptually has lagged behind the techniques used for acute arterial and bypass graft occlusion. Recent experience has demonstrated that a successful outcome can be anticipated with proper catheter positioning.[8, 13–15]

Direct intrathrombus infusion is achieved by placing a catheter from the contralateral femoral vein (Fig 3), the right jugular vein, or both. Interestingly, catheters and infusion guidewires frequently can be advanced

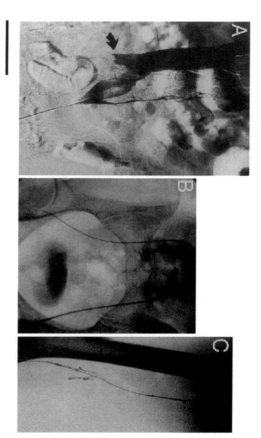

FIGURE 3.

Illustration of catheter placement for iliofemoral-femoral popliteal deep venous thrombosis. **A,** iliocavagram demonstrates proximal extent of iliofemoral thrombosis (*arrow*). **B,** catheter advanced into right iliofemoral segment from contralateral common femoral vein approach. **C,** guide wire advanced retrograde into proximal popliteal vein. Guide wires and catheters in these locations ensure long-segment perfusion of thrombus with plasminogen activators.

distally, through venous valves, allowing infusion of a thrombosed superficial femoral and popliteal vein. Alternative access through an ipsilateral femoral vein catheter or through an ipsilateral popliteal venous puncture performed with ultrasound guidance can be used at the discretion of the physician (Fig 4). If the contralateral femoral vein or the jugular vein is used, a vena caval filter can be placed through the same access before lytic infusion, if indicated. We have not routinely used caval filters for patients treated with catheter-directed thrombolysis for iliofemoral venous thrombosis; however, when nonocclusive or irregular thrombus extended into the vena cava, a filter was placed. If a caval filter is inserted, a subsequent venous thrombectomy, if necessary, becomes more difficult and requires fluoroscopic guidance, because the filter may

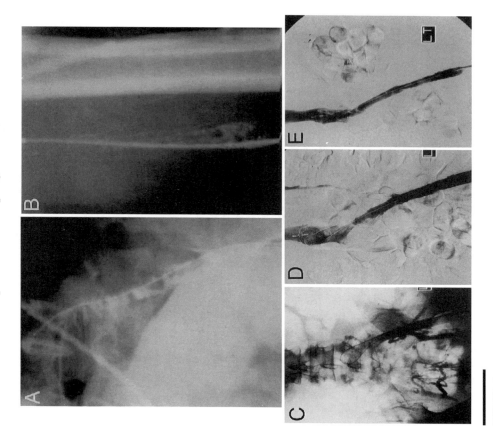

FIGURE 4.

Example of catheter-directed thrombolysis of iliofemoral popliteal deep venous thrombosis via popliteal vein puncture with ultrasound guidance. **A,** occlusion of iliofemoral venous segment. **B,** occlusion of superficial femoral vein with infusion catheter in place. **C,** postlysis phlebogram demonstrating left iliac vein occlusion. **D,** venogram after angioplasty demonstrating residual stenosis of left common iliac vein. **E,** completion phlebogram after venous dilation and stent placement.

be dislodged and malpositioned by the venous thrombectomy catheter. Temporary (removable) caval filters would solve this problem in these patients.[16]

After a guide wire has been appropriately positioned in the thrombus, infusion catheters with multiple side holes are used to infuse systemic doses of plasminogen activators. We have chosen to use urokinase

ALGORITHM FOR CATHETER DIRECTED THROMBOLYSIS FOR ILIOFEMORAL DVT

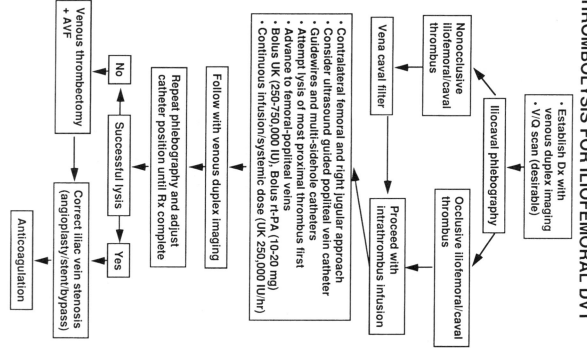

- Establish Dx with venous duplex imaging
- V/Q scan (desirable)

Iliocaval phlebography

Nonocclusive iliofemoral/caval thrombus

Occlusive iliofemoral/caval thrombus

Vena caval filter

Proceed with intrathrombus infusion

- Contralateral femoral and right jugular approach
- Consider ultrasound guided popliteal vein catheter
- Guidewires and multi-sidehole catheters
- Attempt lysis of most proximal thrombus first
- Advance to femoral-popliteal veins
- Bolus UK (250-750,000 IU), Bolus rt-PA (10-20 mg)
- Continuous infusion/systemic dose (UK 250,000 IU/hr)

Follow with venous duplex imaging

Repeat phlebography and adjust catheter position until Rx complete

Successful lysis

No

Yes

Venous thrombectomy + AVF

Correct iliac vein stenosis (angioplasty/stent/bypass)

Anticoagulation

FIGURE 5.

Algorithm for catheter-directed thrombolysis for iliofemoral deep venous thrombosis. *Abbreviations: V/Q,* ventilation-perfusion; *UK,* urokinase; *rt-PA,* recombinant tissue-type plasminogen activator; *AVF,* arteriovenous fistula.

delivered as a 500,000 to 750,000-U bolus, followed by a continuous infusion of 250,000 U/hr. In particularly severe cases, we have added bolus doses of recombinant tissue-type plasminogen activator (10–20 mg), followed by urokinase infusion to take advantage of the synergistic lysis of this combination of agents.[16, 17] We have observed an excellent response in a small number of difficult cases with this method of combined therapy. Repeated phlebography through the infusion catheter is performed at 8- to 12-hour intervals, and therapy is continued until maximal lysis is achieved. The iliac vein thrombi tend to lyse sooner than the more distal thrombi because of the high concentration of plasminogen activators delivered into the proximal thrombus. Venous duplex imaging is used to follow lysis of the infrainguinal clot and as much of the iliac venous system as is accessible to the ultrasound beam. After completion of the lytic infusion, the iliofemoral venous system is examined for a stenotic lesion that may have contributed to the acute thrombosis. If an iliac vein stenosis is present, balloon dilation is performed with a stent placed in patients whose lesions do not respond to dilation alone (see Fig 4). When percutaneous techniques are unsuccessful, a cross-pubic venous bypass provides unobstructed flow from the affected leg. Patients remain anticoagulated with heparin and therapy is converted to oral anticoagulation.

When the infusion catheter cannot be appropriately positioned in the iliac vein thrombus, or when there is a contraindication to thrombolysis, a venous thrombectomy is performed. The principles of catheter-directed thrombolysis for iliofemoral DVT are summarized in Figure 5.

VENOUS THROMBECTOMY

TECHNIQUE

The operative technique of venous thrombectomy has improved considerably since the early reports, when the procedure was usually a blind thrombectomy associated with high operative morbidity and failure rates. The principles of successful venous thrombectomy are listed in Table 1. The surgeon should be prepared to use fluoroscopy to assess adequacy of thrombus removal and examine the iliac veins for a stenotic proximal lesion, which might have contributed to the acute iliofemoral venous thrombosis.

Through an inguinal incision, exposure of the common femoral vein, saphenofemoral junction, superficial femoral vein, and profunda femoris veins is performed. Either a transverse or longitudinal venotomy can be used, depending on location and access to the profunda venous system. A longitudinal venotomy is preferred and offers the best exposure to the orifice of the profunda femoris veins. Because the thrombosed femoral vein is usually dilated, closure is easily accomplished without luminal compromise.

The leg is elevated and exsanguinated with a rubber bandage to expel clot from below. Occasionally, a cut-down to the posterior tibial vein in the lower leg is performed and a No. 3 Fogarty catheter advanced proximally and brought out through the common femoral venotomy. A No. 4

TABLE 1.

Principles of Venous Thrombectomy

1. Define full extent of thrombosis (contralateral iliofemoral phlebography is essential).
2. Obtain blood specimens for full hypercoagulable evaluation (before anticoagulation).
3. Fully anticoagulate with heparin and continue throughout procedure and postoperatively.
4. Prepare operating room for fluoroscopy and radiography.
5. Inguinally incise to expose and control common femoral, saphenous, superficial femoral, and profunda femoris veins.
6. Perform right retroperitoneal caval control and caval venotomy for removal of caval thrombus.
7. Exsanguinate leg with rubber bandage and expel clot from below.
8. Pass venous thrombectomy catheter part way into iliac vein for several passes before advancing into vena cava. (use No. 8 or No. 10 venous thrombectomy catheter).
9. If caval filter in place, use fluoroscopy for thrombectomy with contrast to fill balloon.
10. Cut-down to posterior tibial vein and advance No. 3 Fogarty catheter to femoral venotomy. Attach and guide No. 4 Fogarty catheter retrograde in leg, to allow balloon catheter thrombectomy in selected patients (especially patients with thrombus in or inadequate drainage from profunda) and repeat as needed. Flush leg with high-volume/pressure heparin-saline solution and infuse urokinase, 500,000 U, before ligating posterior tibial vein. (Consider leaving catheter in posterior tibial vein for heparin infusion.)
11. After completing thrombectomy, evaluate iliofemoral system with completion phlebogram/fluoroscopy.
12. Correct underlying iliac vein stenosis (if present) with angioplasty/stent if possible, or cross-pubic venous bypass with 10-mm externally supported polytetrafluoroethylene graft plus arteriovenous fistula.
13. Construct 4-mm arteriovenous fistula with saphenous vein (or large proximal branch of saphenous) end to side to superficial femoral artery. Arteriovenous fistula is considered permanent.
14. Slip piece of polytetrafluoroethylene graft, 5–6 mm in diameter, around saphenous vein before arteriovenous fistula, and leave small loop of O-prolene with clip in subcutaneous wound (in case closure of arteriovenous fistula becomes necessary).
15. Measure femoral vein pressure before and after arteriovenous fistula is open. If pressure increases, band arteriovenous fistula to decrease flow and normalize pressure. If pressure increases with arteriovenous fistula, look for proximal iliac vein stenosis or large arteriovenous anastomosis.
16. Continue full anticoagulation after surgery.
17. Apply external pneumatic compression garment after surgery.

Fogarty catheter is secured and guided distally into the lower leg. This is best achieved by placing each balloon catheter into opposite ends of a 16-gauge plastic IV catheter after amputating its hub. Each balloon is inflated to an infusion pressure high enough to secure the catheters within the plastic sheath, allowing unimpeded retrograde passage of the No. 4 Fogarty catheter. A balloon catheter thrombectomy is then performed by repeating this passage 2 or 3 times. A large-bore infusion catheter is then placed into the posterior tibial vein and large volumes of heparinized saline flushed through the lower leg, aspirating the drainage from the femoral venotomy. It is surprising how much additional acute thrombus can be flushed from the leg with this maneuver. A solution of urokinase (250,000–500,000 U) is infused and the posterior tibial vein ligated. A venous thrombectomy catheter is initially passed part way into the iliac vein and subsequently advanced into the vena cava.

After completing the thrombectomy, the iliofemoral system is evaluated with completion phlebography/fluoroscopy (Fig 6). If an underlying iliac vein stenosis is present, angioplasty and/or stent placement can be performed.

In our early experience of treating an iliac vein stenosis, a cross-pubic venous bypass was constructed with a 10-mm externally supported polytetrafluoroethylene graft, including an arteriovenous fistula (Fig 7); however, operative balloon angioplasty is now the preferred procedure. An arteriovenous fistula is routinely constructed with the end of the proximal saphenous vein sewn to the side of the superficial femoral artery. If a large proximal branch of the saphenous is present, it is used. A 3.5- to 4-mm anastomosis is performed, and the arteriovenous fistula is considered permanent. A small piece of polytetrafluoroethylene graft is placed around the saphenous vein before the arteriovenous anastomosis, and 0-monofilament suture looped around the polytetrafluoroethylene, and left in the subcutaneous space, in case it is necessary to dismantle the arteriovenous fistula in the future. Femoral venous pressure is measured before and after flow through the arteriovenous fistula is restored. If the

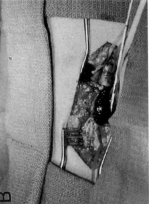

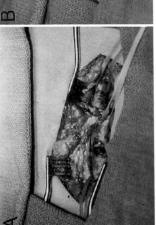

FIGURE 6.

Patient undergoing venous thrombectomy for extensive left leg deep venous thrombosis, involving the tibial, popliteal, femoral, and iliac veins. **A,** operative exposure of left common femoral, superficial femoral, and saphenous veins. **B,** Venotomy demonstrates the clot occluding the entire common femoral vein. **B,** progressive extrusion of clot because of high venous pressure.   *(Continued.)*

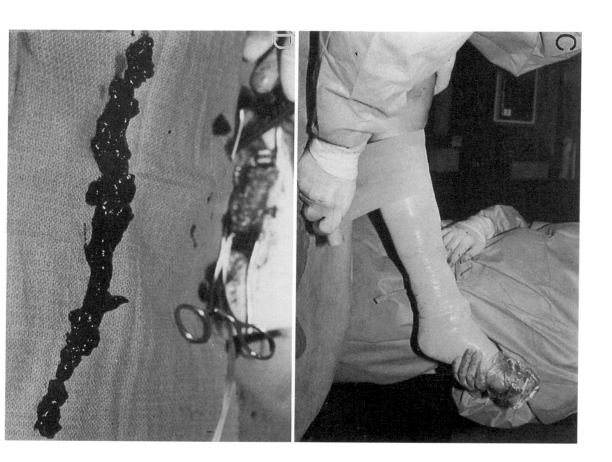

FIGURE 6 (cont.).

C, leg elevated with application of rubber bandage from foot to thigh. **D,** thrombus that was removed from the left iliofemoral venous system.   (*Continued.*)

pressure increases, the arteriovenous fistula is constricted to decrease blood flow through the fistula and maintain a normal common femoral venous pressure. In patients without proximal obstruction, the venous pressure is not elevated when the arteriovenous fistula is opened.

External pneumatic compression garments are applied postoperatively, and the patient is maintained with aggressive anticoagulation therapy, keeping the partial thromboplastic time greater than 100 seconds until therapeutic with oral anticoagulation.

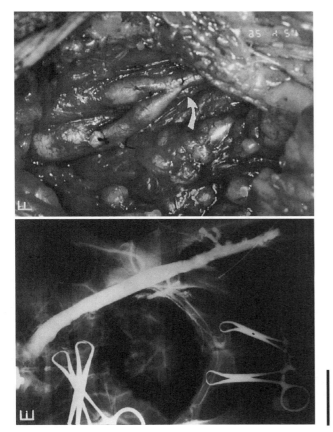

FIGURE 6 (cont.).

E, completion phlebogram demonstrating unobstructed venous drainage from femoral vein to vena cava. **F**, end-to-side greater saphenous vein to superficial femoral artery anastomosis *(arrow)* performed (3.5- to 4-mm anastomosis) to increase venous velocity to reduce risk of rethrombosis. A small cuff of polytetrafluoroethylene is subsequently placed around the saphenous vein segment and looped with 0-monofilament suture, in the event that subsequent closure of arteriovenous fistula is indicated.

CLINICAL EXPERIENCE

During the past 8 years, we have treated 28 patients in this manner. Catheter-directed thrombolysis was performed in 15 patients, venous thrombectomy in 13, and both lysis and thrombectomy were performed in 4 patients.

Of the 13 patients undergoing venous thrombectomy, 10 had a good or excellent clinical outcome, with a poor outcome in 3. One patient had long-standing iliofemoral venous occlusion associated with metastatic pancreatic carcinoma, and attempts at mechanical removal were unsuccessful. Another patient, with an intracranial malignancy, who could not receive anticoagulation therapy, had vena caval thrombosis 3 months after a successful iliofemoral venous thrombectomy. This patient required take-down of a well-functioning arteriovenous fistula. A third patient had a persistent iliac vein stenosis that led to rethrombosis. Although these three patients were not improved, and the results of the surgical procedure were considered to be poor, none of the patients was harmed by the attempted thrombectomy.

Sixteen patients had catheter-directed thrombolysis attempted, with successful catheter positioning accomplished in 14. Of those 14 patients, 12 had successful lysis with patency restored, whereas 2 patients failed

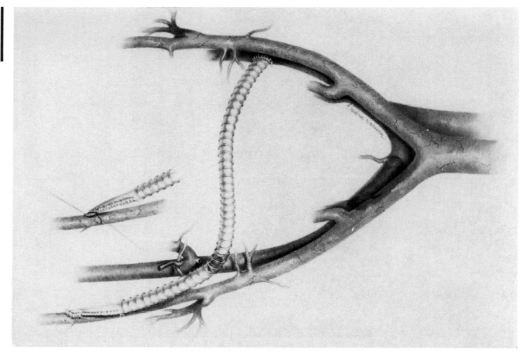

FIGURE 7.

Cross-pubic venous bypass with 10-mm externally supported polytetrafluoroethylene graft. Note: 3.5- to 4-mm arteriovenous fistula constructed to superficial femoral artery **(inset).**

lysis but underwent successful venous thrombectomy. The two patients who did not have successful catheter positioning both failed thrombolysis and underwent venous thrombectomy.

Bleeding complications were limited to puncture-site hematomas. One was extensive, necessitating termination of the urokinase infusion, operative evacuation of the hematoma, and repair of the femoral vein. No patient had a clinically evident pulmonary embolus.

Overall results (Table 2) were categorized according to the Society for Vascular Surgery/International Society for Cardiovascular Surgery clinical classification of chronic venous disease.[18] Outcome correlated directly with patency of the iliofemoral venous segment. Twenty-four patients had a good or excellent clinical outcome, whereas four patients were considered to have a poor outcome.

DISCUSSION

The rationale for aggressive intervention in patients with iliofemoral venous thrombosis is the serious long-term morbidity for many patients. Reasons not to intervene have been the high failure rate reported for both pharmacologic and operative intervention. Thrombolytic therapy for venous thromboembolic disease has traditionally been systemic therapy via IV infusion. Lytic therapy has evolved to catheter-directed techniques, which deliver the plasminogen activator directly into the thrombus. This modification is associated with significantly improved success and the potential for reduced complications.

In patients with iliofemoral DVT, a large volume of thrombus is in the involved veins, with a minimal surface area exposed to circulating blood. Therefore, it is not surprising that systemic thrombolysis frequently fails, because the plasminogen activator cannot reach the thrombus. This problem is overcome by the catheter-directed technique. Lysis can be followed with sequential phlebography, and the catheters can then be repositioned to appropriately treat segments of the venous system with residual thrombus. Interestingly, guidewires can be advanced retrograde in the venous system as far as the popliteal vein, through venous valves that are thrombosed in the open position (Fig 3) (a maneuver that is usually unsuccessful when attempted in the operating room with a thrombectomy catheter). Therefore, direct delivery of plasminogen activators into the popliteal vein and proximally is now the routine rather than the exception.

Molina and colleagues have demonstrated a high degree of success with catheter-directed thrombolysis.[18a] Similarly, Semba and Dake have adopted catheter-directed thrombolysis for both acute and chronic iliofemoral venous occlusion.[14] In 27 limbs with iliofemoral deep venous thrombosis, catheter-directed urokinase was associated with a 72% complete lysis and a 20% rate of partial lysis. Lysis was not achieved in two limbs (8%), both of which were chronically diseased. More than 50% of their patients had an underlying stenosis that required either angioplasty or angioplasty and stent placement. The average duration of therapy in their series was 30 hours (range, 15–74 hours), and the average total urokinase dose was 4.9 million units (range, 1.4–16.0 million U), which is similar to our experience. If treatment can be instituted within 7 days of thrombosis, and the catheter appropriately positioned within the thrombus, successful lysis can be anticipated.

During the past 2 decades, the technique of venous thrombectomy has been refined and therefore results have improved compared with the previously dismal reports. Among the technical improvements are the accurate evaluation of patients preoperatively, including the use of contralateral iliocavography. The performance of fluoroscopy and completion phlebography during the operation ensures the adequacy of the thrombectomy. Correction of underlying venous stenosis with balloon dilation and stenting, and as a last resort, the use of a cross-pubic venous bypass to ensure unobstructed venous drainage, is important. Construction of arteriovenous fistulae and immediate and prolonged therapeutic anticoagulation are important measures that reduce rethrombosis. Postoperative external pneumatic compression further accelerates venous drainage to avoid rethrombosis.

A multicenter, prospective, randomized trial was performed in Scandinavian centers, evaluating venous thrombectomy and arteriovenous fistulae with standard anticoagulation. Significantly better patency and fewer posthrombotic symptoms were observed in operated patients.[19] Six-month follow-up demonstrated complete iliofemoral patency in 76% of the operated patients compared with 35% of those treated with anticoagulation alone. Twice as many thrombectomy patients had patent femoropopliteal segments (52% vs. 26%). Forty-two percent of the patients who underwent surgery were free of posthrombotic symptoms at 6 months compared with only 7% in the anticoagulation group. In a 5-year follow-up study of these patients, radioisotopic phlebographs demonstrated iliofemoral patency in 76% of the operated group compared with 20% in the anticoagulation group.[20] Long-term venous function was normal in 39% of the operated patients compared with 19% of those receiving anticoagulation alone.[21] Fifty-five percent of those who had surgery were free of posthrombotic symptoms compared with 27% of those receiving anticoagulation alone.

Eklof and Juhan recently reported their experience in 230 patients undergoing thrombectomy for iliofemoral venous thrombosis.[22] There were no fatal pulmonary emboli and only one operative death. It is apparent that the application of venous thrombectomy now can be based on the merits of its effectiveness relative to other forms of therapy. Appropriately selected patients have a marked reduction in early morbidity in the late sequelae of iliofemoral venous thrombosis.

Pooled data from a number of contemporary reports on iliofemoral venous thrombectomy (see Table 2) indicate that the early and long-term patency of the iliofemoral venous segment is approximately 80% to 85%, contrasted to 30% patency in patients treated with anticoagulation alone.[19, 21, 23–27] Unfortunately, there is no study comparing venous thrombectomy and lytic therapy. If such a study were to be performed today, catheter-directed thrombolysis should be the technique used.

These data, combined with the natural history studies, underscore the importance of eliminating venous obstruction, especially in the iliofemoral venous segment. A treatment strategy that offers patients the benefits of catheter-directed thrombolysis in addition to operative intervention should yield the best overall results, both in the short-term and long-term. Advances in antithrombotics and ongoing improvement of techniques

TABLE 2.
Iliac Vein Patency After Venous Thrombectomy (Pooled Results)

Follow-up	Patients	No. of Reports	Patent Iliac Veins (%)	References
Early results	421	7	361/421 (86%)	19, 23–25
Late results (mean, 28 mo.)	198	5	156/198 (79%)	21, 23, 24, 26, 27

of thrombolysis and drug delivery systems continue to improve the chances that these patients will achieve a realistically good long-term prognosis.

REFERENCES

1. Comerota AJ: Treatment options for phlegmasia cerulea dolens (letter). *J Vasc Surg* 21:998–999, 1995.

2. O'Donnell TF, Browse NL, Burnard KG, et al: The socioeconomic effects of an iliofemoral thrombosis. *J Surg Res* 22:483–488, 1977.

3. Cockett FB, Thomas L: The iliac compression syndrome. *Br J Surg* 52:816–821, 1965.

4. Shull KC, Nicolaides AN, Fernandes e Fernandes J, et al: Significance of popliteal reflux in relation to ambulatory venous pressure and ulceration. *Arch Surg* 114:1304–1306, 1979.

5. Johnson BF, Manzo RA, Bergelin RO, et al: Relationship between changes in the deep venous system and the development of the post-thrombotic syndrome after an acute episode of lower limb deep vein thrombosis: a none to six year follow-up. *J Vasc Surg* 21:307–313, 1995.

6. Meissner MH, Manzo RA, Bergelin RO, et al: Deep venous insufficiency: The relationship between lysis and subsequent reflux. *J Vasc Surg* 18:596–608, 1993.

7. Killewich LA, Bedford GE, Beach KW, et al: Spontaneous lysis of deep venous thrombi: Rate and outcome. *J Vasc Surg* 9:89–97, 1989.

8. Comerota AJ, Aldridge SA, Cohen G, et al: A strategy of aggressive regional therapy for acute iliofemoral venous thrombosis with contemporary venous thrombectomy or catheter-directed thrombolysis. *J Vasc Surg* 20:244–254, 1994.

9. Haller JA, Abrams BL: Use of thrombectomy in the treatment of acute iliofemoral venous thrombosis in forty-five patients. *Ann Surg* 158:561–566, 1963.

10. DeWeese JA: Thrombectomy for acute iliofemoral venous thrombosis. *J Cardiovasc Surg* 5:703–712, 1964.

11. Lansing AM, Davis WM: Five-year follow-up study of iliofemoral venous thrombectomy. *Ann Surg* 168:620–628, 1968.

12. Karp RB, Wylie EJ: Recurrent thrombosis after iliofemoral venous thrombectomy. *Surg Forum* 17:147, 1966.

13. Hill SL, Martin D, Evans P: Massive deep vein thrombosis of the extremities. *Am J Surg* 158:131–136, 1989.

14. Semba CP, Dake MD: Iliofemoral deep venous thrombosis: Aggressive therapy using catheter-directed thrombolysis. *Radiology* 191:487–494, 1994.

15. Okrent D, Messersmith R, Buckman J: Transcatheter fibrinolytic therapy and angioplasty for left iliofemoral venous thrombosis. *J Vasc Interv Radiol* 2:195–197, 1991.

16. Pieri A, Santoro G, Duranti A, et al: Temporary caval filters: Our experience. Preliminary analysis of 24 cases. *Phlebologie* 46:457–466, 1993.

17. Collen D, Stump DL, Van de Werf F: Coronary thrombolysis in patients with myocardial infarction by intravenous infusion of synergic thrombolytic agents. *Am Heart J* 11:1083, 1986.

18. Porter JM, Moneta GL, and an International Consensus Committee on Chronic Venous Disease: Reporting standards in venous disease: An update. *J Vasc Surg* 21:635–645, 1995.

18a. Molina JE, Hunter D, Yedlicka JW: Thrombolytic therapy for iliofemoral venous thrombosis. *J Vasc Surg* 26:630–637, 1992.

19. Plate G, Einarsson E, Ohlin P, et al: Thrombectomy with temporary arterio- venous fistula: The treatment of choice in acute iliofemoral venous thrombo- sis. *J Vasc Surg* 1:867–876, 1984.

20. Akesson H, Brudin L, Dahlstrom JA, et al: Venous function assessed during a 5 year period after acute iliofemoral venous thrombosis treated with antico- agulation. *Eur J Vas Surg* 4:43–48, 1990.

21. Plate G, Akesson H, Einarson E, et al: Long-term results of venous thrombec- tomy combined with a temporary arteriovenous fistulae. *Eur J Vasc Surg* 4:483, 1990.

22. Eklof B, Juhan C: Revival of thrombectomy in the management of acute il- iofemoral venous thrombosis. *Contemp Surg* 40:21, 1992.

23. Piquet PH, Tournigand P, Josso B, et al: Traitement chirurgical des thrombo- ses ilio-caces: exigences et resultats, in Kieffer E (ed): *Chirurgie de la Vein Cave Inferieur et de ses Branches.* Paris, Expansion Scientifique Francaise, 1985, pp 210–216.

24. Juhan C, Cornillon B, Tobiana F, et al: Etude de la permeabilitie des throm- bectomies veineuse iliofemorales et ilio-caves. *Ann Chir Vasc* 1:529–533, 1987.

25. Einarsson E, Albrechtsson V, Eklof B: Thrombectomy and temporary arterio- venous fistula in iliofemoral vein thrombosis: Technical considerations and early results. *Int Angiol* 5:65–70, 1986.

26. Einarsson E, Albrechtsson V, Eklof B, et al: Follow-up evaluation of venous morphologic factors and function after thrombectomy and temporary arterio- venous fistula in thrombosis of iliofemoral vein. *Surg Gynecol Obstet* 163:111–116, 1986.

27. Torngren S, Swedenborg J: Thrombectomy and temporary arteriovenous fis- tula for iliofemoral venous thrombosis. *Int Angiol* 7:14–18, 1988.

Suction Catheter Embolectomy and Other Primary Treatment Strategies in the Management of Pulmonary Embolism

Samuel Z. Goldhaber, M.D.

Cardiovascular Division, Brigham and Women's Hospital, Harvard Medical School, Boston, Massachusetts

Anticoagulation, the cornerstone of pulmonary embolism (PE) management, is called "treatment" but really constitutes *secondary prevention* of recurrent PE. Pulmonary emboli differ markedly in size and physiologic effect. Therefore, *risk stratification* is crucial to determine when anticoagulation alone will suffice and which patients should be considered candidates for primary therapy with thrombolysis or embolectomy.

INDICATIONS FOR SECONDARY PREVENTION

Echocardiography should play a major role in assessing prognosis and helping determine whether anticoagulation alone will be effective. Patients with normal systemic arterial pressure and normal right ventricular function generally have a good prognosis after PE. For such individuals, secondary prevention is usually adequate with anticoagulation or, if major bleeding from anticoagulation is likely, with placement of an inferior vena cava filter (Fig 1).

INDICATIONS FOR PRIMARY THERAPY

An outdated adage about embolectomy needs fundamental reassessment. It used to be taught that patients who underwent successful embolectomy really did not require the operation because they would have recovered with conservative measures (e.g., anticoagulation plus insertion of an inferior vena cava filter). Conversely, it was argued that patients who died of embolectomy were hopelessly ill by the time they were referred for surgery and therefore should not have undergone surgery. Such circular reasoning was destined to condemn both the referring physician and the operating surgeon, regardless of outcome. This stance, now waning, has

Advances in Vascular Surgery®, vol. 4
© 1996, Mosby–Year Book, Inc.

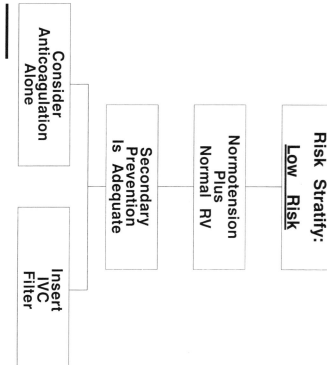

FIGURE 1.
Low-risk patients have normal systemic arterial pressure and normal right ventricle (*RV*) function; they have good outcomes with anticoagulation alone. *Abbreviation: IVC*, inferior vena cava.

impeded progress toward a rational, proactive, but thoughtful approach to pulmonary embolectomy.

I certainly recall two decades ago that patients would not be accepted for embolectomy unless they had prolonged systemic arterial hypotension that was refractory to pressors. This philosophy ensured that the few desperately ill patients who underwent surgery were unlikely to survive. Even with technically superb surgery, such individuals were preoperatively subjected to protracted periods of poor perfusion of vital organs, adverse metabolic effects of released cytokines, progressive heart failure, and arrhythmogenic effects of circulating catecholamines.

Although systemic arterial hypotension (often a manifestation of cardiogenic shock) confers an ominous prognosis, frank hemodynamic collapse is quite unusual. Much more commonly, patients with PE demonstrate normal systemic arterial pressure combined with occult right ventricular dysfunction that is detectable only on echocardiographic evaluation. The presence of moderate or severe right ventricular hypokinesis, even in the absence of systemic arterial hypotension, suggests that primary therapy for PE should be strongly considered (Fig 2).

A contemporary approach toward embolectomy (Fig 3) advocates early intervention once a decision has been made that a patient is experiencing moderate or severe right heart failure. Because peripheral vasoconstriction is often preserved as a compensatory mechanism even among moribund patients in cardiogenic shock, the presence of normal systemic arterial pressure should not by itself delay primary therapy. Embolectomy

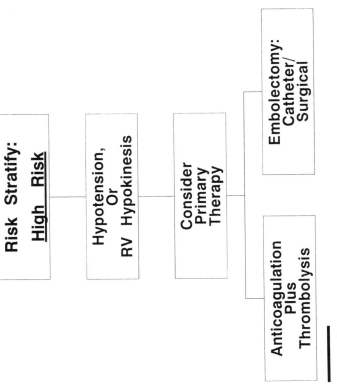

FIGURE 2.

High-risk patients have either systemic arterial hypotension (rare) or, much more commonly, normal systemic arterial pressure in the presence of often occult right ventricular (*RV*) hypokinesis. The clinical outcomes of these patients can improve with primary therapy for pulmonary embolism: thrombolysis or embolectomy.

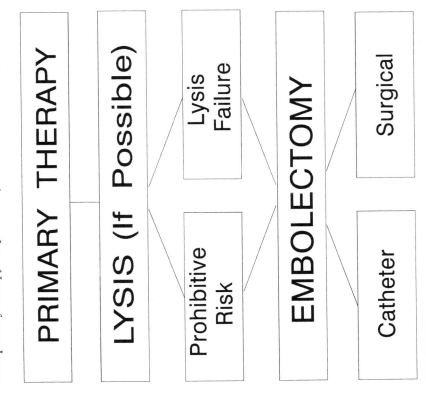

FIGURE 3.

Indications for embolectomy; please refer to the text.

is most appropriate for those patients undergoing intervention who fail to respond to thrombolytic therapy or who have major contraindications to its use.

THROMBOLYTIC THERAPY

Thrombolysis can be considered a "medical embolectomy" that debulks clot and provides primary treatment of PE. This approach appears to be lifesaving in patients with massive PE who have cardiogenic shock and overt right heart failure.[1] Thrombolysis can also reduce the rate of recurrent PE in patients with preserved blood pressure but right ventricular dysfunction.[2] The procedures for administering thrombolytic therapy (Table 1) have been streamlined to improve efficacy, enhance safety, and reduce costs.[3]

SUCTION CATHETER EMBOLECTOMY

Interest has resurged for aggressive interventional management of PE, often performed in the angiography laboratory. Suction catheter embolectomy is ideally undertaken while systemic arterial pressure is preserved,

TABLE 1.
Contemporary Pulmonary Embolism Thrombolysis

Variable	"Old" Concepts	Contemporary Concepts
Diagnosis of PE	Mandatory pulmonary angiogram	High-probability lung scan or suggestive echocardiogram (if hypotensive) or angiogram
Indications for thrombolysis	Systemic arterial hypotension	Hypotension or normotension with accompanying right ventricular hypokinesis
Time window	5 days or less	14 days or less
Thrombolytic agents	SK or UK	rt-PA, SK, or UK
Dosing regimens	24 hr SK or 12–24 hr UK	100 mg/2 hr rt-PA (FDA approved)
Route of administration	Via pulmonary artery catheter	Via peripheral vein
Coagulation tests	"DIC screens" every 4–6 hr during infusion	PTT at conclusion of thrombolysis to help dose heparin
Location	ICU	Intermediate care ("step-down") unit

Abbreviations: PE, pulmonary embolism; SK, streptokinase; UK, urokinase; rt-PA, recombinant tissue-type plasminogen activator; FDA, Food and Drug Administration; DIC, disseminated intravascular coagulation; PTT, partial thromboplastin time.

before the onset of overt cardiogenic shock. This approach is preferable to prolonged observation of patients with progressive deterioration in right ventricular dysfunction until the point where their last compensatory mechanism, peripheral vasoconstriction, is exhausted and frank cardiogenic shock ensues.

The Greenfield embolectomy device (Fig 4) is probably the most frequently used catheter-based method of extracting pulmonary arterial thrombi.[4] It consists of a 10-French steerable catheter with a suction cup attached at the tip. Because of the cup's large size, a surgical venotomy is performed, usually in the right internal jugular vein. A steerable handle controls progression of the catheter through the right cardiac chambers and the pulmonary arterial branches. This device permits the removal by catheter of extensive PE (Fig 5).

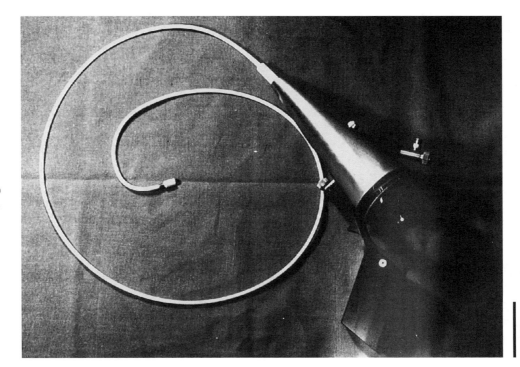

FIGURE 4.

Greenfield catheter embolectomy device. (Courtesy of Meyer G, Tamiser D, Reynaud P, et al: Acute pulmonary embolectomy, in Goldhaber SZ (ed): *Cardiopulmonary Diseases and Cardiac Tumors*, vol 2, in Braunwald E (ed): *Atlas of Heart Diseases.* Philadelphia, Current Medicine, 1995, pp 7.1–7.12.)

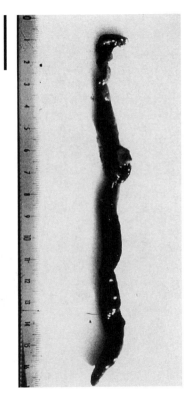

FIGURE 5.

Seventeen-centimeter pulmonary embolus removed via the Greenfield catheter embolectomy device. (Courtesy of Meyer G, Tamiser D, Reynaud P, et al: Acute pulmonary embolectomy, in Goldhaber SZ (ed): *Cardiopulmonary Diseases and Cardiac Tumors*, vol 3, in Braunwald E (ed): *Atlas of Heart Diseases*. Philadelphia, Current Medicine, 1995, pp 7.1–7.12.)

Alternative catheter-based modalities include simultaneous mechanical clot fragmentation and pharmacologic thrombolysis,[5] as well as mechanical fragmentation of thrombus with a pulmonary artery catheter.[6] Currently, a rotating basket catheter is undergoing clinical testing. It consists of a 5-French Teflon catheter in which the distal tip is divided into four 15-mm bends. The high-speed mechanical rotation of the catheter (about 100,000 rpm) causes centrifugal force to open the distal bends and form a soft flexible helical spiral that can pulverize thrombi into microscopic particles within seconds.[7]

EXAMPLE OF SUCTION CATHETER EMBOLECTOMY

We have performed suction catheter embolectomy at Brigham and Women's Hospital *without* angiographic catheters specifically designed for this purpose. For example, a 78-year-old woman was evaluated for marked shortness of breath, persistent hypotension (blood pressure, 78/51 mm Hg), and right ventricular dilatation and hypokinesis on echocardiography.[8] Pulmonary angiography showed massive right pulmonary artery embolism as well as a small left lung volume because of a prior left lung thoracoplasty to treat tuberculosis (Fig 6, A). Heparin was administered, and a Greenfield filter was inserted.

We believed that she required primary therapy for PE rather than secondary prevention alone because hemodynamic compromise and hypoxemia persisted despite ventilatory support. However, our cardiac surgeons thought that she would not survive surgical embolectomy because of the prior thoracoplasty.

Suction catheter embolectomy was undertaken in the interventional angiography laboratory. The right common femoral vein was accessed with a single-wall puncture needle. A guide wire was advanced across the Greenfield filter. A 7-French pigtail catheter with a tip-deflecting guide wire was used to enter the pulmonary artery. The catheter was exchanged for a 9-French multipurpose coronary guiding catheter. Two guide wires were then advanced side by side through the coronary guiding catheter, which was removed and then reinserted over one of the two

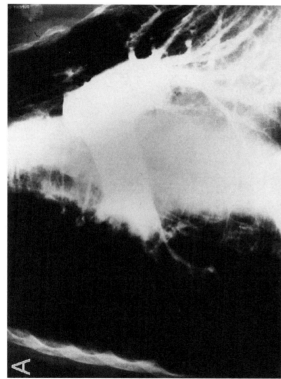

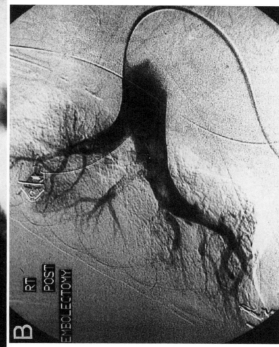

FIGURE 6.

A, massive right main pulmonary artery embolus in the presence of markedly diminished left lung volume as a result of prior thoracoplasty. **B,** digital subtraction pulmonary angiography immediately after combined suction catheter embolectomy and thrombolysis. There is an approximate 30% reduction in overall clot burden as compared with the baseline angiogram (Fig 5, A). (Courtesy of Goldhaber SZ: Treatment of acute pulmonary embolism, in Goldhaber SZ (ed): *Cardiopulmonary Diseases and Cardiac Tumors,* vol 3, in Braunwald E (ed): *Atlas of Heart Diseases.* Philadelphia, Current Medicine, 1995, pp 3.1–3.25.)

wires. The wire for the guiding catheter was then withdrawn, and clot was sucked through the catheter.

She had marked pulmonary hypertension. Pressures were as follows: 18 mm Hg (mean) in the right atrium, 90/18 mm Hg in the right ventricle, and 90/40 mm Hg in the pulmonary artery.

Suction catheter embolectomy removed both fresh and old clot from the pulmonary artery branches of the upper and lower right lobar arteries. However, systemic arterial hypotension persisted, so 50 mg of recombinant tissue-type plasminogen activator (rt-PA) was administered over a 15-minute period through the pulmonary artery catheter. Pulmonary angiography then showed an approximate 30% reduction in the overall clot burden (Fig 6, B).

The procedure was complicated by retroperitoneal bleeding, which was corrected with 12 U of packed red blood cells. Pneumonia and acute respiratory distress syndrome also developed. Nonetheless, her clinical picture gradually improved, and she was eventually transferred to a rehabilitation facility.

I have just received a letter from this patient 2½ years after the suction catheter embolectomy. She states, "I am able to get around with a walker and a portable cannister of oxygen. I celebrated my 80th birthday last year, so I guess I am a tough old bird. I just thought you might want to know I am alive and kicking."

OPEN SURGICAL EMBOLECTOMY

If these strategies fail, acute surgical pulmonary embolectomy can be undertaken.[9] A nonrandomized comparison of rt-PA thrombolysis with surgical embolectomy showed that both approaches can be lifesaving in the majority of patients with massive PE.[10]

PULMONARY THROMBOENDARTERECTOMY

Patients with chronic pulmonary hypertension caused by prior PE may be virtually bedridden with breathlessness because of high pulmonary arterial pressure. They should be considered for pulmonary thromboendarterectomy, which, if successful, can reduce and at times even cure pulmonary hypertension.[11]

The operation involves a median sternotomy incision, institution of cardiopulmonary bypass, and deep hypothermia with circulatory arrest periods. Incisions are made in both pulmonary arteries into the lower lobe branches. Pulmonary thromboendarterectomy is always bilateral, with removal of organized thrombus from all involved vessels. When surgery is successful, one can expect a gradual decline in pulmonary arterial pressure during the first few postoperative months with a concomitant improvement in the quality of life among patients previously debilitated by chronic pulmonary hypertension.

REFERENCES

1. Jerjes-Sanchez C, Ramirez-Rivera A, Garcia ML, et al: Streptokinase and heparin versus heparin alone in massive pulmonary embolism: A randomized controlled trial. *J Thromb Thrombolysis* 2:227–229, 1995.
2. Goldhaber SZ, Haire WD, Feldstein ML, et al: Alteplase versus heparin in acute pulmonary embolism: Randomised trial assessing right ventricular function and pulmonary perfusion. *Lancet* 341:507–511, 1993.
3. Goldhaber SZ: Contemporary pulmonary embolism thrombolysis. *Chest* 107:45S–51S, 1995.

4. Greenfield LJ, Proctor MC, Williams DM, et al: Long-term experience with transvenous catheter pulmonary embolectomy. *J Vasc Surg* 18:450–458, 1993.

5. Essop MR, Middlemost S, Skoularigis J, et al: Simultaneous mechanical clot fragmentation and pharmacologic thrombolysis in acute massive pulmonary embolism. *Am J Cardiol* 69:427–430, 1992.

6. Brady AJB, Crake T, Oakley CM: Percutaneous catheter fragmentation and distal dispersion of proximal pulmonary embolus. *Lancet* 338:1186–1189, 1991.

7. Dievart F, Fourrier JL, Lefebvre JM, et al: Treatment of severe pulmonary embolism by means of a high speed rotational catheter (Angiocor Thrombolizer): First experience of mechanical thrombolysis in human beings. *J Am Coll Cardiol* 474A, 1994.

8. Goldhaber SZ: Treatment of acute pulmonary embolism, in Goldhaber SZ (ed): *Cardiopulmonary Diseases and Cardiac Tumors*, vol 3, in Braundwald E (ed): *Atlas of Heart Diseases*. Philadelphia, Current Medicine, 1995, pp 3.1–3.25.

9. Meyer G, Tamiser D, Reynaud P, et al: Acute pulmonary embolectomy, in Goldhaber SZ (ed): *Cardiopulmonary Diseases and Cardiac Tumors*, vol 3, in Braunwald E (ed): *Atlas of Heart Diseases*. Philadelphia, Current Medicine, 1995, pp 7.1–7.12.

10. Gulba DC, Schmid C, Borst H-G, et al: Medical compared with surgical treatment for massive pulmonary embolism. *Lancet* 343:565–577, 1994.

11. Fedullo PF, Auger WR, Channick RN, et al: A multidisciplinary approach to chronic thromboembolic pulmonary hypertension, in Goldhaber SZ (ed): *Cardiopulmonary Diseases and Cardiac Tumors*, Vol 3, in Braunwald E (ed): *Atlas of Heart Diseases*. Philadelphia, Current Medicine, 1995, pp 7.1–7.25.

PART VII

Issues in Basic Science

Management of Reperfusion Injury in the Lower Extremity

Paul M. Walker, M.D., Ph.D., F.R.C.S.C.

James Wallace McCutcheon Chair, Surgeon-in-Chief, Vice President, Surgical Directorate, The Toronto Hospital, Canada

O ver the course of the past 15 years, much new information has become available regarding the management of ischemia/reperfusion injury to the lower extremity. Most of this information has been gained from animal studies, where careful control of variables has enabled investigators to dissect the mechanisms of injury associated with this syndrome.[1] Application of this information in the clinical setting, however, has been slow to come forward because of a number of different specific aspects of this problem. It is very difficult to define a homogeneous population because it is hard to determine the precise extent of the ischemic injury, the exact duration of ischemic time, and the completeness of the revascularization. End points available for measurement tend to be imprecise, including physical findings of loss of motor and sensory modalities, ankle/arm brachial pressures before and after reconstruction, and the appearance of abnormalities in the postreperfusion period such as muscle dysfunction in the form of footdrop and even frank necrosis requiring débridement or amputation.

The results of management of ischemia/reperfusion of the lower extremities have not noticeably improved overall despite this new information, although there is a trend toward a reduction in the amount of renal impairment associated with this syndrome.[2]

During the course of this chapter, several of the mechanisms of ischemia/reperfusion injury will be discussed in the context of their direct relevance to management strategies in an effort to reduce both local injury and systemic complications.

ISCHEMIC INJURY

During a period of circulatory arrest caused by embolism, thrombosis, or trauma, normal oxidative metabolism is interrupted. Muscle is uniquely adapted to prolonged periods of ischemia by virtue of large stores of creatine phosphate, which contains high-energy phosphate bonds and glycogen that can be metabolized to lactate and culminate in the production of adenosine triphosphate (ATP), in addition to hydrogen ions and lactate.[3] These large intracellular energy stores coupled with the relatively

Advances in Vascular Surgery®, vol. 4
© 1996, Mosby–Year Book, Inc.

low metabolic demand of resting muscle enable muscles to endure up to 3 hours of ischemia without significant irreversible injury. After a 3-hour period, most of the creatine phosphate has been depleted and there is a relatively steady fall in levels of ATP despite rises in lactate and hydrogen ions, which suggests that energy demands cannot be met by anaerobic metabolism alone.[4] The ischemia-induced breakdown of high-energy adenine nucleotides results in a concomitant accumulation of nonphosphorylated precursors. This latter fact is of significant importance because nonphosphorylated nucleotides cross the phospholipid membranes and are easily washed out of the muscle upon return of circulation, thus leaving the muscle depleted of precursors for the resynthesis of high-energy nucleotides.[5]

Many factors determine the tolerance of muscle to ischemia, including the length of ischemic time, the completeness of ischemia, the temperature during the ischemic period, and the muscle fiber types involved as demonstrated in Figure 1. The clinically important range of ischemia of 4 to 5 hours can result in a very significant difference in the degree of ischemic damage related to these independent variables.[6] The end result of the period of ischemia is the depletion of intracellular energy stores and a large accumulation of hydrogen ions and lactate. Reducing agents accumulate in the cytoplasm and mitochondria and are capable of producing toxic oxygen radicals upon the sudden reintroduction of oxygen.

With reintroduction of the circulation, a new set of reactions is initiated locally but also begins to involve the systemic circulation. The net effect of reperfusion may in fact be damaging despite its necessity for any potential salvage of the extremity. Partially injured muscle cells may be

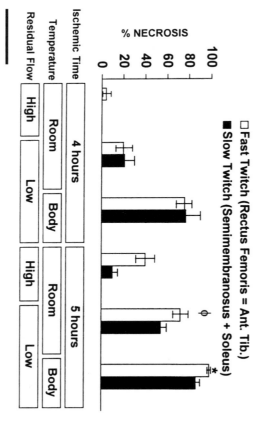

FIGURE 1.

Distribution of muscle necrosis on the basis of muscle fiber type. Predominantly fast-twitch muscle (rectus femoris and anterior tibialis) had significantly greater necrosis than did slow-twitch (semimembranosus proprius and soleus) after 5 hours of ischemia. No significant differences were observed after 4 hours of ischemia. $*P < 0.01$, $\phi P < 0.05$, fast-twitch vs. slow-twitch fiber muscle. (Courtesy of Petrasak PF, Homer-Vanniasinkam S, Walker P: Determinants of ischemic injury to skeletal muscle. *J Vasc Surg* 19:623–631, 1994.)

converted to irreversibly injured and ultimately necrotic muscle.[7] This paradox of reperfusion-induced necrosis may be a therapeutic window open to the vascular surgeon because at the time of surgical repair there is an opportunity to gain control of the reperfusion and to perhaps alter its nature.

When blood flow is allowed to return to an ischemic extremity, a significant reactive hyperemia occurs.[8] The degree and the extent of the reperfusion are not related to the degree of ischemic injury but rather related to the loss of autonomic function as a result of the period of ischemia. The nature of the reactive hyperemia is related to the period of ischemia in a reverse nature; that is, with a prolonged period of reperfusion, the actual degree of hyperemia is blunted, probably because of the alteration in physical properties of the microcirculation.[9]

This large and sudden return of blood flow may result in a number of diverse events. Reactive hyperemia results in a greater availability of oxygen molecules contributing to the increased concentration of oxygen free radicals. Normally, tetravalent reduction of oxygen occurs, with the production of water and carbon dioxide.[10] During the reperfusion phase this reduction may be incomplete and result in the production of oxygen molecules with a single electron in their outer orbit, known as oxygen free radicals. These are highly reactive particles capable of inducing very significant damage on local structures, including both protein and phospholipid-containing molecules.[11] Local scavengers, which can control the normal, small quantity of free radical production, are often overwhelmed by the significant accumulation of free radicals and therefore results in concomitant lipid peroxidation. The sudden increase in blood flow when cell membranes are damaged may contribute to the formation of edema and contribute to myeonecrosis.

The local destruction of phospholipid membranes by lipid peroxidation results in the leakage of many of intracellular substrates into the general circulation.[12] The net effect of this leakage is quite significant. It accentuates the release of intracellular toxic products and the depletion of many necessary intracellular substrates, including cytoplasmic enzymes and larger molecules such as myoglobin. At the same time, these cell wall abnormalities allow the influx of calcium, which has the effect of uncoupling oxidative phosphorylation, thereby leading to continuing loss of energy stores.[13]

Therefore in summary, at the point of early reperfusion, cellular membranes have been damaged by oxygen free radical–mediated injury. The intracellular products that have accumulated are in the process of being washed out of the cells, and further local injury is possible because of cell swelling. Lactate, potassium, and hydrogen ions are being released from inside cells, as well as larger molecules including myoglobin and necessary cytoplasmic enzymes because of continuing cell wall damage; in addition, calcium is accumulating intracellularly.[14]

This local injury sets the stage for a very significant systemic response resulting in remote complications, the timing of which might be quite variable. We have previously demonstrated that ischemia/reperfusion injury can significantly influence complement stores and result specifically in complement activation through the alternative pathways.[15] Comple-

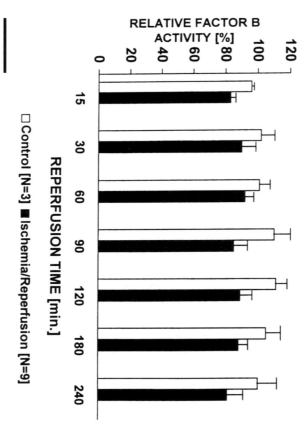

RELATIVE FACTOR B
ACTIVITY [%]

REPERFUSION TIME [min.]

□ Control [N=3] ■ Ischemia/Reperfusion [N=9]

FIGURE 2.

Systemic factor B activity during reperfusion. The decline in factor B activity with time ($P = 0.023$ by random measures–analysis of variance) demonstrates the ischemia/reperfusion potentiated activation of the alternative complement cascade. (Courtesy of Rubin BB, Smith A, Liauw SK, et al: Complement activation and white cell sequestration in postischemic skeletal muscle. *Am J Physiol* 259:H525–H531, 1990.)

ment activation may represent the first mediator elaborated inasmuch as we showed a significant reduction in systemic factor B activity within 15 minutes of reperfusion in an animal model (Fig 2).

In addition, the cytokine interleukin-1 has been measured after severe muscle ischemia/reperfusion injury, and it may well play a role in development of the subsequent systemic response. These humoral factors lead to an upregulation of ligands in neutrophils as well as on the endothelial surface.[16] The accumulation of white cells within reperfused skeletal muscle has previously been documented and the time course noted. White cell accumulation starts early, and this process builds for hours over the course of the reperfusion. In order to have white cells accumulate in the area of reperfusion, a number of events must occur. The first aspect of neutrophil accumulation is slowing of the streaming and the beginning of neutrophils rolling along the endothelium. This results from an upregulation of certain selectins, a subgroup of the ligand family. Activation of these ligands results in the characteristic rolling action of neutrophils seen in the intravital microscopy representations of early reperfusion.[17] With the conformational change or upregulation of neutrophil adhesion receptors such as CD11b or CD18, in conjunction with the upregulation of intercellular adhesion molecule type 1 (ICAM-1), the receptor on the endothelium, the neutrophils begin to adhere firmly to the endothelium.[18] With the progressive accumulation of more and more neutrophils as a result of this reaction, plugging of the capillary bed occurs and results in slowed and in fact complete obstruction of blood flow, again seen with intravital microscopy. These ligand interactions may not be permanent, however, and in areas where reperfusion has been blunted because of the accumulation of neutrophils, after a relatively short period of time the neutrophils often become freed and are washed away and the circulation is restored.[19] However, adherence of neutrophils also causes them to be activated, as a result of which some of the neutrophils migrate into interstitial areas and release their intracellular stores of elastases and proteinases, as well as produce more oxygen free radicals. The process of oxygen free radical production is related to surface enzymes, nicotinamine adenine dinucleotide and its reduced form, which produce free radicals locally; this results in the formation of hypohalous acids[20] and further phospholipid membrane damage. In previous studies we have demonstrated that the myeloperoxidase content of the interstitial space, which is a clear marker of neutrophil sequestration, is maximal at 48 hours, thus indicating that this is a prolonged process that may result in increased injury over time and further muscle damage[21] (Fig 3).

We have detailed some of the basic mechanisms of injury that have been separately elucidated during the process of ischemia/reperfusion of the lower extremity. Understanding these injury processes will lead to more focused therapeutic interventions. Unfortunately, until now there has been little in the way of application of this information except in animal models. The toxicity of some of the agents and the lack of availability of appropriate quantities of therapeutic agents (such as specific monoclonal antibodies) because of prohibitive cost have reduced the application of this information. Nevertheless, there may well be significant advances in our therapeutic interventions in the near future.

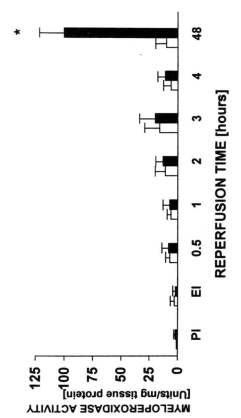

FIGURE 3.
Myeloperoxidase activity in surface tissue biopsy specimens during the initial 48 hours of reperfusion in vivo. *Abbreviations: PI,* preischemia; *EI,* end ischemia; $P = 0.0004$ by random measures–analysis of variance; *$P = 0.00001$ vs. time-matched, nonischemic control by unpaired test. (Courtesy of Rubin BB, Smith A, Liauw SK, et al: Complement activation and white cell sequestration in postischemic skeletal muscle. *Am J Physiol* 259:H525–H531, 1990.)

THERAPY

With repair of the arterial injury and restoration of normal blood flow to the extremity, the process of reactive hyperemia is initiated. Depending on the adequacy of perfusion of all the muscle cells and the length of time of ischemic injury, the immediate washout of the intracellular stores of lactate and hydrogen ion is perhaps the first and may potentially be the most lethal intraoperative event. Lactate is a small molecule and is easily washed out of the cells. There may be a large store of lactate with associated hydrogen ion, and the sudden appearance of a large concentration in the circulation may significantly affect myocardial contractility and irritability. In the presence of underlying coronary artery disease, this may result in malignant arrhythmias or even cardiac arrest. Therapeutic interventions that have been demonstrated to be successful in this area are maintenance of blood pressure, hydration, and adequate oxygenation.[22] The addition of IV bicarbonate has been proposed as a means of modulating the immediate acid-base imbalance. With normal liver function, this lactate load is actually relatively easily metabolized, and evidence has shown that this is a short-lasting phenomenon with most of the lactate washed out within 15 to 30 minutes. The long-term systemic consequences of the immediate washout and other metabolic by-products is not clearly understood, and its significance may in fact be greater because of stimulation of the release of various other components, perhaps not yet fully identified.

The progression of local injuries with increasing phospholipid membrane destruction allows the egress of larger molecules such as myoglobin and other cytoplasmic structures, including creatine phosphokinase. A number of interventions directed at preventing free radical–induced lipid peroxidation have been used in animal studies to reduce membrane damage, often measured by changes in the permeability index. Oxygen free radical scavengers used in animal and in vitro experimentation include superoxide dismutase, catalase, dimethyl sulfoxide, and dimethylphyorea.[7]

Specific inhibitors of xanthine oxidase include allopurinol and oxypurinol. Deferoxamine has been used to prevent Fenton chemistry, which produces dangerous hydroxy radicals capable of significant damage to phospholipid membranes.

Depletion of xanthine oxidase with tungsten-supplemented diets attenuated postischemic deficits in microvascular function.[23] Decreasing the availability of oxygen in the immediate reperfusion area has also been shown to decrease postischemic necrosis. This has been found in myocardial ischemic studies as well and suggests that the overabundance of oxygen during the immediate reperfusion phase is not beneficial and in fact may be deleterious. However, the contribution of locally generated free radicals to overall tissue injury likely remains small in human skeletal muscle, and the greatest free radical damage may be related to neutrophil oxidase production.

The neutrophil's contribution to ischemic/reperfusion injury has been identified, and a number of strategies are available to specifically minimize the injury they initiate. These include delaying the entry of neutrophils into the circulation by mechanical means. Research work has demonstrated that this is an effective modality in the experimental situation, and indeed, preventing neutrophil penetration in the early period alone may be sufficient to reduce the degree of overall ischemic damage.[24]

An alternative strategy is directed at preventing neutrophils from undergoing the characteristic series of events in the microcirculation leading to sequestration, blockage of capillaries, and release of reactive oxygen metabolites and cytotoxic enzymes. Inhibition of leukocyte adhesion and oxidative metabolism with a number of agents has been demonstrated, including ATP magnesium chloride, adenosine, and fructose 1,6-diphosphate.[25]

A number of agents have also been identified that reduce the activation of hydrolytic enzymes stored within the granules of neutrophils. These include the elastin inhibitors eglin C or L-658758, which also significantly decreases leukocyte sequestration, and L-658758 alone, which decreases leukocyte adherence.[26]

Specific evidence implicating neutrophils locally in muscle damage relates to the effectiveness of monoclonal antibodies to specific glycoprotein adherence complexes such as CD11 and CD18. Experiments with antineutrophil serum or anti-CD18 monoclonal antibodies demonstrated significantly attenuated changes in vascular permeability in comparison to controls.[27]

In reperfusion myocardial necrosis, anti-CD18 antibodies decreased adherence and neutrophil migration in the post-ischemic mesentery and decreased skeletal muscle contractile dysfunction. In addition, CD18 antibody treatment appears to be effective in our rabbit model of hindlimb ischemia in preventing necrosis. In fact, it was as successful as a fasciotomy alone in reducing myocyte necrosis, but the two factors were in fact additive in reducing postischemic muscle necrosis. This combined intervention of fasciotomy and anti-CD11 monoclonal antibodies suggests that successful intervention must be multifunctional. In this setting, fasciotomy definitely reduced the ultimate degree of necrosis (measured at 48 hours), which suggests that there is a mechanical component of compressive myonecrosis that requires decompression and may be specifically necessary in the early phases of reperfusion. The significant additional salvage as a result of the prevention of neutrophil adherence suggests that ongoing necrosis may be related to neutrophil activation and release of destructive properties over the more prolonged phase of reperfusion.[28]

The role of these specific monoclonal antibodies in the human situation remains experimental, particularly because of the large quantities of these monoclonals that would be necessary. At this moment there is no good source of monoclonals in appropriate quantities that would enable them to be given in a therapeutic regimen.

Similarly, in the subendothelial layer, ischemic reperfusion causes significant structural changes that lead to further local damage. They can be attenuated by the addition of such molecules as phalloidin, which has been found to stabilize the F-actin in endothelial cells.[29] However, again none of these experiments have proved effective in the clinical setting and are probably toxic in appropriate clinical doses.

The mechanisms of complement activation have been discussed previously. Clearly, if it is possible to decrease the extent of this systemic response, there may be an improvement or attenuation in the entire cascade of the reperfusion injury. The administration of recombinant soluble complement receptor type 1, which acts by displacing the catalytic subunits from both C3 and C5 convertase, was capable of reducing leukocyte sequestration and myocardial necrosis in experiments in which reperfusion followed left coronary occlusion.[30]

Despite the recognized importance of adenine nucleotide metabolism, no particularly successful modality has been identified that reduces the degree of ischemia-induced adenine nucleotide degeneration. Several hypotheses to prevent dephosphorylation have been suggested, specifically by inhibiting the 5-nucleotidase enzyme, but no successful experimental work has proved this methodology.

A number of experimental and several isolated clinical reports have suggested that there may be some advantage to reducing the postischemic microvascular plugging caused by the accumulation of thrombotic material. The use of fibrinolytic agents perfused down the lower extremity has been suggested as a means of decreasing the no-reflow phenomena associated with reperfusion.[31] In recently published results, pulmonary changes (as measured by the lung permeability index) were identified in the early phases of reperfusion of the lower limb extremities.[32] These changes correlated with increased neutrophil sequestration in the lungs as measured by myeloperoxidase concentrations. These findings support the concept that remote organ injury is associated with reperfusion of ischemic muscle and that the mediators may be neutrophils. The magnitude of the systemic response may be related to the quantity of muscle that has been rendered ischemic, a hypothesis that agrees with the clinical observation of high complication rates associated with management of an acute aortic occlusion.

A recent review of our own results demonstrated a 20% mortality rate associated with a simple femoral embolectomy under local anesthesia, with the rate of limb loss less than 5%. Therefore, although attention has been focused on reducing the degree of muscle necrosis, the systemic effects may in fact be the most significant.

A recent report has suggested a new approach to preventing muscle damage through systemic modalities. We reported that pre-exposure of muscle to ischemia induces the production of heat shock proteins (HSPs) capable of preventing muscle necrosis at a remote site. In these experiments, one gracilus muscle was rendered ischemic and then harvested at 48 hours, followed by the induction of a similar period of ischemia in the contralateral muscle. When harvested at 48 hours, the second muscle had a 60% reduction in the degree of muscle necrosis. Analysis showed that ATP depletion was spared in the second muscle. In addition, there was clear evidence that HSPs 90, 72, and 42 were induced. The presence of a 42-kd protein was identified in the second muscle, before ischemia/reperfusion.[33] This finding suggests that a humoral mediator elaborated by the first ischemic muscle triggered a cytoprotective effect in the second muscle. These findings are of particular interest because they offer new insight for potential systemic intervention capable of reducing the organ injury associated with an ischemia/reperfusion injury.

Surgical management of this ischemia/reperfusion may be relatively straightforward, but the systemic consequences are quite systematically profound. We have demonstrated that despite a relatively straightforward operation, the morbidity and mortality rate of this operation remains extremely high. In a recent publication, our group has demonstrated the impact of ischemia followed by reperfusion of the lower extremities on lung vascular permeability in an acute model. In a relatively short time there is significant evidence of changes in pulmonary vascular permeability associated with an increase in the neutrophil count in this area.[32] These findings are compatible with what is seen clinically when pulmonary edema complicates even a relatively mild degree of ischemia.

In summary, although a great deal of work has been done on understanding the mechanisms of injury in postischemic skeletal muscle necrosis, there are many gaps in the application of this work to the clinical model.

In order for greater progress to be made in the area of control of ischemic damage, there must be an improved method of influencing reperfusion injury by control of local factors known to be significant contributors to this injury.

REFERENCES

1. Walker PM: Ischemia/reperfusion injury in skeletal muscle. *Ann Vasc Surg* 5:399–402, 1991.
2. Blaisdell FW, Steele M, Allen RE: Management of acute lower extremity arterial ischemia due to embolism and thrombosis. *Surgery* 84:822–834, 1978.
3. Haljamae H, Enger E: Human skeletal muscle energy metabolism during and after complete tourniquet ischemia. *Ann Surg* 182:9–14, 1975.
4. Harris K, Walker PM, Mickle D, et al: Metabolic response of skeletal muscle to ischemia. *Am J Physiol* 250:H213–H220, 1986.
5. Lindsay T, Liauw K, Romaschin A, et al: The effect of ischemia/reperfusion on adenine nucleotide metabolism and xanthine oxidase production in skeletal muscle. *J Vasc Surg* 12:8–15, 1990.
6. Petrasek PF, Homer-Vanniasinkam S, Walker P: Determinants of ischemic injury to skeletal muscle. *J Vasc Surg* 19:623–631, 1994.
7. Korthuis R, Granger D, Foronsky M, et al: The role of oxygen derived free radicals in induced ischemia increases in canine skeletal muscle vascular permeability. *Circ Res* 57:599–609, 1985.
8. Forrest I, Lindsay T, Romaschin A, et al: The rate and distribution of muscle blood flow after prolonged ischemia. *J Vasc Surg* 10:83–88, 1989.
9. Carden DL, Smith JK, Korthuis RJ: Neutrophil-mediated microvascular dysfunction in postischemic canine skeletal muscle. *Circ Res* 66:1436–1444, 1990.
10. McCord J: Oxygen derived free radicals in post ischemic tissue injury. *N Engl J Med* 312:159–163, 1985.
11. Lindsay T, Walker P, Mickle D, et al: Measurement of hydroxy conjugated dienes after ischemia/reperfusion in canine skeletal muscle. *Am J Physiol* 254:H578–H583, 1988.
12. Romaschin AD, Rebekya I, Wilson GJ, et al: Conjugated dienes in ischemic and reperfused myocardium: An in vivo chemical signature of oxygen free radical mediated injury. *J Mol Cell Cardiol* 19:289–302, 1987.
13. Nayler WG, Sturrock WJ: Calcium channel blockers, beta blockers and the maintenance of calcium homeostasis. *Adv Exp Med Biol* 194:535–556, 1986.

14. Smith A, Hayes G, Romaschin AD, et al: The role of extracellular calcium in ischemia/reperfusion injury in skeletal muscle. *J Surg Res* 49:153–156, 1990.

15. Rubin BB, Smith A, Liauw SK, et al: Complement activation and white cell sequestration in postischemic skeletal muscle. *Am J Physiol* 259:H525–H531, 1990.

16. Bevilacqua MP, Sengelin S, Gimbrone MA, et al: Endothelial leukocyte adhesion molecule 1: An inducible receptor for neutrophils related to complement regulatory proteins and lectins. *Science* 243:1160–1165, 1989.

17. Bevilacqua M, Butcher E, Furie B, et al: Selectins: A family of adhesion receptors. *Cell* 67:233, 1991.

18. Granger DN, Russell JM, Arfors KE, et al: Role of CD18 and ICAM-1 in ischemia/reperfusion induced leukocyte adherence and emigration in mesenteric venules. *FASEB J* 5:1753A, 1994.

19. Jerome SN, Smith CW, Korthuis RJ: CD18-dependent adherence reactions play an important role in the development of the no-reflow phenomenon. *Am J Physiol* 264:H479–H483, 1993.

20. Carden DL, Smith JK, Korthuis RJ: Neutrophil mediated microvascular dysfunction in postischemic canine skeletal muscle: Role of granulocyte adherence. *Circ Res* 66:1436–1444, 1990.

21. Rubin BB, Liauw S, Tittley J, et al: Prolonged adenine nucleotide resynthesis and reperfusion injury in post ischemic skeletal muscle. *Am J Physiol* 262:H1538–H1547, 1992.

22. Haimovici H: Muscular, renal and metabolic complications of acute arterial occlusions: Myonephropathic metabolic syndrome. *Surgery* 85:461–468, 1979.

23. Kvietys PR, Inauen W, Bacon BB, et al: Xanthine oxidase–induced injury to endothelium: Role of intracellular iron and hydroxyl radical. *Am J Physiol* 257:H1640–H1646, 1989.

24. Rubin BB, Smith A, Tittley J, et al: A clinically applicable method for long term salvage of postischemic skeletal muscle. *J Vasc Surg* 13:53–63, 1991.

25. Hayes G, Liauw S, Smith A, et al: Exogenous magnesium chloride–adenosine triphosphate administration during reperfusion reduces the extent of necrosis in previously ischemic skeletal muscle. *J Vasc Surg* 11:441–448, 1990.

26. Zimmerman BJ, Granger DN: Reperfusion-induced leukocyte infiltration: Role of elastase. *Am J Physiol* 259:H390–H394, 1990.

27. Korthuis RJ, Grisham MB, Granger DN: Leukocyte depletion attenuates vascular injury in postischemic skeletal muscle. *Am J Physiol* 254:H823–H827, 1988.

28. Petrasak PF, Liauw S, Romaschin AD, et al: Salvage of postischemic skeletal muscle by monoclonal antibody blockade of neutrophil adhesion molecule CD18. *J Surg Res* 56:5–12, 1994.

29. Korthuis RJ, Carden DL, Kvietys PR, et al: Phalloidin attenuates postischemic neutrophil infiltration and increased microvascular permeability. *J Appl Physiol* 71:1261–1269, 1991.

30. Lindsay TF, Hill J, Ortiz F, et al: Blockade of complement activation prevents local and pulmonary albumin leak after lower torso ischemia-reperfusion. *Ann Surg* 216:677–683, 1992.

31. Quinones-Baldrich WJ, Chervu A, Hernandez JJ, et al: Skeletal muscle function after ischemia: "No reflow" versus reperfusion injury. *J Surg Res* 51:5–12, 1991.

32. Lindsay TF, Walker PM, Romaschin AD: Acute pulmonary injury in a model of ruptured abdominal aortic aneurysm. *J Vasc Surg* 22:1–8, 1995.

33. Liauw SK, Rubin BB, Lindsay TF, et al: Sequential ischemia/reperfusion results in contralateral skeletal muscle salvage. *Am J Physiol* 270 (Heart Circ Physiol) 39-4:H1407–H1413, 1996.

Index